COMMUNITY MENTAL HEALTH

COMMUNITY MENTAL HEALTH

A Sourcebook for Professionals and Advisory Board Members

Edited by

Wade H. Silverman

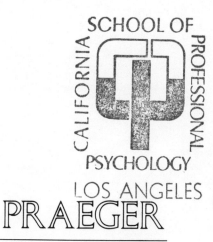

CALIFORNIA SCHOOL OF PROFESSIONAL PSYCHOLOGY

LOS ANGELES

PRAEGER

PRAEGER SPECIAL STUDIES • PRAEGER SCIENTIFIC

Library of Congress Cataloging in Publication Data

Main entry under title:

Community mental health.

    Includes bibliographies and indexes.
    1. Community mental health services--Administra-
tion. 2. Mental health boards. 3. Community
mental health services. I. Silverman, Wade H.
RA790.5.C62   362.2'2'068   80-25984
ISBN 0-03-057006-9

Published in 1981 by Praeger Publishers
CBS Educational and Professional Publishing
A Division of CBS, Inc.
521 Fifth Avenue, New York, New York 10175 U.S.A.

123456789 145 987654321

Printed in the United States of America

To Fred, who taught me the difference between paternalism and advocacy.

FOREWORD BY
George W. Albee

Recently a friend of mine said she would know when the millenium had arrived: public schools and mental health centers would have more money than they needed, and the Air Force and Navy would be sponsoring bake sales and bingo parties!

We are a long way from that millenium. Mental health centers and agencies have watched their funding sources dry up as a new wave of fiscal conservatism has swept the country. Limited state and federal funds are earmarked for direct treatment services which means one-to-one therapy and rehabilitation. Centers are eliminating staff positions that do not bring in third-party payments, and harassed directors and boards must constantly evaluate programs on the basis of whether they can pay for themselves and not whether they are needed or worthwhile.

Recently John Ambrose told the assembly at the annual meeting of the National Council of Community Health Centers in San Francisco that he has found a number of centers operating businesses in order to plow their profits into service activities. He discovered that one center is operating a hamburger franchise and another is manufacturing fork-lift trucks. This evokes a déjà-vu feeling in some of us oldtimers. It was not so long ago that state hospitals operated large farms, with the labor of inmates providing most of the muscle power; the use and the sale of vegetables and dairy products supplied a significant part of the cost of running the institution.

In some ways I feel like Rip Van Winkle awakening from a 20-year nap. Way back in 1959, I wrote a book on mental health manpower that examined the nation's needs and resources in the mental health delivery field. I concluded with the observation that mental health professionals would continue to be in short supply, with psychiatrists having the thinnest ranks. The book was one of a series published by the Joint Commission on Mental Illness and Health (JCMIH). The final report of the commission, Action for Mental Health, led to a whole new national approach for helping emotionally disturbed people. The JCMIH recommended that no new state hospitals be built and that the patient population of existing state hospitals be drastically reduced. The report led to the decision that a large number of new community mental health centers be built so that early treatment could prevent unnecessary hospitalization. A young senator, Jack Kennedy, who later became president, read the report. He sent the first mental health message from a president to

Congress with recommendations that the federal government become involved in funding mental health programs. Ultimately, Congress appropriated funds to build community mental health centers, but there was always great ambivalence and reluctance about providing federal funds to staff the centers. Meanwhile, the National Institute of Mental Health was pouring money into the training of psychiatrists, psychologists, social workers, and psychiatric nurses. The thrust of the commission report had been its emphasis on early treatment. By intervening early, the reasoning went, prolonged and extensive hospitalization might be avoided for large numbers of people. The financial savings would more than compensate for the increased cost of early treatment. (It did not escape the notice of sharp-eyed state budget people that federal tax dollars could replace state tax dollars if people were released or kept out of the state hospitals.) This shift of tax support accounts for the massive discharge of people from the state hospitals in the past 25 years. Psychiatry credits "breakthroughs in drug therapy" but this is nonsense. People not on drug therapy—like the elderly senile—are also pushed out and onto the federal dole!

While nearly 800 centers were built or are now in operation, the whole movement has been hampered from the outset by the chronic lack of funds to pay staff salaries. Especially acute has been the shortage of psychiatrists. Despite the large amounts of money paid to train psychiatrists, very few have been willing to throw in their lot with tax-supported and salaried agencies. Most prefer private office practice, although many are willing to give a few hours a week to signing forms for agencies.

A kind of curious paradox has been developing. Medicine and psychiatry continue to have great political clout and have been able to demand allegiance to the medical model for explaining emotional disturbances. Every client (called patient) coming to a center must have a diagnosis taken from the greatly expanded new Diagnostic and Statistical Manual of the American Psychiatric Association (DSM III) and everyone must have a treatment plan. This means that every user of a center must be found sick and, therefore, eligible for third-party medical payments. At the same time that the medical model has been placed in the center of the stage a serious and chronic shortage of psychiatrists has developed.

Recently I reviewed the human resources situation in psychiatry and compared it with the situation 20 years ago. My analysis (published in Hospital and Community Psychiatry, November 1979, Vol. 30, Number 11, pp. 783-86) finds that the serious shortage of psychiatrists continues and grows even worse. Well over half of all psychiatrists in the country are to be found in five states—New York, Massachusetts, Pennsylvania, Illinois, and California—and the

District of Columbia. Rural and poor states have few psychiatrists. Very few American-trained psychiatrists take jobs in public hospitals or tax-supported clinics and centers. These places have long depended on foreign-trained physicians to fill their psychiatric vacancies. Now, with a change in the federal law controlling the admission of foreign-trained physicians, this supply is rapidly drying up. This situation affects other branches of medicine in addition to psychiatry, but because of the vast demand for psychiatrists to staff state hospitals the situation is more critical in our field.

As a consequence of the shortage of psychiatrists, mental health centers have been forced to appoint as directors qualified people from other disciplines and to hire people from these other disciplines as their front-line intervention personnel. So we see the strange situation where people who do not believe in the medical illness model for mental disturbance are forced to use it, and forced to abandon programs aimed at resocialization, day care, consultation and education, and primary prevention because none of these are reimbursable under the existing illness model.

We are a long, long way from meeting the identified needs for intervention. Reports from the President's Commission on Mental Health and the head of the Alcohol, Drug Abuse, and Mental Health Administration concur in estimating that 32 to 34 million people constitute the hard core of the emotionally disturbed in the United States. These people have been identified repeatedly, and include those with serious depression, alcoholic addictions, incapacitating neuroses, mental conditions associated with old age, and the serious forms of psychoses. In any given year, the entire mental health system is able to see only about 7 million persons! But not all of these 7 million come from the hard-core group. Many individuals being seen in our centers and private offices have "problems in living"—those undergoing marital disruption, identity problems, and life crisis concerns that bring them to the therapist's chair or couch. So we are actually seeing many fewer than one in five of the seriously disturbed people.

In spite of 20 years of intensive effort since the report of the Joint Commission on Mental Illness and Health, and many millions of federal dollars poured into the support of federal training, the construction of centers, and the support of research, we are still falling behind.

Is there any real hope? Not if we continue our mental health business as usual. Over and over again, surveys have found that individual psychotherapy and individual "treatment" represents the backbone of the efforts being made in our centers. As long as we walk that particular treadmill, the situation will remain hopeless.

Two strategies make sense for resolving our shortfall of people and service. The first of these is to find alternatives to one-to-one intervention by a highly trained professional. We need to develop group programs and mutual aid groups, to encourage and develop self-help programs, to find workers who want to get out into the community, and to use existing networks and support systems.

The second strategy is to put significantly more of our efforts into primary prevention. We must recognize the fact that no mass disorder afflicting large numbers of human beings has ever been controlled or eliminated by attempts at treating each affected individual. This is not only sound public health dogma, but it is as applicable to the field of mental health as to the field of public health.

What stands in our way? Why can't we offer more group programs and use more self-help and mutual help efforts of the sort that have been demonstrated to be effective? Why can't we put more energy and effort into primary prevention? The answer is deceptively simple. None of these approaches fits the medical model that dominates our field. This illness model, which stresses diagnosis, treatment, and one-to-one intervention, discourages efforts by non-professionals and lay persons, and its proponents have taken to arguing vehemently against primary prevention. The arguments of the illness model adherents have a sort of boring consistency. They warn that only highly qualified health professionals can be entrusted with the responsibility of treating sick patients. Diagnoses are urgently required. And just around the corner, it is promised, new drugs and organic treatment methods will soon make dramatic changes in the number of people seen. Furthermore, these people argue, we really don't know enough about the specific causes of each specific illness to do anything significant about prevention. These tired old arguments would not be worth considering were it not for the fact that they are advanced by senior and respected people in the field.

Why, we ask ourselves, is the medical model defended with such vehemence? Why is primary prevention so strongly rejected? Why are lay groups not welcome as helpers?

The answer is again deceptively simple. Changing models means threatening the status quo. Primary prevention efforts lead inevitably to an examination of the role of social forces in the production of human emotional distress. The first step in any effective primary prevention program is an examination of the epidemiology of the disturbances in question. We quickly learn that poor people are far more likely to be affected than are the affluent. Women are more frequently depressed than men. Children, adolescents, and elderly people were all identified in the President's Commission on Mental Health report as being among the unserved and underserved.

Migrant farm workers, the rural and urban poor, the handicapped—all of these groups have emotional problems that reflect social injustice. The medical model (mental illness is an illness like any other) is a bulwark against public recognition of the social and class origins of mental and emotional disturbance.

It is time for another mental health revolution!

This revolution will emphasize social changes aimed at improving the quality of life and reducing avoidable stresses. It will challenge the authority of the mental health establishment and attack the ritualistic devotion to one-to-one intervention. It will expose the fallacies of the illness model.

For the past year and more, I have been reading the literature on revolutions. I would like to suggest some characteristics of all revolutions—something that might help identify the anatomy of a social revolution. I am especially concerned with fomenting this revolution in the human services field.

First of all, for a revolution to begin there must be widespread injustice. I suggest that this is the case today. The President's Commission on Mental Health identified a gap that will only get wider and will never be closed. So injustice is a condition that widely prevails. Service is inequitably available.

Second, a revolution always calls for an overt challenge to authority. I believe that the number of voices criticizing medical hegemony in human emotional problems has become a large chorus. We are beginning to converge in our theories in the various human service professions that emotionally disturbed people are not sick, that the defect model that sees personal taint and genetic or biochemical defect as the causes of all human mental problems is an invalid model, and this insight is leading us to suggest social change rather than medical treatment as a solution.

Third, a revolution needs a clear-cut political position that everyone can understand. The position that I see gaining prominence suggests that no mass disorder afflicting humankind has ever been eliminated through one-to-one intervention, but only as a result of successful prevention. Related to this position is the recognition that powerlessness is a major cause of emotional distress, and that the only resolution for powerlessness is a redistribution of power. So the revolutionary political position is that the poor, the minorities, children and youth, women, and other powerless groups must benefit from a redistribution of power.

Fourth, revolutions need a core of dedicated leaders with a clear vision of the goals. We have learned a great deal from our brothers and sisters doing one-to-one case work and psychotherapy. People involved in attempting to help individually distressed and disturbed human beings have given us a great deal of insight into the

xi

social origins of their clients' problems. From these one-to-one interventionists we need to recruit a cadre of leaders who will dedicate themselves to the cause of prevention through redistribution of power.

Fifth, we need to anticipate and be prepared for strong resistance from those whose power would be reduced or usurped. The Establishment is ruthless in its defense of the defect (illness) model. Enormous power and resources are at stake in this struggle. We can expect continued resistance from the mental health establishment to any suggestion that there are not a number of separate and discrete mental illnesses, each with an individual cause, cure, and possible prevention. Our suggestion that human stress results from the injustice and unfairness of the present economic system will result in a powerful counterattack. We already see that funds available for prevention are going to relatively meaningless and trivial projects. It is clear that a great deal of noise will be made about the importance of prevention to cover the fact that little significant work in this area is being supported by the Establishment.

Finally, revolutions occur when there is an unstable power structure. Again, my reading of the current situation within the helping professions suggests growing instability. Clearly, psychiatry is decreasing in its power and control largely because it is unable to recruit young people into residency training.

In short, conditions are ripe for revolution!

ACKNOWLEDGMENTS

I would like to thank Marsha Silverman for her invaluable assistance and advice and Sam James for his excellent work and dedication in completing the typing of this manuscript.

W.H.S.

INTRODUCTION

Since the first community mental health centers (CMHCs) opened their doors in the mid-1960s, dramatic changes have taken place in the way mental health services have been organized and delivered. The initial aims of the community mental health movement were to make services more available by localizing them and making them affordable. An allied goal was deinstitutionalization, gradually de-emphasizing the large mental hospital as the major public service provider. Finally, there were those mental health professionals who saw the movement as an opportunity to focus their energies on the tasks of primary prevention and early detection of emotional disorders rather than exclusively on psychotherapy and rehabilitative care.

During the last two decades, new administrative concepts and evaluative tools have increased the quantity and types of services while reducing their relative costs. Comprehensiveness, continuity of care, networking, and accountability are all administrative goals that did not formally exist prior to the movement either in operational terms or as mental health principles. Factors affecting emotional disorders have been systematically studied and used in planning services. These include demographic variables, support systems, professional and client values and beliefs, and community control.

A myriad of evaluative tools now exist to assess the availability, accessibility, and validity of mental health services. We are able through the use of management information systems to analyze quickly and thoroughly complicated questions regarding the functioning of CMHCs. Standards for evaluating CMHC performance have been established by the National Institute of Mental Health (NIMH) and the Joint Commission on Accreditation of Hospitals.

In any field of endeavor, a rapidly expanding knowledge base necessitates a strong commitment to inservice training and continuing education of its practitioners. This is particularly essential to such a new field as community mental health in which the vast majority of employees received their basic training from mental health professionals who had no knowledge in the field. Through its Continuing Education Branch and now through its Division of Manpower and Training Programs, NIMH has developed interdisciplinary training programs to disseminate knowledge in community mental health.

As executive director of the NIMH-sponsored Continuing Education Program (CEP) in Mental Health at the School of Public Health, University of Illinois, I have had the opportunity to address the training needs of over one thousand mental health professionals and advisory/governing board members. These trainees and their colleagues have continually complained to me about the dearth of training opportunities for mental health professionals beyond entry level. The training needs of citizen advisory/governing boards have been particularly neglected, since they must depend on their own agencies and local governments for support. However, as government presses for continuing education as a precondition to relicensure, and as citizen participation mandates become more strictly enforced, the number of available programs will inevitably increase. Hand-in-hand with the scarcity of training programs has gone the lack of well-designed curricula and training materials.

At the beginning of the CEP in 1974, the staff was faced with the challenge of planning training programs for a variety of roles, agencies, and communities. We decided to take a grass roots planning approach in which the trainees would design all aspects of their program, including content, format, intensity, and discussion leaders. Three initial training groups—administrators, advisory/governing board members, and trainers/supervisors—devised and participated in their own programs. Subsequent programs were modifications of these initial efforts. The legacy of all the trainees who designed, attended, and evaluated the CEP, and of all the trainers who researched, taught, and consulted is this sourcebook.

The purpose of the sourcebook is to provide an overview of current knowledge in community mental health. It is biased toward the practical rather than the theoretical and is most useful to those who desire to work or are already engaged in applied settings. As such, three groups will find this text particularly useful. The first group is advisory/governing board members, primarily nonprofessional volunteer laypersons who are increasingly responsible for making policy decisions to determine the direction of their centers. These citizens need a basic sourcebook to build skills and understand community mental health concepts. The second group, mental health administrators, will find useful information pertaining to such key responsibilities as evaluation, planning, and funding. The third group, university students and faculty interested in applied settings, need an introductory text for understanding new concepts and practices. The sourcebook is both comprehensive and informative. Others who will find useful information include citizens interested in mental health services and policy, direct service providers, consultation and education staff, and inservice and continuing education providers.

The organization of the sourcebook takes into account the preeminence of active citizen participation and sound fiscal management in the success of any CMHC. Thus, Part I, Board Organization and

Roles, includes discussions on the philosophy of citizen participation, different kinds of boards, methods of organizing an effective board, relationships between the board and executive director, interrelationships among the board, administrators, professionals, and host community, and the use of volunteers. Part II, Funding, considers all the possible sources of funding and how to work with them. Also included is a chapter on effective spending. Part III, Mental Health Services, is comprised of chapters on services required by the Community Mental Health Centers Act and its Amendments. The rationale for Part IV, Special Populations, is to acquaint the reader with the mental health needs of those groups that have been traditionally underserved by both the private and public sectors. Unfortunately, it is not possible to describe all such groups so that the chapters here present information on only the largest. Part V, Planning and Accountability, is concerned with topics on planning for and monitoring of clients' rights and center effectiveness.

CONTENTS

I

BOARD ORGANIZATION AND ROLES

Community control and citizen participation in decision making is the bedrock of our democratic tradition. During the 1960s, these themes were highlighted because of concern that the rights of the poor and minorities were not fully represented by government. Many programs, including Head Start, Volunteers in Service to America, and Model Cities, were instituted to promote equal opportunity for all citizens.

It was in this climate that the community mental health movement was fostered. Public mental health services became available and accessible by placing programs in neighborhoods. Citizen input was encouraged primarily through the creation of boards that served as advisors to federally funded community mental health centers (CMHCs).

The principle of citizen control of CMHCs was codified into law with P. L. 94-63, the Community Mental Health Centers Amendments of 1975. Along with their new formal governing power was a legal responsibility to offer quality care in an unbiased manner. Board members quickly realized that they required knowledge and skills in administration, funding, politics, and service delivery. Much has been learned by those citizens who have given their time and energies to community mental health. Similarly, professionals have had to learn to be partners with and employees of their communities.

This section will provide an overview of citizen participation in community mental health. It focuses on the effective development and functioning of boards, and the interactions among board, professional and volunteer staff, and the community. Cravens gives an historical account of citizen involvement in CMHCs, and he identifies three current trends in board involvement: greater acceptance of responsibilities, more formal working agreements with executive directors, and greater need and demand for training. He predicts that in the future boards will increasingly concentrate on prevention, on securing alternative sources of funding, and on providing service to underserved population groups including children, the elderly, and racial and ethnic minorities. Management and accountability will be among the highest priorities, as will be "networking" service systems to avoid costly duplication.

Robins argues that board participation in community mental health has not been particularly successful. Professional acceptance

of boards has been grudgingly slow, as has been government recognition of their authority. His basic point is that competent board
participation must rely on objectively measured functioning rather
than on meeting quotas for demographic representation. A schema
for board participation is presented in which "effectiveness areas"
are defined, objectives are described, and tasks are enumerated.
Robins is skeptical about the usefulness of advisory boards. He
notes that they are in the untenable position of exercising responsibility without authority.

Nowlen describes the nuts and bolts of building a well-function-
ing board. Among his many practical suggestions are how to recruit
and maintain membership, how to use committees, how to execute
agenda, and how to keep minutes.

The political thicket in which boards operate is explored by
Chiarmonte. Unlike Robins, he thinks that advisory boards bolster
the strength and confidence of their members and that they can truly
influence local government. In a colorful description of his experiences as a board president in Chicago, he offers suggestions, warn-
ings, and encouragement to citizen participants in community mental
health.

In the format of a dialogue and from the perspective of an executive director, Eaddy examines the relationship between the director and the board. The nature of their interaction varies from center to center as a function of the background and experience of the
involved parties, and the kind and extent of external controls; it depends, too, on whether the center is free-standing or hospital based.
These parameters form the arena in which the director and board
sort out their responsibilities in policy making and implementation,
fund raising and expenditure, public relations, and service delivery.

Silverman discusses the role of volunteers in mental health.
She describes their backgrounds, the types of tasks they perform,
reasons for their use, and the frequency with which they are used.
A seven-step progression for building an effective volunteer program
is presented.

1

GRASS ROOTS PARTICIPATION IN COMMUNITY MENTAL HEALTH
Richard B. Cravens

It is probably easier to form a cabinet, especially a
coalition cabinet, in the heat of battle than in quiet
times. The sense of duty dominates all else, and
personal claims recede.

(Churchill, 1949, p. 8)

HOW IT BEGAN

In 1961 the Joint Commission on Mental Illness and Health
questioned the quality of treatment for the emotionally disturbed,
focused attention on the archaic state hospital system, and created
a sound basis for developing accessible mental health services.
Their final report recommended a national mental health program of
community centers that would each deliver services to a population
of 50,000 (JCMIH, 1961). Immediately following the report of the
Joint Commission, federal grants were awarded to each state to support comprehensive mental health planning. The heavy involvement
of citizens in planning was an important bridge between the Joint
Commission and the community mental health centers (CMHC) legislation that soon followed. Many CMHC applications were a direct
result of this early citizen participation in the nationwide planning
effort. Three years after the Joint Commission completed its work,
the Community Mental Health Centers Act of 1963 (P. L. 88-164) was
enacted with the full support of President John F. Kennedy (CMHCA,
1963). This statute initiated the first steps, underwritten with federal funds, toward creation of a national mental health program that
ultimately led to the federal funding of 763 CMHCs through Fiscal
Year 1979.

Several unique and important elements were contained in this landmark legislation. Foremost was the implication of a new philosophy of mental health service. A comprehensive program going beyond the traditional inpatient and outpatient programs of the past would make services totally accessible to the population. Thus, the concept of the catchment area came into being, making it possible to control the size of population to be served. Today, the average catchment area has a population of 150,000.

Another concept of importance was that of continuity of care. Consumers should not only have access to a range of services, but they should enjoy unrestricted movement or easy transition from one treatment modality to another, depending on their mental health needs.

Also vital to the CMHC program was the notion that mental health services should be available where people live and work. This was in direct contrast to the state hospital, which typically was located in an isolated rural setting far from the community. The separation of the individual from the familiar and necessary ego supports of family, home, job, church, and friends contributed greatly to the state of chronicity that so often characterized the resident population of state hospitals. Perhaps the most far-reaching requirement of the CMHC program was the stipulation that citizens be advisors to the designated state agency having responsibility for administering the program in the state. The CMHC Act required that a state advisory council be established to review CMHC applications for funding. This council consisted of providers and private citizens. In addition, each private not-for-profit CMHC had an incorporated board that served as the legal entity to apply for and receive the grant.

EARLY CITIZEN INVOLVEMENT

Until the early 1960s the major effort to involve citizens in mental health issues was channeled through limited activities encouraged by various mental health organizations. These activities often highlighted the need for increased state hospital budgets for salaries and construction, and promoted public education typically through pamphlets and talks by professionals. Volunteer programs collected clothing for state hospital patients or sponsored Christmas parties with gifts and refreshments. Lobbying efforts commonly took the form of directly approaching state legislators and holding annual luncheons in conjunction with seminars on mental health and the need for legislation. Such organizations usually employed a small paid staff who carried out the work through the year with citizen members coming together periodically for committee, board meetings, and annual conventions. Citizen involvement was valuable, for it contributed to a heightened public awareness of mental health issues and maintained varying degrees of pressure on state legislatures to improve the lot of emotionally disturbed persons.

With the passage of P.L. 88-164, the role of the citizen was changed from one of passive supporter to one of dynamic catalyst who participated actively in the decision-making processes of the CMHC. In the 16 years following the passage of P.L. 88-164, the citizen's role has not only become one of great power, but it continues to undergo strengthening and change through new responsibilities.

In the early days, little was known about how to work with private citizens in the cause of mental health. Professionals were accustomed to being authorities, and citizens had been programmed to behave with deference toward them. Furthermore, professionals tended to conceptualize problems as solvable if only there were sufficient funds. They frequently turned to citizens to provide the money; however, this relationship was not reciprocal because the professional seldom shared administrative responsibility. The early and surprisingly vigorous attempts to take advantage of the provisions of the CMHC Act often were made by clusters of private citizens with minimal professional participation. Most often, the initial citizen group was small in size and generally consisted of the community decision makers. The community might be defined as one or more towns or counties. The group always met at night, as was the custom when busy people turned from their respective occupations to attend to the perceived needs of their community. There were many other cases, to be sure, in which professionals participated actively and would form an entity that was eligible to apply for CMHC grant funds.

The decision-making groups were predictably similar from state to state. A newspaper publisher or editor, attorney, business person, banker, physician, Mental Health Association member, public school official, and hospital administrator often comprised the nucleus of concerned citizens.

The first task for the group was to obtain information about the CMHC Act and to tie its provisions to local needs. In many cases there was more than passing awareness of local mental health problems and, without exception, it was this knowledge that fueled the desire to initiate a local mental health program.

The 1963 legislation (P.L. 88-164) provided funds only for construction; it was not until passage of the 1965 Amendments that personnel costs were supported by staffing grants (CMHCAA, 1965). Although there was resistance among professionals for limiting federal support only to construction rather than to staffing, in retrospect it seems that efforts to initiate an accessible program were facilitated more than if staffing support had occurred first. The ideal would have been to give both construction and staffing funds from the beginning.

In hindsight, the advantage of starting with a construction program was that citizens could become excited about a new community building. An idea took shape with a few quick strokes of an architect's pen; the rough sketches soon became a symbol around which the community could rally. Funds could be raised, and a building site was located and frequently donated. Further, it was a simple task to raise large sums of money for construction (P.L. 88-164 called for matching local funds to federal dollars), an activity that many community decision makers had undertaken with success on countless previous occasions. The building became a visible symbol of accomplishment and, of course, there were plaques scattered liberally throughout such a structure that bore the names of local contributors.

In these early days, the community decision makers were comfortable in identifying a local problem, then organizing to form an incorporated board or identifying an existing body to pursue the federal CMHC dollar. This nucleus group was not necessarily representative of the community to be served. Racial and ethnic minorities were not present; neither were women, unless they were physicians or elected officials; and, likewise, the poor were left out of the picture. If planning took place in a rural setting, the farmer was a member only if he were wealthy or happened to be an elected official.

Much time was spent in planning fund raising programs and plotting the future financial soundness of the enterprise. In passing, it must be said that the nation's economy was healthy and optimism ran high. In contrast, little time was devoted to planning the services to be provided. In some cases, decision makers were totally lacking in mental health resources or personnel, and it was soon realized that such professionally trained people would necessarily have to be recruited. When one reflects on this state of affairs, one cannot avoid being impressed with the mixture of enthusiasm, naivety, gutsiness, sense of social responsibility, and pioneering qualities that characterized the earliest citizen involvement in the CMHC movement.

Once a decision was made to apply for CMHC construction funds, the local planning group became aware of the need to share this decision with the community and to broaden the base of support for such contemplated action. This was accomplished through word of mouth, newspaper articles and editorials, talks before civic groups (an absolutely vital activity), and radio and television programs. It was also at this time, and not always before, that political authorities were contacted at the municipal, county, and state levels. However, representatives of the state mental health authority and the regional offices of the Department of Health, Education, and Welfare had customarily been actively involved with the local decision makers from the beginning.

Despite sharing of information and the growth of broad-based support for a CMHC project, the power, authority, and responsibility still tended to be maintained by the nucleus of decision makers. This phenomenon sometimes took the quality of possessiveness or ownership. Even with the necessity for the decision-making group to become representative of the catchment area, new additions were seldom more than token symbols of rural residents, minority groups, or the poor. The age of consumerism, activism, and participatory management was still some years away.

There was one facet to planning for the CMHC that was delegated with confidence and relief. With the excitement and responsibility accompanying the task of fund raising and construction planning, the actual work of designing a program, preparing a budget, and working with an architect were activities easily delegated to a professional. Such an individual, if not supplied by the state, was the first employee and often became the fledgling center's first director. In those days, the professional was less well equipped to take on the design of such a project (which today amounts to an average budget of $2.5 million) than were the community leaders who were accustomed to identifying problems and pointing the way for the community to resolve issues.

During the time of federal funding for CMHC construction, 478 centers were built. As they were constructed, staff was recruited, services were put in place, and problems of managing a center began to emerge. The decision makers and early board members were faced with new challenges. Rather than dealing with the issue of raising $500,000 to build a center, the problem became one of generating revenue to support the center, purchasing malpractice insurance, developing personnel policies, and approaching the state legislature for a mental health services act. Sometimes an unanticipated need for additional space to house services surfaced.

These new problems, demands, and challenges meant a swing away from the early excitement of building construction to the more complex issues of center management. This process was also accompanied by increased public visibility of the centers and a willingness, later a demand, on the part of citizens for greater and more meaningful participation in CMHC affairs. A new board composition evolved as different talents were required to address newly emerging center problems. In short, many of the early members lost interest or were debilitated from the strenuous efforts of constructing a center which often required a gestation period of several years. This was coupled with a new era in which citizens aggressively sought participation in organizations that affected community life.

CITIZEN INVOLVEMENT AND THE CMHC STAFF

The usual arrangement for a CMHC was to incorporate a board of directors under the state law as a not-for-profit entity, thereby making it eligible to receive grant funds or to become a unit of municipal, county, or state government. No federal law or regulation required that the board be representative of the catchment area until May 1966, at which time a federal policy was developed. In 1971, this policy was published and read as follows:

> Community mental health centers must involve the community in the planning, development, and operation of the program. Community involvement is required to assure that the center's program will be responsive to the mental health needs of the community, have visibility, optimal utilization, and a public base of support. The exact form such involvement takes will vary from one center to another to achieve the goals stated above. Community involvement may be formal or informal, and may include representation on policy and advisory boards. In any case, the participating citizens must include board representation of all elements of the community such as professionals, lay persons, appropriate consumers, persons from the range of socio-economic groups, cultural groups, age groups (youth, adults, and aged) and geographic and political subdivisions. Applicants for community mental health center staffing and/or construction grants must describe the nature and extent of community involvement in the center program, past, present and future. [NIMH, 1971, chap. 2, p. 28]

With the formal establishment of governing or advisory boards, a long period of courtship began between center directors and boards. The most commonly observed relationship was one of an unstated division of labor. CMHC directors tended to view boards as a necessary evil that dealt with crises often involving money. The board was a body that met once each month and would show polite interest in the operations of the center. In many cases, the board expected the director to deal with problems in a way that required minimal attention of the board. Among many directors, however, there was an awareness that the board could serve as the eyes and ears of the center and the community. Thus, attempts were made to provide educational opportunities: typically, a portion of each board meeting was devoted to a presentation about operations. Only much later did more highly structured and ambitious training activities for board members come into being, and it was later still that CMHC directors and boards began to fashion their working relationships in a way that resembled that of the chief executive officer and board of a corporation.

As initially passed, the CMHC Act called for a service delivery model that would be responsive to the mental health needs of all people residing in the catchment area. The concept of comprehensiveness was, thus, created for use in mental health service delivery. Federal policy later required that there be a provision for citizen input, and it is this early expectation—one that predated other federal programs requiring citizen participation—that serves to underscore all that is implied in the word "community." The CMHC is responsive to needs of local citizens because of their long-term involvement at the grass-roots level. In the 1960s, these citizens not only became aware of mental health problems, but were also cognizant that the traditional public mental health model was not a responsible answer to current needs. Citizen enlightenment coupled with action brought badly needed services to the people. For the most part, it was only after public awareness of mental health issues was generated that the professional became involved as a part of the community planning effort.

CITIZEN INVOLVEMENT TODAY

In one sense, the roles of the citizen and board evolved without much guidance. Both center directors and board members became concerned with board/center relationships, and boards tended to become organized into working committees, for example, personnel, finance, and membership. As the 1970s approached, however, citizens began to accept a larger and more clearly defined role. This upsurge of renewed citizen involvement was consistent with citizen involvement in other public programs that required citizen/consumer participation and planning.

Not until P.L. 94-63, the Community Mental Health Centers Amendments of 1975, was the requirement of a governing board set forth along with certain basic duties (CMHCA, 1975). Provisions for an advisory board were also specified. Throughout the history of the

CMHC movement, conflict and uncertainty over the concepts of incorporated governing boards and advisory boards had always been present. With the passage of P. L. 94-63, CMHCs were required to have governing rather than advisory boards. The only exception to this requirement occurred with respect to CMHCs operated by a government agency and funded with a staffing grant prior to the enactment of P. L. 94-63 (and, later, hospital grantees as provided for in P. L. 95-622). P. L. 94-63, Section 201(c)(1)(A) states:

> The governing body of a community mental health center (other than a center described in subparagraph [B]) shall (i) be composed, where practicable, of individuals who reside in the center's catchment area and who, as a group, represent the residents of that area taking into consideration their employment, age, sex, and place of residence, and other demographic characteristics of the area, and (ii) meet at least once a month, establish general policies for the center (including a schedule of hours during which services will be provided), approve the center's annual budget, and approve the selection of a director for the center. At least one half of the members of such body shall be individuals who are not providers of health care.

The intent of this section is quite clear: to give the citizen a defined role in the operation of the center. In the past when citizen boards met infrequently, they often floundered over what responsibilities to assume and agonized over center costs. The Act clearly mandated their assumption of major duties and responsibilities.

In Section 206(c)(1)(A) and Section 206(c)(1)(B), P. L. 94-63, the following may be found:

> The community mental health center for which the application is submitted will provide, in accordance with regulations of the Secretary (i) an overall plan and budget that meets the requirements of section 1861(z) of the Social Security Act, and (ii) an effective procedure for developing, compiling, and reporting to the Secretary statistics and other information (which the Secretary shall publish and disseminate on a periodic basis and which the center shall disclose at least annually to the general public) relating to (I) the cost of the center's operation, (II) the patterns of use of its services, (III) the availability, accessibility, and acceptability of its services, (IV) the impact of its services upon the mental

health of the residents of its catchment area, and (V)
such other matters as the Secretary may require;
(B) such community mental health center will, in consultation with the residents of its catchment area, review its program of services and the statistics and
other information referred to in subparagraph (A) to
assure that its services are responsive to the needs of
the residents of the catchment area.

Although P. L. 94-63 does not specifically require that these functions be assumed by the board, it would appear that the board is in
an ideal position to represent the CMHC in dealing with the general
public and to participate in carrying out the aforementioned provisions.

As board members have gained more experience in CMHC management, they have realized that specific kinds of knowledge and
skills are needed. These needs have been addressed in a variety of
ways, such as the use of 2 percent technical assistance funds to
sponsor training workshops. (P. L. 94-63, Section 206[e] provides
for 2 percent technical assistance.) Other efforts have been directed
toward compiling printed materials ranging from journal articles to
training manuals. Journal articles seem to have limited value because of their inaccessibility and because many are written from the
viewpoint of CMHC staff vis-à-vis the board. One training manual,
developed specifically for the CMHC board member as the reader,
represents a joint project of professional mental health personnel
and CMHC board members (Ragland & Zinn, 1979a). The value of
this type of publication is great because it is designed to meet a
variety of board member needs. Material may be found on procedures
for holding a meeting, the goal being efficiency and orderliness in
conducting business. In addition, specific information about the CMHC
program, including the CMHC Act, is contained in the booklet. Another publication developed by NIMH for both CMHC personnel and
board members presents an annotated bibliography on board functioning (Ragland & Zinn, 1979b).

For years, CMHC board members have participated on CMHC
monitoring teams and, more recently, have become involved with
program evaluation activities. In order to carry out some of the requirements of P. L. 94-63, Section 206(c)(1)(A) and 206(c)(1)(B),
NIMH has prepared a manual written for board members on how to
participate in program evaluation (Peters, Lochtman, & Windle,
1979).

On a different level, and one that suggests growing cohesive-
ness, is the rapid growth of formal workshops that draw board members from throughout the country. An example of the popularity for

such formal training occurred in 1979 when the annual meeting of the National Council of Community Mental Health Centers was held in Washington, D.C. Premeeting workshops for CMHC board members provided training on such topics as public relations, program evaluation, and urban, small town, suburban, rural, clinical, and legislative issues. The workshops attracted 200 people, all CMHC board members who attended with enthusiasm. The annual meeting drew another 100 board members. This kind of group behavior is usually the first step toward the establishment of a formal organization with officers, dues, and annual meetings. Should this occur, there will be a new and extraordinarily powerful constituency group in the CMHC arena, one that will have a powerful impact on the federal mental health legislative process. The influence of such an organization is of great importance because private citizen groups are not encumbered with the aura of professional vested interest and self-enhancement that frequently characterize professional organizations.

CITIZEN INVOLVEMENT AND THE FUTURE

Predictions about future citizen involvement must take into consideration the many forces that have influenced the development and functioning of CMHCs. Federal support for the creation of new CMHCs has declined since 1975, with the demand for the funding of new centers outstripping the amount of federal dollars available. With the present high rate of inflation and competing priorities of the federal budget, it is unlikely that significant amounts of federal money will be funded into the CMHC program. The high spending days of the 1960s are not likely to be enjoyed again. Even with amendments to the current CMHC Act or passage of a new mental health systems act, appropriations are expected to be limited. Such are the fiscal realities of the 1980s.

Even so, it is possible to make some forecasts, with CMHC boards as the reference point. First, there are a growing number of CMHCs that have completed basic federal support, that is, they have exhausted the eight-year staffing grant. At the close of Fiscal Year 1979, 325 centers had completed basic federal grant support. Another 167 CMHCs received no CMHC grant support; they had completed basic grant support along with other assistance such as consultation and education (C&E), conversion, and financial distress funding. These centers continue to operate and provide services but with several major differences. Nonrevenue producing activities have been reduced or eliminated, staff size has been cut, and inpatient service has been used as a source of revenue. Quite clearly, CMHC boards will increasingly have to face the problems encountered with the loss of a major source of funding (Naierman, 1977).

A new and badly needed focus will be on providing services to priority population groups such as children, the elderly, chronically emotionally disturbed, racial and ethnic minorities, rural residents, and the poor. Concentrating services on these high-risk groups will pose new demands for the CMHC boards: recruitment of specially trained staff (including racial and ethnic minorities who are professionals); agreements with other agencies to provide the necessary support systems on a catchment areawide basis; and designing outreach programs to individuals who do not come to the attention of the mental health system. Attending to the needs of priority population groups could well bring about a change in the composition of CMHC boards as well.

Accountability has been part of the jargon of the mental health profession for the past few years. Interest in accountability has helped to speed the program evaluation movement; in many cases, though, a concerted effort to relate program evaluation results to the decision making has been lacking. Accountability and more focused evaluation efforts will be forthcoming. Very precise objectives will be expected, with performance indicators set forth in applications for funds and annual evaluation reports. It is conceivable that continued federal support will be contingent upon a CMHC's meeting stated objectives in a quantifiable manner.

The role of the state mental health authority will be enhanced as a major provider of mental health services, with an emphasis on total state system networking. The objective will be to maximize available services, to avoid duplication and fragmentation of services, and to build a single delivery system that will be made up of the public and private not-for-profit sectors. Such a state system will call for carefully worded and honored cooperative agreements between a variety of health, social, mental health, and support system agencies. Many efforts to coordinate and link mental health services with health programs already exist. Indeed, P. L. 94-63 requires that CMHCs develop cooperative agreements with health maintenance organizations.

It is anticipated that in the future the focus will be on those people who suffer serious emotional disturbances, rather than on those who experience problems of daily living. This focus will come about in part because of scarcity of resources and the belief that the seriously disturbed person poses the greatest need and in part because of the drain on resources if concentrated care is not forthcoming.

There has been a renewed interest in prevention, precipitated primarily by the President's Commission on Mental Health (PCMH, 1978). Prevention cuts across service, training, and research. Although CMHCs have offered prevention services throughout the course of the program, even more aggressive prevention activities are predicted.

An increased emphasis on good management of CMHCs as well as improvement of the management capacity of administrators will occur. This thrust will affect both board members and directors as a part of the administrative-governance structure.

A FINAL THOUGHT

Over the past ten years CMHCs have evolved from relatively simple service provider systems to complex enterprises that resemble businesses. One essential ingredient of any business operation is the quality of administration. The management of a business is usually a responsibility that is shared by the executive officer and the board of directors with a defined division of labor. The relationship between the executive officer and the board must be one of dedication and commitment to the product. CMHCs, particularly those receiving reduced federal support, will survive and continue to offer greatly needed mental health services at the community level only if the management is maintained at a high qualitative level. One key to this level of excellence is the nature and degree to which stewardship for center operations is assumed by the board.

REFERENCES

Churchill, W. S. Their finest hour. The Riverside Press, 1949.

The Community Mental Centers Act of 1963 (CMCA), Title II, P.L. 88-164.

The Community Mental Health Centers Act Amendments (CMHCAA). P.L. 89-105. 1965.

The Community Mental Health Centers Amendments of 1975 (CMHCA). P.L. 94-63.

Joint Commission on Mental Illness and Health (JCMIH). Action for mental health. New York: Basic Books Inc., 1961.

Naierman, N. An evaluation of community mental health centers in their 10th and 11th years of operation. Contract No. HEW 100-76-0205. Abt Associates, 1977.

National Institute of Mental Health (NIMH). Community mental health centers program operating handbook part I: Policy and standards manual. Washington, D.C.: Department of Health, Education and Welfare Public Health Service, 1971.

Peters, S., Lochtman, S. A., & Windle, C. Citizen roles in community mental health center evaluation: A guide for citizens. Department of Health, Education and Welfare Publication # (ADM) 79-789. Washington, D.C.: Superintendent of Documents, U.S. Government Printing Office, 1979.

President's Commission on Mental Health (PCMH). Report to President (Vol. 1). Washington, D.C.: U.S. Government Printing Office No. 040-000-00390-8, 1978.

Ragland, S. L., & Zinn, H. K. Orientation manual for citizen boards of federally funded community mental health centers. Department of Health, Education and Welfare Publication # (ADM) 78-759. Washington, D.C.: Superintendent of Documents, U.S. Government Printing Office, 1979(a).

Ragland, S. L., & Zinn, H. K. Citizen participation in community mental health centers: An annotated bibliography and theoretical models. Department of Health, Education and Welfare Publication # (ADM) 79-737. Washington, D.C.: Superintendent of Documents, U.S. Government Printing Office, 1979(b).

2

MENTAL HEALTH BOARDS: DIRECTIVE AND ADVISORY
Arthur J. Robins

The purpose of this chapter is to suggest a frame of reference for understanding the role of the citizens' board in a mental health agency. In order to identify the appropriate areas of responsibility and authority of the board, be it directive or advisory, one must first specify all of the expected outputs of the community mental health center (CMHC) and the programs pertinent to those outputs. Also, one must differentiate board responsibilities from those of the staff. Such an assignment of responsibility should consider not only program demands but legislative mandates as well.

Once responsibility has been allocated to any unit, it is important that the appropriate authority be given to that same unit. Failure to observe this old principle is one of the most common explanations of conflict among governing bodies, advisory committees, and professional staff. Responsibility can be defined as accountability for the achievement of an objective. Authority is the power, legitimated by one's position, to influence the actions of others in the organization. Authority must be commensurate with responsibility because responsibility without authority leads to frustration; authority without responsibility leads to tyranny. Neither condition contributes to productivity. A brief account of the revival of interest in governing bodies may provide some perspective on the problem of task definition.

THE PROFESSIONAL AND HIS PATRONS: FROM PROTÉGÉ TO ENTREPRENEUR

Much of the literature on boards derives from the experience of private charitable agencies, many of which were founded by citizens

18

who had both the concern with some social problem and the financial capacity to support it. They often applied their entrepreneurial capabilities to establishing and administering a social agency. The founders had complete administrative responsibility and authority, that is, they either "owned" the agency or represented the majority interest. This was true not only of philanthropic agencies, but also of types that could be antecedents of the mental health center, such as family service, mental hygiene, and aftercare clinics. As the agencies became more complex, some of the authority was delegated to professional staff. In this manner, greater attention was given to the role of the board and its relationships with executive and staff. This evolution was not unlike that which occurred in industrial and business organizations as the family-ruled enterprise gave way to a system that shared managerial power with employees.

In contrast to those early days, funding sources in recent years have been directly accessible to professionals in the human service field. This has enabled professionals to establish and sustain the delivery of services. An outgrowth of this recent trend, the term "grantsmanship" has entered the language. The protégé no longer needed his patrons, as the federal "angel" supplanted the philanthropist. Professionals became the entrepreneurs, planning the organization, obtaining the funds, producing the services, and locating the clients. The issue of ownership of the enterprise was no longer as clear as it had been in former days. In terms of mental health matters, professionals formulated the application for federal funds, and it was through their efforts that the payroll was met. Despite rhetorical statements of legislative intent and lip service paid to them, citizen participation was often viewed as a burden laid on by federal requirements that could be satisfied simply by establishing a subservient board.

By 1968, state-imposed requirements for CMHC governance could be considerably more rigorous than federal requirements. Despite the fact that a state could require a formal board structure complete with bylaws, it is doubtful that the board carried out the notion of community ownership of the center. Five years after the legislation establishing the community mental health program, a national professional organization still found it necessary to issue a statement directed at curbing the arrogance of professional power. The statement warned about the possibility that a professional elite might develop a proprietary attitude toward a center.

As more and more centers approached the time when federal funding was due to be replaced by other sources, professionals were distressed to discover that local sources of support could not be counted on to substitute for diminishing federal support. Many CMHCs were rescued by the state and by new federal programs, but those that had not cultivated local constituencies realized that their neglect was costly. As Connery (1968) pointed out:

> Federal grants-in-aid offer short-term grants for long-range problems. The federal program asks the state and local government to make a long-range commitment to support each community mental health center constructed without a similar commitment on the part of the federal government, even though mental health is declared to be a national problem. In this situation, the political power structures in the states are understandably loath to place a long-term lien on their financial resources in the interests of a low-priority program (p. 586).

One may speculate that it is the revival of interest in fund raising, one of the governing body's traditional functions, that has led to a spate of articles on CMHC governance. This interest may also account for the more specific, although still not stringent, federal requirements on governance. Even though the decade of the 1960s brought a great interest in citizen participation, there has been no widespread move on the part of citizens to gain control of mental health centers. In some poverty areas, interest groups have engaged center management in heated struggles over center operations. The demand for power was probably as much attributable to awareness of the potential for patronage, particularly in paraprofessional positions, as to concern for increasing the responsiveness of services. By and large, however, no effective pressure has been exerted by the community to exercise its equity in the local center.

Early federal guidelines required that the state mental health authority be assisted in planning for centers by an advisory council whose membership represented all interests concerned with the production and consumption of mental health services. Responsiveness to need was to be assured by the specification that at least one half of the council members represent consumers. Each state was enjoined to set standards to assure responsiveness and was urged to require each center to organize advisory groups for that purpose. The guidelines further suggested that those groups have more than an advisory role in establishing policy and that there be meaningful consumer input to the day-to-day operations of the center.

The current requirements, stated in P. L. 94-63, specify that the governing body of a CMHC, except for those operated by governmental agencies,

> shall be (i) composed, where practicable, of individuals who reside in the center's catchment area, and who, as

a group, represent the residents of that area taking into
consideration their employment, age, sex, and place of
residence, and other demographic characteristics of
the area, and (ii) meet at least once a month, establish
general policies for the center (including a schedule of
hours during which services will be provided), approve
the center's annual budget, and approve the selection
of a director for the center. At least one-half of the
members of such body shall be individuals who are not
providers of health care.

While these requirements do not apply to centers operated by governmental agencies, such centers are, nevertheless, directed to
appoint a committee to advise it with respect to the operations of
the center. The composition of the committee is guided by the same
criteria as for governing bodies.

The primary rationale for the requirements of the governing
body seems to be that such a body will maximize the program's responsiveness to community needs. We can deduce, then, that the
various criteria concerning the composition of the board and the
authority specified in the requirements are somehow related to responsiveness. The criteria seem to assume that the specific mental health needs of a community are related to employment, age,
sex, and "other demographic characteristics." If we try to analyze
the reasons for the other specific requirements, it would appear
that convening a meeting at least once a month will assure that the
board keeps in touch with what is going on. The specification of its
authority to set the center's schedule will assure that availability of
services is related to the particular constraints imposed by the
unique nature of the community's employment and other characteristics. The power to approve the budget and select a director provides assurance that the program is satisfactorily responsive to
community needs and will be implemented by the staff. The requirement that at least half of the governing board members will not be
providers of health care is an attempt to curb the power of professionals whose vested interest in health services presumably limits
their concern with responsiveness.

The recent guidelines do little more than require that there be
a governing body; they probably have had minimal impact on the function and structure of existing governing bodies. They require less
than what most centers already have. Authentic community participation in the governing of a center will not emanate from the enforcement of the regulations. It will come only with recognition that the
governing body possesses areas of effectiveness different from those
of the staff, that it has unique goals it must strive to achieve, that

it must develop programs to achieve these goals, and that it must have the appropriate value base and data base for decision making.

Finally, the governing body must be accountable. The more we rely on objective confirmation of these goals, the less faith need be placed in the ephemeral quality of representativeness. It is fatuous to assume that the needs of a given community will be met if the demographic characteristics of that community are represented in the governing body, for one would then have to believe that a small sample of persons, stratified on those characteristics, is ipso facto competent to evaluate the extent to which a program responds to those needs. I reiterate the belief that underlies this chapter; namely, that

> . . . the effectiveness of boards is not insured by provisions regarding composition and constitutional authority; rather, effectiveness is probably a function of the clarity of objectives assigned to a board, the competence of a board to achieve the explicit objectives, formulation of objective criteria to measure achievement, and the tying of tenure of board members to achievement. (Robins & Blackburn, 1974, p. 38).

EFFECTIVENESS AREAS

The first task is to define the general areas within which center outputs fall. Given the plethora of output-oriented terms used so nonuniformly by writers, I eschew debate as to whether effectiveness area means purpose, mission, aim, goal, objective, or key factor. In arriving at the outputs of a governing body, the most complete analysis would start with identifying the mental health needs of catchment area clients. The center's overarching objective is to meet those needs.

I shall not attempt to settle the question of what constitutes a mental health need, but am suggesting a general approach based upon a set of assumptions. For our purposes, it is not necessary to agree on a single definition of a mental health need. These vary as a function of the observations and values of each community.

Recognizing that the service delivery process begins with need identification, we then consider the current outputs of a CMHC. This stage is preparatory to allocating responsibility and authority for producing the outputs to the professional staff, the governing body (directive or advisory), or to both. I have addressed some of these issues elsewhere (Robins, 1972, 1974; Robins & Blackburn, 1974). The public health model provides one frame of reference for categorizing objectives. Undoubtedly there are alternative approaches. Historically, the community mental health movement has identified itself with the public health model. It is applicable to mental health problems and is comprehensive in its approach to problem solution.

In accordance with the public health model, the various outputs of a CMHC could be classified in the following effectiveness areas:

Health promotion. The objectives in this area strengthen health producing environmental factors and prevent the development of health inhibiting factors.

Specific protection. These objectives establish a defense against disorders by the elimination of essential causative factors.

Detection and treatment of disorders. These objectives concern the introduction of remedial measures.

Disability limitation. These objectives concern the arrest of deterioration and the preservation of normal function.

Rehabilitation. These objectives concern restoration of the individual to the highest level of independent activity of which he/she is capable.

Another effectiveness area is comprised of that which Spaner and Windle (1971) have referred to as process objectives. All objectives are related to the requirement that centers demonstrate responsiveness to community need; the effectiveness area that encompasses those objectives is "responsiveness to community needs." Outputs concern the offering of effective services that are accessible, adequate in volume, appropriate to the catchment population's priority needs, and acceptable and known to the population. Each of those characteristics makes a contribution to the concept of responsiveness.

Responsiveness to community need is a broader characteristic than program effectiveness. An illustration of this point was provided by one community that complained that individuals with alcohol abuse problems spent unusually long periods of time on its center's waiting list, while a considerable amount of therapeutic service was being expended on assertiveness training of clients whose primary complaint was their shyness. The community was indifferent to the success claimed for the training program, having assigned the problem a low priority compared to alcoholism. A second process effectiveness area is local funding. Although a center that is responsive to community need may, thereby, enhance its claim on local financial support, the local funding objectives do not necessarily contribute to responsiveness.

In addition to the effectiveness areas that concern the outcomes of service programs and process, there are general tasks that are related to every effectiveness area and the goals subsumed under each. We refer here to the administrative process that applies to every program. The major steps of this process are planning, organizing, staffing, directing, and controlling. Each of these steps may be viewed as representing an effectiveness area. Planning refers to objectives concerned with creation of a design for achieving a program or process objective. Organizing consists of objectives concerned with the arrangement and relationship of work units pertinent to the plan. Staffing includes objectives related to the collection, orientation, training, and development of competent individuals who are placed in the work units. Directing is concerned with eliciting the best efforts of the individuals in those work units. Controlling is concerned with collection, analysis, and evaluation of the data relevant to the task of maintaining an effective effort toward the goals of the plan.

Figure 2.1 represents the combination of administrative process with program and process effectiveness areas.

The task of determining allocations of responsibilities and authority to the professional staff and to the governing body must consider not only what columns are assigned to each but also what rows. This is a complex procedure because every work unit in the organization follows the administrative process in carrying out its performance program. For example, the planning process is related to the identification of effectiveness areas, and all aspects of the planning process are related to the overall effectiveness areas. Within each effectiveness area, there is a planning process related to programs carrying out individual objectives. Within any one program established to achieve an objective, there may be individual work units, each of which has subobjectives.

OBJECTIVES WITHIN EFFECTIVENESS AREAS

Program Objectives

Having identified the effectiveness areas, the next step is to develop a series of objectives within each of those areas. These objectives must be specified in terms of realistic expectations of what is to be achieved within a given period of time and how the degree of achievement will be assessed. (See Robins & Blackburn, 1974, for a discussion of the application of Management by Objective (MBO) to community health programs.) Space does not permit the presentation of all possible objectives that may be developed within each

FIGURE 2.1

Effectiveness Areas for a Mental Health Center

Administrative Areas	Program or Service Areas					Process Areas	
	Health Promotion	Specific Protection	Early Recognition and Treatment	Disability Limitation	Rehabilitation	Responsiveness to Community Needs	Local Funding
Planning							
Organizing							
Staffing							
Directing							
Controlling							

25

effectiveness area; we mention only a few for illustrative purposes. Under the health promotion effectiveness area, for example, can be placed a number of goals that centers try to achieve under the rubric of consultation and education. The expected outcomes of a program to introduce mental health principles into school classrooms would fall in this effectiveness area. An objective within the specific protection area might concern a program designed to help older people understand the relationship of nutrition to mental well-being and to help them develop good eating habits. An objective under the early detection effectiveness area might be an educational program directed toward helping general practitioners identify persons who might benefit from psychiatric services.

Since the specific mental health needs of communities vary, there may be substantial variety among centers in the formulation of program objectives. It should be noted that the criteria for federal funding of CMHCs require that a specified set of services be in place rather than that a set of objectives be achieved. A center, for example, can be eligible for consultation and education funds based on the fact that it offers a service, whether or not health promotion or any other objective is effectively met by that service. The requirement that services be responsive to community needs demands, inter alia, that the service be effective and not simply that it exist. We shall return to this point when we discuss the allocation of responsibility and authority for evaluation of services.

Process Objectives

Responsiveness to community need comprises a set of objectives which the National Institute of Mental Health has attempted to define operationlly so that the achievement of those objectives can be measured. For example, Bass (1972) has developed an operational definition for continuity of care and indicated which data are required for measuring it. A quantitative measure facilitates assessment of achievement and program improvement. Bass' work provides a model for developing operational definitions of other process concepts, but none has been developed so completely. Also, Mager (1972) has described a technique of goal analysis that produces operational definitions of mental health concepts.

Another objective related to responsiveness to community need is accessibility of services. This may be broken down into five dimensions: temporal, geographic, financial, psychological, and sociocultural. Each of these dimensions can be written as a subobjective related to accessibility. When different performance programs are required, for example, the programs for temporal versus geographical accessibility, the objectives should be individually stated.

Availability of services is a third objective in the area of responsiveness. It has been defined as the amount of various types of services that the center can provide at any given time, expressed as a ratio of items of service per specified number of catchment area residents. Subobjectives may be specified in any particular type of service. Obviously, some standard must be applied to determine whether any given level of availability is adequately responsive.

Awareness of services is another objective under the rubric of responsiveness. If the catchment area's population, both potential patients and referral sources, do not use the services because they are unaware of them, then those services are not achieving the requisite degree of responsiveness.

Acceptability of services is another area of concern. It refers to the predisposition on the part of the catchment population to use the services of the center, and, therefore, refers to responsiveness by the community rather than the delivery system. The CMHC, however, bears the onus of producing services that will be used. If consultation to a school system is unacceptable, the consultant's program, not the school, has failed.

Another component of responsiveness is provision of effective services, meaning that the objective of the service program has been achieved at a satisfactory level. This objective is a necessary but not sufficient condition for the achievement of responsiveness to community need. Programs must not only be effective, but they must also be relevant to need as defined by the community.

Shifting the locus of care to the community is another objective. It is defined as reduction in the use of state hospital facilities and the development of alternative care arrangements in the community. The assumption is that such programs would be responsive to community need. Since the zeal with which the policy of community care has been implemented has frequently outstripped the establishment of satisfactory community care facilities, the assumption of responsiveness has not necessarily been valid.

While there is some question as to whether a second effectiveness area is called for by those outputs associated with local care options, there is no question that the final set of process objectives we will mention compose a separate effectiveness area—namely the development of local sources of financial support. Local support is a federal requirement for each CMHC and is extrinsic to the quality of mental health service. Compliance with federal guidelines has not ipso facto enhanced the quality of care nor the responsiveness of CMHCs, for federal standards are concerned with effort, not effectiveness, and with seeing whether programs exist rather than what programs accomplish.

Administrative Objectives

The following outline, adapted from an excellent diagram of
the management process (Mackenzie, 1969), presents briefly the objectives under each of the effectiveness areas defined earlier:

A. Objectives in planning area—
    1. Forecast: establish where present course will lead in rela-
       tion to need.
    2. Set objectives: determine desired end result.
    3. Program: establish priorities and activity sequences.
    4. Budget: allocate resources.
    5. Set procedures: standardize methods.
    6. Develop policies: make standing decisions on important re-
       curring matters.
B. Objectives in organizing area—
    1. Establish structure: arrange work units and their relation-
       ships.
    2. Establish physician qualifications.
C. Objectives in staffing area—
       Fill positions: recruit, select, appoint, orient personnel.
D. Objectives in directing area—
    1. Delegate: assign responsibility and accountability.
    2. Conflict management: resolve interorganizational differences.
    3. Change management: stimulate creativity and innovation.
E. Objectives in controlling area—
    1. Gather information: establish system for collecting relevant
       data.
    2. Evaluate: ascertain effectiveness and efficiency.
    3. Revise policy, programs, or resource allocations: take ac-
       tion based upon evaluation.

We have presented for each category of effectiveness area
(service, process, and administrative) a number of objectives. For
each objective, there is a set of tasks which, when carried in satisfactory accordance with some standard of performance, is expected
to achieve the objective. Competent implementation of any task at
the appropriate level rests upon the knowledge, values, and skills
of the actor in the situation. We are now at the point when we can
consider what roles to assign to which group: staff, governing body,
or advisory committee.

TASKS IN THE SERVICE EFFECTIVENESS AREAS

The professional mental health worker is the primary person
who has the competencies that are requisite to effective and efficient

performance of programs related to objectives in the service areas. It is conceivable that members of the governing body who are providers may have the same competencies. However, the time demands of giving direct service preclude their involvement with what the jargon frequently refers to as day-to-day operation. It is assumed that the requisite technology has been or should have been mastered in the course of professional or paraprofessional education. Professional staff should have the responsibility and authority to develop and implement service programs, provided that the objectives have had prior approval by the directive body, as shall be discussed below.

The development of a performance program involves the administrative process. Staff must have authority to carry out the steps of the process at the level of service programs, from planning, to evaluation, to modification of the relevant program activities.

TASKS IN THE PROCESS EFFECTIVENESS AREAS

Regardless of the competencies required by the tasks, these objectives must be the responsibility of the governing body because of state and federal regulations. This is not to say that there is no staff involvement. For example, staff can assess mental health needs and report evaluation data without making the policy decisions based upon those assessments. The roles of the staff in relation to the governing body on issues of process effectiveness may be consultative, persuasive, or simply assistive. In some instances, staff may be exclusively assigned to the governing body, a situation more likely at the state or regional level than at the community level. This practice reflects the importance of the governing body effectiveness areas and the stress on its accountability to achieve the stated objectives.

The governing body not only has administrative effectiveness responsibilities in relation to all programs and objectives in the process effectiveness areas, but also has administrative outputs in the service effectiveness areas. Obviously it must be able to plan relative to the appropriate balance among the five effectiveness areas of the public health model. It recruits and selects the executive, and its budgetary authority indirectly affects staffing and service program characteristics. The budgetary authority is the ultimate and pervasive power in any organization. A university president expressed this idea as follows: "The guy who controls the budget is the guy who controls the direction the institution is going to take." (Silber, 1980, p. 17) In universities, faculty controls student admission standards, curriculum, teaching, evaluation, and recruitment and selection of faculty, but its lack of control over the budget severely constrains its legitimate authority. Similarly, CMHC staff control admission, service delivery, evaluation, and staff selection, but not the purse strings. The resolution of the incongruence between program authority and budgetary authority must rest on mutual trust, understanding, and compatibility of values.

This leads us to a consideration of the responsibility and authority of advisory committees. In an earlier day, this designation usually referred to a group of volunteer experts who advised the governing body and the staff on professional service programs. With whatever motivation, they served as unpaid consultants. Their influence over their consultees rested on the authority of their ideas. The prestige and experience of the advisors gave weight to their advice.

There is probably less reason for this consultative type of advisory committee today. Most mental health centers have sufficiently qualified staff to minimize the need for consultation, federal and state technical assistance is readily available, and funds may often be available to purchase consultation as required. Further, since up to 50 percent of the governing body may be health providers, professional consultation is available through that means.

The provisions for P.L. 94-63 on advisory committees do not suggest the consultative role. The governmental agency that operates the center is instructed to appoint an advisory committee composed of residents in the center's catchment area. Since the government agency cannot give away its statutory authority, the advisory committee is in the untenable position of acting as a directive body whose authority rests upon a weak mix of their position vis-à-vis the statutory governing body and whatever source of local power they may possess. The tenuous basis of their authority probably accounts for the frequency of abortive efforts to establish and maintain viable advisory committees. They not uncommonly have an "off-again-on-again" history. Although the statutory authority can enforce as its own the recommendations of an advisory committee, it seems unlikely that a governmental agency will override its staff in any test of will between the staff and the local advisory group. Since their meager authority is based neither on position nor knowledge, advisory committee members who take their responsibility seriously are vulnerable to high levels of frustration. If they do not take their responsibility seriously, then accountability will be irrelevant to them. It would appear that the only way to avoid high turnover of advisory committee members is to select only those who can accept low responsibility and low authority, a combination that is not compatible with serious achievement of process effectiveness area objectives.

The section of P.L. 94-63 dealing with this issue does not seem to have been thought through. It seems almost mischievous to enjoin the advisory committee to become concerned with day-to-day objectives. The wording of this section is ambiguous, leaving unclear whether the advisory committee advises the center or the governmental agency that operates the center. The lack of clarity, perhaps, reflects the confusion that results when the committee may technically be advisory to the superordinate governmental agency but is de facto advisory to the local center's staff.

ACCOUNTABILITY OF THE GOVERNING BODY

The allocation of responsibility for the performance of tasks and the achievement of objectives must be accompanied by the obligation to report and justify levels of effort and effectiveness in specific areas. There must be a mechanism for controlling the performance of all work units, taking corrective action when responsibilities have not been fulfilled, and responding appropriately to success as well as to failure.

The staff is accountable for performance to supervisors throughout various levels in the center hierarchy and, ultimately, to the director. The organizational structure depicts the chain of accountability. The director is accountable to the governing body or, if the center is a component of a larger system, to some higher level in that system.

The governing body should be accountable to the funding agencies, which support the center on the condition that it complies with regulations and guidelines. The government body is also subject to accrediting agencies whose approval or disapproval is vital to the operation, and to the catchment area's total population. Fiscal accountability—the documentation and reporting of the expenditure of income—has long been required of human service agencies. In contrast, program accountability, having to do with goal attainment, is a relatively new concept. In recent years, management systems have been developed that combine fiscal with program accountability (Carter & Newman, 1976). Use of such systems requires that organizational goals be formulated in a way that facilitates assessment of the degree of achievement.

Until governing bodies apply such techniques to their own effectiveness areas, the aspiration for citizen participation in the planning, implementation, and evaluation of mental health services will remain a pious hope. As Stanton (1970) put it in her delightfully acidulous study of volunteers in a mental health association: "Instead of experiencing meaningful involvement, he (the administrative volunteer) is provided a 'sense of participation'" (p. 20). The difficulty of establishing viable controls on the members of the governing body is reflected in the greater security of tenure in the governing body relative to that of center directors and senior staff. The heads that roll because of performance problems, whether in service effectiveness areas or in process effectiveness areas, are much more likely to belong to the professional staff than to members of the governing body.

Advisory committees labor under an even greater handicap than directive bodies in achieving meaningful involvement. They are the weakest component in a triad, the other elements of which are the statutory governing body and the agency staff. The advisory committee's power can be enhanced by forming a coalition with another member of the triangle, a tactic that surely will divert everyone's energies from client service objectives. Until viable accountability procedures are established, both directive and advisory bodies must formulate a scheme for self-evaluation, utilizing reliable and valid measures of performance wherever possible. This chapter, I hope, has provided a guide for an effort at performance self-analysis.

REFERENCES

Bass, R. D. A method for measuring continuity of care in a community mental health center. Department of Health, Education and Welfare Publication # (HSM) 72-9109. Washington, D.C.: Superintendent of Documents, U.S. Government Printing Office, 1972.

Carter, D. E., & Newman, F. L. A client oriented system of mental health service delivery and program management. Department of Health, Education and Welfare Publication # (ADM) 76-307. Washington, D.C.: Superintendent of Documents, U.S. Government Printing Office, 1976.

Connery, R. H. The politics of mental health: Organizing community health in metropolitan areas. New York: Columbia University Press, 1968.

Mackenzie, R. A. The management process in 3-D. Harvard Business Review, 1969, 47, 80-87.

Mager, R. F. Goal analysis. Belmont, Calif.: Fearon Publishers, 1972.

Robins, A. J. Administrative process model for community mental health centers. Community Mental Health Journal, 1972, 8, 208-219.

Robins, A. J. Management-by-objectives for community mental health programs. Hospital and Community Psychiatry, 1974, 25, 228-231.

Robins, A. J. , & Blackburn, C. Governing boards of mental health centers: Roles and training needs. Administration in Mental Health, 1974, 2, 37-45.

Silber, J. Cited by S. Arons. The teacher and the tyrant. Saturday Review, March 1980, 16-19.

Spaner, F. , & Windle, C. The perspectives of national program development and administration: Program needs and evaluation activities. Paper presented at the 79th annual meeting of the American Psychological Association, Washington, D.C. , 1971.

Stanton, E. Clients come last: Volunteers and welfare organizations. Beverly Hills, Calif.: Sage Publications, 1970.

3

DEVELOPING AN EFFECTIVE BOARD ORGANIZATION
Philip M. Nowlen

INTRODUCTION

Effective boards are perhaps more like successful marriages than anything else. Like successful marriage partners, effective board members are people who, while not without problems, confusion, and crises, somehow grow through both success and failure. They improve their understanding of what is expected of them and how to achieve it. Unfortunately, there appear to be no greater number of effective boards than successful marriages.

Organization for What

Some important questions have to be answered by your board. Though difficult, if clear answers can be found, the task of designing an effective board organization is made quite simple.

1. For whom is your board acting? Whom does the board represent? Neighborhoods? Neighborhood institutions or agencies? Ethnic or racial constituencies? The old, middle-aged, or young? Those served by your mental health agency? Those served, plus all others eligible to be served? Some larger public, such as a city-wide or state-wide mental health board? Some combination of the above?

2. How frequently and in what manner should your board report to those it believes it represents?

3. Is yours a governing board or an advisory board? Whom do you govern or advise? What does it mean, concretely, to govern or advise?

4. Does everyone on your board have the same understanding you do of

        (a) whom you represent (another way of saying "to whom you should be accountable");

        (b) how you communicate with those you represent;

        (c) your governing authority or advisory responsibilities;

        (d) the distinction between policy and procedure.

5. What is the range of ways in which the board governs or advises? What information does it need in order to govern or advise? Is such information easily understood by the board?

GROUNDWORK

Accountability, clarity of purpose, and a shared perception of both by the board are the foundations upon which organizational questions can more easily be addressed.

The answers to the questions above, validated by the consensus of the board, should be widely available. They could form the key introductory material in a notebook provided every board member. There is no use carrying on any board function until the board can succinctly explain itself to itself.

In light of the board's answers, it should adopt each year a set of objectives that are realistic, that is, "do-able" within a 12-month period.

There should be no meetings, no committees, no individual assignments, no agenda items and no plans unless the board first states how they relate to the year's objectives.

Therefore no committees should have lives of their own—going on year after year with increasingly vague duties. Specific task forces should be appointed with concrete, explicit objectives; a plan of operation; and a timetable for completion of the task. Upon completion, the task force should be recognized for their effort, then disbanded.

Once task forces are formed based on the year's objectives, the locus of important board work shifts from meetings of the full board to gatherings of task forces and individuals. These activities can be coordinated by a small executive committee. Unless something vitally important and unforeseen occurs, no meetings of the full board are needed until it is time to review the year's objectives or set new goals. It is at such a time that new members can be welcomed and officers elected. The principle: No meetings for the sake of having meetings!

Action suggestion: Look at your constitution and bylaws and change them, if necessary, in order to (1) identify whom the board represents, (2) state clearly how the board governs or advises, (3) facilitate the setting of objectives and creating task forces to achieve them, and (4) have no meetings for the sake of meetings.

MEMBERSHIP

Getting and keeping effective members takes constant work. Unfortunately, it is a task usually relegated to one night a year. The effective board identifies the significant factors, characteristics, and personal qualities that ought to be present in the mix of board members.

Some of the following variables may be important for forming or strengthening your board:

> representative geographic distribution of board members throughout area served by agency;
> representative mix of age, sex, race, ethnic origin, income, and level of education achieved;
> special skills in management, health planning, grantsmanship, accounting, public relations, languages other than English, adult education;
> connections with other community organizations and institutions, including churches, schools, recreation programs, political parties, banks, newspapers, public transportation, and major employers;
> effective leadership experience: solid interpersonal skills, effective chairing and interaction at meetings, record of productive committee work, success at fund raising;
> certain personal qualities, such as reasonable patience, even-temperedness, humor, confidentiality, and the shunning of gossip.

Usually the factors considered significant are presented by a task force to the executive committee for recommendation to the board. Either the task force or the executive committee assigns the qualities priority rankings. When ratified by the board, the factors selected become the criteria for nominations by task force on new board membership. This task force keeps a file of possible nominees as names come to mind, or (for example) as articles on potentially good nominees appear in newspapers. When recommended nominations are due, the task force will typically have more possible candidates than positions to be filled. Therefore they can solicit agreement to be nominated from those who would add the most to the board.

Three members should seek an appointment with the prospective nominee, sending him or her in advance the printed introduction to the board's purpose, customary operating style, accountability channels, organization, and the previous 12 months of minutes. At the interview with the possible nominee the materials sent can be summarized. It is more important to get to the point, that is, to invite the person's interest in serving a term of "so-many" years on the board, estimating the number of evenings or weekends probably requiring his/her time and stating frankly what the person's qualities are that recommended him/her to the board.

The task force will have a better chance to persuade the person to interest himself/herself in board membership to the extent that the interview is brief and to the point, and the advance materials have been well organized. Remember, persons nowadays are more inclined to join an activity when their involvement and obligation are spelled out in detail. No one is inclined to take on open-ended or ill-defined commitments. The chance of misunderstanding is too great.

Listen carefully during the interview and make note of anything the prospective nominee expects to get out of his/her board involvement. For example, "I'm fairly new in town" or "I'm recently divorced" may suggest that he/she is looking for social contacts. If so, you had better use that person—if nominated and elected—in ways that satisfy his/her desire for a wider social circle. Your chance of retaining his/her active membership depends in part on recognizing and responding to such needs.

When a new person is elected, he/she should be provided with a carefully prepared handbook detailing the board's history, constitution and bylaws, a directory of member names, addresses, and telephone numbers, the structure and purpose of the task forces, pertinent information relating to the agency governed or advised, and the short-range objectives set for the current year.

When a new person is elected, he/she should be provided with a specific assignment—on one of the task forces, for example. No one on the board should be without specific tasks for longer than a month.

When a board member appears to "drop out" of activity, two or three members should have an informal meeting with him/her. They can inquire whether some special circumstances or perhaps some disaffection with another board member is the cause. A different assignment might solve the problem. Failing resolution in this way, the member should be strongly invited to resign.

Action suggestion: Try to identify membership gaps that your board should try to fill. Make a grid with the present board members' names on one side and the factors you consider essential on the other.

FIGURE 3.1

Board Members: Sample Grid

Board Members 1980	Geographical Representativeness, by Quadrant				Age				Special Skills				
	NE	NW	SE	SW	18-25	26-35	36-50	51+	Management	Accounting	Public Relations	Ability to Speak Spanish	Health Planning
Abrams	X						X						
Barker	X							X					
Delaney			X							X			
Dellums				X		X							
Fortier			X				X				X		
Hayes	X							X					
Kirk	X				X								
Martino		X										X	X
Otis				X			X						
Reynolds			X			X							
Sullivan				X			X		X				
Trebocic			X				X						
Varner	X							X					
Warren			X					X					

38

Note with an "X" the factors already present on the board and see by contrast where there are gaps. You might try something like the example given in Figure 3.1.

If you use such a grid, the board should be looking for a young person 18 to 35 from the northwest quadrant of the neighborhood. The board should also be on the watch for someone qualified in health planning or someone who speaks Spanish, since the loss of Martino at some point in the future will leave two key qualities missing.

BOARD OPERATIONAL PROCESS

To attract or retain useful board members, time wasting and ineffective board practices must be identified and abandoned. Plan and implement realistic objectives.

Before each meeting, members should receive the agenda and all reports of a strictly informational character. This should happen at least several days before each meeting.

With rare exception, meeting schedules should be set for a year ahead with a pattern that's easy to remember.

Each meeting must begin on time.

Meetings shouldn't run over an hour and a half. That's the limit of the average person's ability to concentrate his/her attention in one sitting.

If the board is large, or must pass on something with legal implications, or has one or more disruptive types—parliamentary procedure should be used. If the board is small or works very easily, less formal conduct of the meeting is in order.

Unless there is an objection, no one should be forced to listen to the minutes of the previous meeting. A special note here about minutes. Neither posterity nor even the board secretary is interested in minutes in the way they are traditionally kept, that is, a blow-by-blow description of what occurred at a meeting, to be read at the meeting following. The only use of such a process is to remind forgetful board members of what their assignments were. Why not transform the minutes into an action information system?

Meeting notes should be taken under two headings: (1) status of projects, and (2) action decisions. For example:

1. Status of projects
    1.1 Budget review: completed
    1.2 Sidewalk repair: no report from City.
2. Action Decisions
    2.1 Jane Murphy to oversee printing and distribution of budget analysis before next meeting.

> 2.2 <u>Jose Benitez</u> to press city for action on sidewalk.
> Specific completion date is desired. Report due next
> meeting.

The minutes, then, consist of <u>brief</u> statements describing
progress on old projects and new actions to be undertaken. After
each brief description, the board members responsible for carrying
out some specific task in behalf of advancing a project or starting a
new effort should have their names and assignments listed with target dates for completion. In order for this system to spur on the
members, the minutes in the new form should be distributed by mail
no later than 48 hours after each meeting.

Under "old business," no show-and-tell, please. Be brief and
to the point. Leave nonessential details out. For example, if assigned to pursue sidewalk repair by the city's department of streets,
report on the status of the project, for example: "A bid has been
selected and work is scheduled for next month." Do not try everyone's patience by reporting, "Well, first I called the city, then they
sent me the application. I filled it out and showed it to the Executive Committee"—and so forth. Only questions based on the written
reports, circulated before the meeting, should be invited.

"New business" should not be the blank space after old business to be filled in by sudden flash ideas or large questions like
"What should we <u>really</u> be doing?" Items for the new business portion of the agenda should be submitted in advance or permitted for
discussion only by consensus of the meeting.

Indeed some important issues can be raised in this way, although it is unlikely that a response worthy of the issue's importance
can be generated by the board in the short time available. The appointment of a task force will accelerate a board decision, as well
as insure that it is an informed decision. Members appointed should
be articulate. They should be charged with reporting in writing the
pros and cons of the issue to the entire board prior to the next meeting.

<u>Action suggestion</u>: Take careful note of the next occasion when
you find yourself bored or angry at what seems to be a waste of your
time at a meeting. Reread this section of the handbook and see if
you can identify the cause of which your irritation is only the symptom. Then seek to change that one procedure that is inadequate or
introduce a corrective procedure if none exists. If your recommendation turns out well, it may lead to a more general reform of board
practices. You will have an important influence on the process.

Handbook for leaders of organizations. Publication Q-2 (Spanish F-23), 1965.

How to give a speech. Publication Q-20, 1977.

Introduction to parliamentary procedure. Publication Q-6 (Spanish F-29).

Job description of the treasurer. Publication Q-18 (Spanish F-19).

Know your community (making a survey). Publication Q-8, 1972.

Leader's guide for workshops on effective organization. Publication Q-7, 1975.

Membership handbook, a guide for membership chairmen. Publication Q-22.

Responsibilities of delegates. Publication Q-19, 1977.

Sample report of a secretary. Publication Q-11 (Spanish F-18).

Simplified parliamentary procedure. Publication Q-1 (Spanish F-5), 1977.

So we're organized: Now what? (How to tackle community problems). Publication Q-13, 1976.

Steps in writing a proposal (how to write for funding). Publication Q-16, 1977.

Suggestions for chairmen. Publication Q-12 (Spanish F-15).

Ways and means handbook. Publication Q-21, 1964.

Whys, whats & whos of bylaws. Publication Q-9 (Spanish F-20).

4

THE CONSTANT BATTLE:
THE POLITICS OF ADVISORY BOARDS
Fr. Francis Chiarmonte

Citizens should strive for maximum feasible community participation. Without it, they will find it difficult to work for their own welfare, promote their own interests, or control what local government does to them. When citizens abandon their political affairs to a few, the welfare of the community tends to be identified with the welfare of the few.

There are many ways for a community to involve itself in its own government. Elections, demonstrations, community meetings, membership in civic organizations, and use of the media are all ways to express public opinion and influence local policy. Knowledge of the community's unique circumstances can help decide which of these methods is the most advantageous. However, more important than the method of community involvement is the question of whether people want to be involved. Very often, a willingness to be involved in its own affairs is a sign of a community's maturity in that it feels competent enough to manage its own life.

This chapter will address one form of community participation that has proved to be effective, the community advisory board. Suggestions for citizen involvement are gleaned from my 15 years of affiliation with Chicago's oldest and largest voluntary community mental health advisory board. I was a charter member of the board, its founding vice chairman, and three-term chairman. I am currently serving as Chairman Emeritus. Since my experience is as a community person, I will speak strictly from the community's perspective and will give examples and draw conclusions based on the experience of this board of ordinary citizens.

The chapter is divided into six sections, the first discussing the value of citizen involvement and the nature and importance of community advisory boards. The second section examines the environment in which the advisory board functions, paying particular attention to the political context in which the board must operate. The next three sections focus on common political situations that any board may encounter: understanding local politics and politicians, recognizing the differing priorities of professionals, governments, friends, and staff, and avoiding pitfalls that may sidetrack the board. I conclude with my personal evaluation of whether citizen participation is worth the constant effort and occasional discouragement that accompany it.

THE CHALLENGE OF THE PEOPLE: ADVISORY BOARDS

A community must realize that unless it is willing to become actively involved in the development of its own mental health services, its services are apt to be more pretense than real. Actions can easily be hidden from the people; unscrupulous politicians can dominate the program and keep the public ignorant by hidden budgets, hiring procedures, and vacant positions. They can push patronage instead of merit. Programs will become dependent on political need; there will be no dialogue with the community and no accountability to the voter. New services will not be developed and existing ones will deteriorate. This is convenient for the politician who may not want to support mental health, but who cannot afford to be against it. If there is active, aggressive citizen involvement, self-serving politicians are quickly recognized and secrecy is broken. Job placements will be earned and programs will serve community needs.

An advisory board is a good way for the local community to speak to its governing body on issues and needs. Its size is manageable and, if composed of a cross section of the community, the advisory board can objectively articulate local needs. The following discussion is intended to give the reader some insight into the nature, role, and importance of advisory boards.

Organizing the Community

The Community Mental Health Centers Amendments of 1965 mandated advisory boards for all mental health centers receiving federal aid. This was the first step in a long journey to bring dignity to the mentally ill. They had been spoken of in hushed tones, secluded in out-of-the-way places, and joked about in bizarre ways.

Much of this was probably due to the general misconception surrounding mental illness. Once the general populace was invited to
join in the care of the mentally ill through the vehicle of community
advisory boards, people began to ask questions, seek advice, and
even make demands on behalf of patients. As community people became more knowledgeable about mental illness, stereotypes began
to disappear. They seriously took up the cause of the mentally ill
by insisting that whenever possible patients be treated in their respective communities, that patient rights be safeguarded, and that
constructive programs replace custodial care.

In Chicago, citizen participation coalesced over the lack of
services to the mentally ill. Knowledgeable citizens joined with a
few professionals in counseling neighborhood people in ways to fund
community mental health centers. As interest and support grew,
so did the number of centers, until 19 in all were built through indigenous efforts. As each center was funded, citizens remained
actively involved by forming advisory boards. Each board consisted
of approximately 25 people who either worked or lived in the community.

As the boards came to know one another, they began to realize
that they shared such common problems as red tape in hiring staff,
political interference, and funding difficulties. Everyone concerned
agreed that a combined effort of all the individual boards would be a
more efficient and effective approach to the problems. Thus, an
umbrella board was formed by electing two representatives from
each board; the new board was called the Community Mental Health
Board of Chicago or, as it was more commonly known, the All-City
Board.

Boards Need Allies

A community advisory board must realize that it is not alone
in its responsibility for the growth and development of mental health
services. While most problems are naturally referred to the board,
solutions must involve other sources. Although the All-City Board
relied on the expertise and prestige of professionals, different alliances are feasible.

Alliances can serve community needs. For example, the
Director of the city's Mental Health Division recruited a professional
advisory council. Most of its members enjoyed far-reaching professional reputations. Mental health programs were presented to them
for their advice. Often the Commissioner of Health, a politician
under whose authority the Mental Health Division fell, would speak
for the community when he met with the professionals, and for the

professionals when he met with the community. Consequently, the professional board and the All-City Board set up a joint committee. When the mental health program reached an impasse in the form of excessive delays, budget discrepancies, or undue political tinkering, the joint committee convened to meet with the appropriate politician. The joint committee gave status and credibility to the opinions of both boards. When confronted by the joint committee, the Health Department found great difficulty explaining away its political machinations without looking absurd.

An Advisory Board Is Not a Board of Directors

An advisory board can be tempted by pressures, frustrations, or even successes to become a board of directors. However, it should not assume an unauthorized role, as this will only provide ammunition to those who want it removed.

On occasion, an advisory board has the opportunity to seize control of its agency. It may be that a weak director succeeds a strong one, or that the board, frustrated by agency resistance, musters sufficient political strength to impose its will upon the agency. However, there is no justification for an advisory board to run an agency, for whenever such a board controls or attempts to control an agency, it creates bitterness and discord. Energy is wasted in power struggles, board members fight among themselves, and staff and board members resign. Neither the agency nor the board accrues permanent gain. Mistrust is rampant and it is difficult to devote time to human services. This is because when the board controls, the agency searches for ways to recover its authority, whereas when the agency controls, the board plots to get rid of individuals standing in its way. Every objection or suggestion is suspiciously viewed by both sides as an attempt to gain points rather than to solve problems.

While it is best for a board to avoid confrontation, it is also important that it not be controlled by the agency. As illustrated earlier, self-defense necessitates the formation of alliances to develop and maintain political power. Confrontation should not be used to control the agency, but only to deliver better services to clients.

What Is a Strong Advisory Board ?

A strong board is a lonely board. Unlike a board of directors, an advisory board has no authority to mandate change. It must rely mostly on itself—its power of persuasion, its knowledge of a situation, its tenacity, its resolve not to be seduced by attractive promises, its ability to judge tactics used by the opposition, its sense of timing, and, ultimately, its ability to create acceptable alternatives as well as develop resources.

Going it alone gives an advisory board both inner and outer strength. Inner strength is the confidence and assurance that moves the board to act against external opposition, particularly when it is threatened. Inner strength makes the board more decisive, more steadfast in the face of smooth talk and exaggerated politeness and gives the board a more realistic sense of the magnitude of problems it faces. In a word, it is courage. Outer strength, on the other hand, is the advisory board's muscle. It is the board's experience, alliances, clout, and ability to create and use resources. Any board that intends to endure has to develop inner and outer strength.

THE BOARD ENVIRONMENT

Is the Board Wanted?

Because an advisory board is often seen by an agency as a necessary evil, it is advantageous for the board to know its position relative to the agency it advises. Generally speaking, it is easy to determine if a board is wanted. The signs are manifest: is the board's role well defined; are training programs available to members; is secretarial help given; are program, budget, and staff information shared? Where these circumstances exist, boards and agencies are disposed to cooperate, even on controversial matters. In all too many cases, boards are only selectively wanted to put on a show of citizen participation in order to impress some outside bureaucrat or funding source. There is nothing wrong with putting on a show as long as a board has the right to advise on substantive issues.

Where's Home?

When a politician or an agency makes a decision favorable to board requests, study it thoroughly before celebrating. Although federal legislation requiring advisory boards was introduced to the communities with a lot of publicity, it soon became evident that its practical application faced serious problems. While the "Feds" were willing to mandate the use of boards in their centers, they were not willing to define how the board should operate. Local governments turned out to be just as unhelpful.

In effect, federal legislation gave boards a home, but refused to give them an address. This forced them to move into any role they thought was home. The landlord, most often a hostile agency, promptly accused them of trespassing and tried to evict them. Boards frequently had to move on, but each time they came closer to defining their responsibilities and functions.

It's Better Not to Ask

If a board wants to help an agency, it must maintain its independence. The board should feel free to step forward and offer advice when it recognizes a problem; it should not have to ask or to be given an invitation. Assertiveness avoids being manipulated by an agency into dealing with "safe" issues. While an agency often wants to avoid controversial issues, particularly those that are self-serving, the board's role is to articulate community needs and help the agency effectively meet these needs. Consequently, when the efficiency of an agency is in question, the board has the right to request information and offer advice. When the board steps forward uninvited, it must realize it will compel the agency to react. However, the subsequent confrontation between the agency and its board can serve to improve a service because what was hidden has now been made public.

Board initiative also clarifies for the agency how the board perceives its role. One word of caution may be appropriate here. An adversary role should be temporary and used only to defend board independence. More positively, the board should attempt to establish procedures for a continual dialogue with the agency.

An example from my experience will illustrate this point. The All-City Board planned monthly meetings with the Health Commissioner and other important personnel. It negotiated annually with the state for additional money and with the "Feds" for special programs in drug abuse; it developed liaisons with federal, state, and private agencies, which eventually helped to establish a city-wide network of services. The All-City Board challenged the Health Department when necessary, supported it when appropriate, but always served as its liaison with local communities. The All-City Board assumed its advisory role on its own authority, as city government would never have offered this opportunity for fear of losing control over finances and patronage.

UNDERSTANDING LOCAL POLITICS AND POLITICIANS

Sometimes an advisory board may feel as though it is getting nowhere. Problems may be overwhelming and the board may feel powerless to act. In such cases, learn to pay close attention to activities in the local political environment. Some people call this being street-wise. In every town or city, there are formal ways in which people are told to address issues. These are usually ineffective. There are less formal ways that get results. For example, one might officially be encouraged to testify before a committee to register an objection, but in reality the best way is to see the "man" about it. If the board does not recognize this, it will be swallowed up by vested interests, hidden agendas, and power plays. To further clarify this point, I have chosen three examples from the Chicago situation. They underscore the importance of understanding the difference between formality and reality.

Clout City

An advisory board should study the methods by which the local government operates. There are simply certain matters to which it will respond and others to which it will not, despite its public posturing. In Chicago, for example, very little matters besides clout. Protocol may open doors, but clout keeps them open. The City Council may discuss ordinances, but clout passes them. People may need a program, but clout gives it to them.

From the early 1960s, Chicago's Democratic Party controlled the most powerful political machine in the country. The party controlled city and state governments and had influence in the nation's capitol. Occasionally, Downstate politicians tried to fight the city by using mental health as a political football, but it was never a contest. Chicago's clout was too strong. The city owned most of the players and called most of the plays.

Published state guidelines demanded community involvement in the planning, operation, and funding of mental health centers as a prerequisite for state funding. Although the State Director of Mental Health referred to these guidelines in his negotiations with the city's mental health division, he could not enforce them in a single city agency. To qualify for state aid, all mental health agencies in Illinois had to demonstrate successful community involvement, except for the Chicago Board of Health. While refusing to submit to this policy, the city continued to receive its money. The All-City Board and many agencies around the state objected to this flagrant violation of state policy, but the state people shrugged their shoulders, while the city people smiled. The city controlled the legislature.

The Mayor's Puppets

It helps immeasurably when a board knows who controls the power. There is frequently a big difference between the way a local government is organized and the way it works. Do not be distracted by appearance.

In Chicago, it was the supposed responsibility of each city department head to ask for new programs in his/her annual budget request, which was then forwarded to the City Council for final approval. When a community wanted to start a new center, it asked the Commissioner of Health. However, because he systematically denied every request, the communities had to turn elsewhere for help, the alderman's office being the most logical place. The more one learned about city politics, however, the more pathetic seemed that option. Except for a few independents, these men and women were machine politicians who owed their political lives to the party and could not afford to incur party disfavor. The mayor, as head of the party, controlled their ward patronage. Thus, a strategy evolved in which a halfhearted formal appeal was made to the alderman—a gesture the system required to save face—and then an appeal went directly to the mayor. Once his consent was given, Council approval was automatic. Apart from a few brave but relatively powerless individuals, a City Council meeting was like a puppet show with one difference. These puppets not only responded quickly and smoothly when their strings were pulled, but, in addition, once they sensed they were pleasing their master, they were able to carry on the show independently. After the center was funded, the alderman's importance increased somewhat. His/her knowledge of city government and departmental bureaucracy enabled him/her to cut the red tape responsible for delayed hiring and spending.

"Political Animals"

Public administrators are often forced by the political structure in which they work to become "political animals." It's up to the community advisory board to recognize this and not to be influenced by their exaggerated sympathy, dazzling eloquence, and empty promises. Many administrators depend more on charm and polish to influence people than on facts. When politics rather than professional expertise rule an agency, the advisory board must become the watchdog of agency integrity because agency decisions are more apt to be based on politics than on human need. It best protects the agency by being aware of the political vulnerability of the administrator and his/her political party. The rule is that since public image is preeminent in politics, leverage is maintained when the board musters broad community support.

The All-City Board learned to be particularly sensitive to appointments made after the election of new political leaders. In the Health Department, the first and most important appointment was not the professional head but the party representative. His job was to protect the party's interests, and he had the authority over finances and patronage to do it. On one occasion, the Board was engaged in a serious struggle with the Health Commissioner not to consolidate local mental health centers with comprehensive health centers. The Deputy Commissioner recruited a psychiatrist to lecture the board on the advantages of consolidating health care. The All-City Board knew that the real issue was community participation, not consolidation. The Commissioner wanted to eliminate a significant number of mental health people and weaken the local boards. The All-City Board recognized this ruse and organized so much public protest against consolidation that the city failed in its efforts. Afterward, the psychiatrist was given an important position in one of the comprehensive health centers.

DISAPPOINTING LESSONS

Not Everyone Wants the Same Thing

Sometimes advisory boards seek support from organizations and people whose stated goals and interests appear similar. They may logically assume that mental health professionals or organizations, because of their common interests, would willingly assist the board in serving the mental health needs of the community. Such an assumption is often invalid. While their interests in mental health are indeed common, their priorities may differ markedly. It is vital for a board to learn about a person's or organization's practices as well as their interests before trusting them.

The All-City Board could not be effective in dealing with the Chicago Board of Health without allies, for the department was a party stronghold for patronage workers and political deputies. The All-City Board went to the most logical places for friends—the federal and state monitoring agencies, voluntary mental health organizations, mental health professionals, and center staff.

While those contacted were interested in helping the advisory board, they did not consider assistance high on their list of priorities. Some were afraid to confront a city agency because of personal consequences, while others were more interested in ingratiating themselves with powerful political forces. In a couple of instances, individuals felt indebted to the mayor for past favors. Still others became so institutionalized over the years that they no longer cared. The All-City Board would have saved time and energy if it could have anticipated these responses, but instead it felt needlessly betrayed and angry.

Government Is Not Necessarily for the People

Since the idea of community mental health boards was a federal brainchild, one would assume that federal representatives would want to see them work. However, boards have often been disappointed because the "Feds" have tended to abandon them in their struggle for recognition and acceptance. The federal government was interested in advisory boards, but gave them a low priority.

In Chicago, we knew that the federal government wanted to reduce the tight control of the machine, and consequently we thought that the "Feds" would support the All-City Board in its struggle with the Mental Health Division. It denied board requests because the issue was not big enough to incur the wrath of Chicago's powerful machine. In effect, the "Feds," in order to protect their own interests, ignored citizen participation.

Local government might be expected to have a greater investment in the welfare of its citizens, but somehow their investments tend to become misplaced. On one occasion, the Commissioner of Health decided that the mental health program needed better structure and organization. He insisted on a medical model of service delivery even though the current system had the sanction of three different local departments of psychiatry. Reorganization was needed because he was under pressure from political sources to initiate services for drug addiction, hypertension, and immunizations. He needed resources to effect these services and decided to use the local mental health centers not only for their available manpower but also for their strategic locations around the city. The All-City Board objected to turning the mental health centers into primary care health centers. The Commissioner appointed a new director to carry out this policy in the name of good mental health. Thus, for a period of time, nonmedical mental health staff were used as health technicians in taking blood pressure, running errands, and delivering vaccine around the city.

Professionals Are Not Always Professional

It is foolhardy to assume automatically that mental health professionals have the same priorities as citizen boards even though

they live in the same environment and are subject to the same pressures and temptations. The All-City Board had a particularly traumatic experience learning this lesson. Although a mayoral appointee
to the Chicago Board of Health, one particular psychiatrist was
greatly respected by the Board. He befriended board members,
mediated problems with the Health Department, and publicly declared himself sympathetic with the Board. When he became the
Director of the State Department of Mental Health, the Board was
elated. He knew the problems community boards were having with
the city and was now in a strong position to support them.

The All-City Board's greatest leverage was its authority to
oversee state money allocated to individual city mental health centers. This money could not be as easily manipulated by the city
since it required consent of the local advisory boards. Shortly after
his appointment as director, the psychiatrist was "influenced" by
his city connections. He wrote a new contract with the city that dis-
continued the practice of earmarking funds for each center and replaced it with a lump sum grant awarded directly to the Health Department. Despite the unanimous dissent of all 19 local boards, the
All-City Board, and many professional, state, and private mental
health agencies, the Health Department now had complete control
over all of its city and state funds. This disastrous setback almost
ended community mental health and citizen participation in Chicago.

Friends Are Not Always Friendly

After losing its advisory position vis-à-vis state money, the
All-City Board was particularly vulnerable to political pressure.
The Commissioner of Health pressed his advantage by administering
a civil service exam to the temporary mental health staff that was
designed to fail over 50 percent. The All-City Board met with the
Commissioner and then appealed to the mayor to no avail. As an
expression of solidarity and sympathy with the staff, the Board
donated $200 to its legal fund. The employees were suing the Board
of Health. The Commissioner was furious and "fired" the Board.
This act aroused widespread community support against him and
news media across the country carried the story.

The Commissioner soon realized his mistake and attempted
to save face. When he asked to meet with the "fired" board to discuss the formation of a new board, everyone knew it would be a
token board and refused. He persevered for months. Finally, in a
move that flabbergasted the All-City Board, the Mental Health Association of Greater Chicago came to his rescue. The president of
the Association was a former state governor with interests under

the control of the Board of Health. In essence, he made a backroom deal to supply the Commissioner with enough Mental Health Association members to organize an interim board. However, the All-City Board ultimately prevailed by aligning itself with a mayoral candidate who defeated the machine.

Staff Is Not Always Supportive

Until the victories of the All-City Board, the Health Department had never been successfully challenged, so word of even its modest achievements spread rapidly throughout the city. There were those among the staff at the local centers who were emboldened by its success and wanted to use the board to their advantage. They beseeched the board to fight for selfish issues. Insubordinate staff asked the board to save their jobs, ambitious staff played off the Health Department and the board for political gain, and weak administrators wanted board protection for personal positions on policy.

Unfortunately, because the All-City Board did not distinguish between personal and public issues, it felt compelled to act in inappropriate areas and unnecessarily to assume adversary positions with the Health Commissioner. Before this could change, the board had to clarify its role as advisor on public needs and not as champion of individual ones. With this new understanding as a guide, the board was able to refuse inappropriate staff requests easily. It readily referred discontented employees to the city's personnel code to resolve grievances, adamantly refused to advance individual ambitions, and comfortably permitted weak administrators to stand alone on personal positions.

DIRTY TRICKS AND WHAT TO DO ABOUT THEM

Public agencies are often motivated solely by political gain. Consequently, they can be satisfied with maximum public recognition for minimum service. In this manner they consume resources for agency promotion rather than for services to the people. An agency often uses diversionary tactics on its advisory board to neutralize it, while the agency continues to shortchange the public. The following examples will demonstrate some of the more concrete ways in which agencies and governmental bodies sidetrack citizen boards.

In-depth Studies

Advisory boards must be especially careful to distinguish between subterfuge and genuineness, or they end up jousting with

windmills. Sometimes the subterfuge is cloaked in social acceptability. For example, in an attempt to delay or evade an issue, an
agency may announce the need for an "in-depth study" or announce
the appointment of a "committee of knowledgeable people." They
claim to be "working on the matter," with decisions to come "shortly."

Once the board sees through this pretense, it must be concerned about whether or not to denounce it publicly. The public may
perceive a critical stance as unreasonable, thereby increasing the
vulnerability of the board's position. In the case of the All-City
Board, the Health Commissioner delighted in publicly denouncing it
as a group of self-appointed agitators. Until a board is strong
enough for open confrontation, it must join in the bogus committees
and the phony studies to gain time to document its case.

"Give Him/Her a Chance"

An advisory board may be required to work with an administrator who has been appointed without its input. The board is asked
to trust the new man/woman, share information with him/her, and
give him/her time to implement needed reform. If it hesitates to
give its trust, the board may be accused of bias. Even if there is
overwhelming evidence to suspect the appointment, the board may
still be vulnerable to this charge. Since the first impulse is to give
the new administrator a chance, the following suggestions may be
helpful. Closely observe the administrator's stance toward the board
and thoroughly examine his/her ability. Does he/she encourage
regular meetings between himself/herself and the board, or does
he/she assign other staff? Does he/she have power over the supervisor, administrator, deputy administrators, budget directors, and
staff? At a minimum, he/she must control the use of his/her budget and have the right to hire and fire. An executive who has limited
authority in such matters can never make significant changes. A
board should be wary of any administrator who is in a weak position
because he/she is there to do what is ordered.

The advisory board is the community's only hope against administrators who take orders from politicians. Therefore, it must
continue to pressure him/her on behalf of the community by object-
ing to unreasonable delays, exposing subterfuge, and insisting upon
needed change. Throughout all this struggle, it helps to keep in
mind that confrontation is not against the person of the administrator as much as against the system oppressing both. Once it is evident the administrator can't or won't do anything, the board should
not waste time. Go to the politician with the power and address the
problem to him/her in the name of the community.

"Meeting the Needs of the Patient"

A public agency often uses noble language to cover up its ig-
noble moves prompted by underlying political concerns. "Meeting
the needs of the patient" is just such an example. Because of its
close relationship with the agency, an advisory board is in the best
position to judge its motives and to expose any underlying political
issues. On one occasion, the Health Department cited patients'
needs as ostensible justification for a proposal to reorganize its
Mental Health Division. The All-City Board knew the underlying
motive was to eliminate effective community advisory boards and
decided to fight fire with fire by proposing its own plan to meet the
patients' needs. It convened the joint committee of professionals
and community people and proposed an alternate reorganization plan
that favored community boards. At no time during the discussion
between the advisory board and the agency was the question of eliminating community input discussed, although that was the real issue.
The entire discussion centered on meeting the patients' needs most
appropriately. Ultimately, the strong professional and community
support prevailed and no reorganization occurred.

What You Don't Know Will Hurt You

Without information a board cannot work any better than machinery without fuel. Often agencies conceal or distort vital information so that they will not be held accountable. Important facts
about budget, hiring, vacant positions, and unspent funds are unob-
tainable. If the agency is dominated by politics, the public's right
to information is easily disregarded. Formal channels of communication are closed to the board, appeals to higher authority are usually ineffectual, and most boards cannot afford to go to court.
Under these circumstances, community boards must not waste
their time fighting for information they will never receive. By expending valuable time in fruitless pursuit, the board serves the purpose of the agency. A board must develop its own sources of information. This is essential even if the agency does not deprive it of
information. Independent information serves as a reliability check
on that received from the agency and is also helpful in making alliances with the agency's funding sources. These sources typically
want to assure maximum return on their dollar.
Unchecked fiscal mismanagement or political meddling can
have disastrous consequences. In the case of the Health Department,
the All-City Board was able to document that over $300,000 ear-
marked for mental health was spent elsewhere.

The Name of the Game Is Help Yourself

Politicians have a knack for making people think they are interested in them. We tend to think of them as "nice guys." However, advisory boards cannot afford to be distracted by appearances.
Always remember that these "nice guys" make decisions based on
what is good for themselves, while public need remains secondary.
Average politicians mark their intentions by indicating that their
priority is helping people. In reality, politicians do not respond to
public need unless they can also increase their own prestige or party
strength. Mental health is a low profile service that may easily be
sacrificed for political ends.

Another fact is that control over jobs is top priority because
it is essential in building an army of loyalists. In Chicago, every
job applicant, professional or not, has to have a political patron who
is usually a ward committeeman. Who you know counts more than
what you know. It also means that city services are unavailable
during some campaigns and on voting days.

Advisory boards cannot afford to be lulled into inactivity because federal, state, or local politicians give them some attention,
nor should they be fooled by loud protests of indignation at their
shabby treatment. Judge politicians by the results they achieve for
the board, because in the end this is what matters. To get results,
the All-City Board found it helpful to publicize what politicians did
and did not do for them. While the latter did not necessarily encourage support for the board, it did earn the board respect and
discouraged feigned political support. Insofar as it helped their
public image, favorably disposed politicians continued helping the
board.

Having Your Cake and Eating It: A Chicago Phenomenon

"Beware of Greeks bearing gifts" is as true today as it was in
ancient Troy. Avoid being distracted by what you get, because local
governments are good at conning the public.

In Chicago, each celebration of a new center was shortlived
because community people found out that getting the funds was only
part of the problem. Spending them was a bigger problem. Few
centers managed to spend as much as 50 percent of their budget.
Why? Because the city held back its funds while the State Department of Mental Health was providing matching grants. How was the
city able to have its cake and eat it too? Each year the city would
fund a new center in a corporate budget to qualify for state matching
funds. Then the Health Department proceeded to jam the new center

with so much red tape that it took a year or more to get it opera-tional. In the meantime, the city was free to spend the available state funds to provide mental health services. Two other favorite city tactics to bottle up spending were to delay up to two years the renting of office space and to prolong hiring procedures for as long as 18 months per position.

IS THE EFFORT WORTH IT?

The time will inevitably come when an advisory board ques-tions its usefulness. It may occur when the board is promoting an unpopular cause, when it is in an advisory relationship with the director, or when it is ignored or publicly attacked by the agency. These events take their toll. Board members tire of neglect or dis-respect, and may doubt their usefulness. Some may even resign. It is important during these crises to review the history of the board to gain a proper perspective.

The All-City Board had to function in one of the most blatantly political cities in the nation. With all our doubts and frustrations, we continued to survive and eventually to succeed because we exam-ined our record over time and did not succumb to temporary set-backs. Each year we gained at least one additional center. Mental health services grew in direct proportion to community involvement, patient referrals multiplied, and a network of services developed. The board's help gave staff the security to develop innovative and creative programs.

The thrust of this article has been to offer some general prin-ciples for advisory boards with no apparent clout or advantage to work successfully with powerful antagonistic agencies and govern-mental bodies. The detailed examples from the experience of Chicago's All-City Board were offered to add color, depth, and flavor to the problems other boards will encounter with government and agency politics. Boards face strong opposition and can easily become frustrated and disappointed.

If this article can aid boards by forewarning and forearming them against political pitfalls, I will be happy to have made the con-tribution. One can safely assume that problems encountered by the All-City Board are similar in kind to those of many community ad-visory boards across the country. In my many years of experience working with boards, the problems have never changed, only the faces.

5

THE EXECUTIVE DIRECTOR AND THE BOARD
Morris L. Eaddy

The successful or unsuccessful operation of a community mental health center (CMHC) can often be traced to the relationship between the CMHC's executive director and his/her board of directors. This relationship can be one that results in a clear understanding and acceptance of the roles and responsibilities of each, or one in which constant conflict and territorial battles between the two detract from the true mission of the CMHC. The clarification of these roles and responsibilities and the sharing of mutual expectations can lay the groundwork for a relationship that is positive, constructive, and in the best interest of the CMHC.

What is the nature of a healthy, effective interaction between a CMHC executive director and a CMHC board? In the following hypothetical conversation, a new member of a CMHC board of directors talks to the executive director concerning this relationship.

Board Member: What do you feel is the ideal relationship between an executive director and a board?

Executive Director: The answer to that question is both simple and complex.

Board Member: Start with a simple answer and ease into the more complex.

Executive Director: Well, a simple answer to the ideal relationship between an executive director and a board is "the board sets policy and the executive director implements this policy." This statement, or some variation of it, implies a simple and clear distinction between the roles of board and executive director, and a clear definition of the responsibility of each.

Board Member: That makes sense to me.

Executive Director: Yes.

Board Member: But there is more to it than that.

Executive Director: Yes, that's right. The truth of the matter is that the roles are seldom initially well-defined. These roles tend to evolve as the CMHC changes over a period of time. These roles are also influenced by a wide variety of factors.

Board Member: What sort of factors?

Executive Director: Let's look at a few. First the roles of the board and the executive director are influenced by the unique characteristics of the CMHC.

Board Member: I'm not sure I know what you mean by that. Is one CMHC so greatly different from another?

Executive Director: CMHCs vary organizationally a great deal. Some CMHCs are organized as private, nonprofit corporations. These CMHCs may contract directly with the state and local government as well as receive federal funds. While they are certainly influenced a great deal by governmental regulations and priorities, legally these CMHCs are not governmental entities.

Other CMHCs, however, are administered as units of state government. The staff of these CMHCs are state employees. State control may exert a greater influence in these CMHCs than in CMHCs that are operated as private, nonprofit corporations.

Some CMHCs are administered and governed by hospitals, whereas others are "free-standing" and contract for necessary inpatient or other hospital services. The hospital-based CMHC may be faced with a number of issues that are peculiar to hospitals. For example, services may be more closely tied to what has been called the "medical model" than might be the case if the CMHC were not part of a medical institution.

The location of a CMHC influences its plan for service delivery and the style of board leadership needed. Some CMHCs are located in urban areas, and others are located in predominantly rural areas. The rural CMHC has problems and needs that may be quite different from a CMHC located in a more densely populated area.

Some CMHCs are relatively small and organizationally simple, while others are responsible for quite large budgets and are extremely complex organizations requiring sophisticated management staff and board members with special areas of expertise.

Board Member: Therefore, the type of relationship that develops between an executive director and a board of directors may differ considerably from one CMHC to another.

Executive Director: Yes. While there will be many similarities in this relationship from one CMHC to another, there will also be distinct differences, depending upon the unique characteristics of a particular CMHC.

Board Member: You mentioned other factors in addition to the type of CMHC. What other factors did you have in mind?

Executive Director: One factor that is quite important in determining the type of relationship that will exist between a board and an executive director is the developmental stage of the board—that is, whether the board consists of people who are experienced in functioning as a policy-setting group, or of persons who have little experience and will require a period of time to understand their proper role and be comfortable with it. The readiness of a board to function smoothly and effectively depends upon the level of sophistication the board has obtained concerning the primary mission of the CMHC, its understanding of the CMHC's service priorities, and its understanding of the complex relationships between the CMHC and external controls and influences upon CMHC operations.

Board Member: External controls?

Executive Director: By external controls and influences I mean the direction given to CMHCs by governmental service priorities, governmental rules and regulations that affect CMHC policies and procedures, and the rules and regulations of various other funding sources. CMHCs are financed through a multiplicity of funding sources. Each funding source sets certain priorities, and these change over time. There is an ever-increasing need for the executive director and board to anticipate future changes and constructively prepare for them through short- and long-range planning efforts (Mazade, 1978). Board sophistication in such matters is closely related to how good a job the executive director and his/her staff have done in the area of continuing inservice education with the board, the length of time the CMHC has been in existence, and the experience background of the board members prior to serving on the CMHC board. In many cases, CMHCs find it desirable to plan for some specific training in governance to help board members function more effectively (Morrison, 1977b; Howell, 1979; Robins & Blackburn, 1974).

Board Member: Are there other factors?

Executive Director: I would say there is one other extremely important factor. Just as a board of directors may vary tremendously from one CMHC to another, depending upon the factors I have mentioned, it is also true that all CMHC executive directors are not cut from one mold. The community mental health movement is still fairly new in this country. There is at this time no common agreement about the best "type" of chief administrator for a CMHC. Most CMHC executive directors come to their jobs with a background in psychiatry, clinical psychology, or psychiatric social work. In the beginning of the CMHC movement, almost all executive directors were people whose past experience had primarily been that of clinical work with patients. For one reason or another, they had become interested in mental health administration. In more recent years, a larger number of people with primarily business or administrative backgrounds have started assuming leadership responsibilities in CMHCs.

Board Member: You say there is no common agreement concerning the best experience background for a CMHC executive director. Has this issue been studied?

Executive Director: Yes. There has been considerable debate over the issue (Hinkle & Burns, 1978). There are those who feel strongly that only the clinician-administrator has the experience background necessary to understand the mental health system and to deal effectively with mental health practitioners. They feel that the clinician-administrator has the broad background in human behavior that is necessary to deal with the issues that exist in mental health. They assert that this background is also necessary to have credibility with mental health professionals and representatives from related human service agencies. On the other hand, there are many who point out that the CMHC of today is a very complex organization responsible for expending millions of dollars each year. They feel that the effective administration of a modern CMHC therefore requires a specific administration and business background. This is an experience background that few clinicians have.

Board Member: Are there specific personality traits or personal characteristics needed by a successful CMHC executive director?

Executive Director: That, too, is unclear. One study looked for such individual characteristics and considered the possibility that "the traits that characterize successful industrial administrators would also characterize administrators in effective CMHCs" (Howell, 1976). Much to the surprise of many, this study did not find that such traits were necessarily linked to effective CMHC administration. Let me quote a few lines from the results of the study: "The predictions were derived from previous findings in other types of organizations—mostly industrial firms. CMHCs are unique organizations in many ways. Their objectives, sources of funding, manpower, clientele, location, and political and legal restrictions are only a few of many possible factors that influence their functioning and are largely beyond their control. The common performance criterion used in business organizations (i.e. profitability) is not easily applied in this setting. . . . It may be that the unique nature of CMHCs (especially their objective and clientele) requires an equally unique type of administrator—one who bears very little resemblance to the effective administrator in other organizations" (Howell, 1976, pp. 131-132).

Board Member: What is the answer to this dilemma?

Executive Director: There is probably no single answer at this time. What seems to be occurring is that clinician-administrators are increasingly recognizing their need for additional training in all areas of management in order to administer CMHC programs effectively. This includes standard business procedures, personnel matters, business law, accounting and budgeting, skills in negotiation and conflict resolution, and long-range planning. During the past few years, opportunities for this additional training have started to develop. There are workshops and courses in various aspects of community mental health management being made available through the Staff College of the National Institute of Mental Health, several universities, and through some state organizations whose membership is composed of community mental health centers. In my view, there is probably a need for the development of specialized, advanced academic degrees in community mental health administration or human service administration (Buntz, 1977). In any case, the CMHC executive director needs to have knowledge of both the mental health system and of sound management practices. However, there is simply no way that the executive director in a CMHC can have an adequate experience background in all areas of responsibility. This means that the executive director and the board need to agree upon a plan for continuing professional education of the executive director in "deficit" areas of knowledge or experience.

Board Member: All right. We must then assume that the relationship between the board and the executive director will vary from one CMHC to another, depending upon the type of CMHC involved, the background and experience of the board, and the background and experience of the executive director. Still, there must be some common elements of the relationship that exist even with these variations from one CMHC to another.

Executive Director: Yes, there are common elements, but I wanted to make sure that several key factors influencing that relationship were pointed out at the beginning because they are important in understanding the discrepancy that may exist when looking at what might be termed an ideal relationship as opposed to the more common or actual structural and functional relationships.

Board Member: Well then, let's look at some of these more common areas of the relationship.

Executive Director: We first began talking about the setting of policy. Why don't we look at that in more detail?

Board Member: Fine.

Executive Director: The role of the board in establishing policy seems to be generally agreed upon. A recently published orientation manual for citizen boards of federally funded CMHCs (Citizen

Participation Program, 1979) states: "major areas of conflict between board and staff frequently revolve around the issue of authority. Clarifying the roles and responsibilities of each group must be an ongoing effort based on sound and consistent principles rather than a matter of whim or expediency. There is general agreement that the basic distinction between the role of board and staff is summarized in a phrase—the board makes policy; the staff implements policy." The manual further states that "board policy should be expressed in the broadest terms wisdom permits. Staff are then able to consider options and determine the appropriate method of implementation."

Board Member: Is that how it is done?

Executive Director: Broadly speaking, yes. However, the executive director is usually involved to a great extent in formulating policy issues, preparing position statements concerning policy options, and making recommendations based upon his/her perception of programmatic or funding implications for various policy options.

Board Member: Could you state that a little more clearly?

Executive Director: Well, policy does not suddenly develop in a vacuum. While the board has the responsibility for "making policy," the executive director and his/her staff have the responsibility for assisting the board in several ways. First, they can be of help in determining areas where it is important that policy be developed. Areas of necessary policy development would certainly include the formulation of clear personnel policies, a policy concerning acquisition or leasing of CMHC facilities, a policy concerning review and evaluation of CMHC programs, as well as policies in many other areas of CMHC operation. The executive director should provide whatever staff assistance is necessary for the board to properly address policy issues. This may include developing position papers, providing staff input concerning problem areas that require policy determination, and providing information about the likely consequences of adoption of specific policies.

I believe the important thing here is that the board and executive director work collaboratively in the development of CMHC policy. The executive director must clearly see his/her function as that of acting in an advisory capacity and in providing staff support to the board. There should, at no time, be any misunderstanding concerning the separation of roles. It should always be clear that the board has the responsibility and the sole authority to set CMHC policy.

Board Member: So that's the way it should work.

Executive Director: That's the way it should work, and in most instances, it does work that way. It is true, however, that some CMHCs may operate for many years with implicit policies as opposed to explicit policies. Where board policies are not explicit—in written form—there may be considerable confusion on the part of staff concerning the intentions of the board. In some cases, where the CMHC has a relatively weak board and a strong executive director, the CMHC may operate over a period of years with implicit policies originated by the executive director. Where clear policies are not developed by the board, then implicit or "unwritten" policies will fill the gap by default. The CMHC will continue to operate—for better or worse—whether or not there are explicit board-originated policies concerning CMHC operations. In the absence of such policies, staff evolves "common understandings" that permit the CMHC to operate on a day-to-day basis even with the lack of official board guidance. Let me mention that there are several publications currently available that can assist in orienting new CMHC board members so they can better know what is expected of them. One publication is entitled "Manual on Governance and Policy-Planning for Board Members" (Price, 1977), and another is the "Orientation Manual for Citizen Boards of Federally Funded Community Mental Health Centers" (Citizen Participation Program, 1979). These publications provide a helpful historical perspective on the community mental health center movement, as well as effective presentations on board organization, duties and responsibilities of board members, and policy planning. There are also several journals that many CMHCs receive on a regular basis, and there are often articles in these journals that are relevant to board members. Administration in Mental Health and the Community Mental Health Journal are two such publications. Both journals address important community mental health topics.

Board Member: Before we go much further, let me ask you to make a distinction between a board of directors and an advisory board. As I understand it, the CMHC has, in addition to a board of directors, both an advisory board and a professional advisory committee.

Executive Director: That's a good point. Let me see if I can clarify some important differences, responsibilities, and functions between them.

I think it would help to begin by substituting the term "governing board" for "board of directors." The CMHC board of directors is the governing body of the CMHC. As a governing board, it is fully responsible and accountable for all CMHC operations and for the actions of CMHC employees, volunteers, and students in training. The governing board is the grantee; it receives the money for CMHC operations and is therefore responsible for the proper expenditure of that money. The governing board is legally responsible for all aspects of CMHC operations, including both administrative and clinical services. The governing board is where the buck stops.

Advisory boards, on the other hand, do not normally have this legal responsibility. They do not have the statutory authority to make binding fiscal or programmatic decisions, even though they may advise in most matters pertaining to CMHC operation. Advisory boards can be extremely helpful and give important feedback to the governing board. They should certainly not be viewed as inconsequential and, in fact, may play a powerful role in the direction taken by a CMHC. Considerable influence and power may be exerted by advisory boards, since they may present to their governing board points of view that might otherwise be lacking. These groups can assume a number of important responsibilities assigned by the governing board.

I should mention that CMHCs established by a governmental agency—such as county government or the state—prior to the 1975 amendments are allowed to function with an advisory committee, representative of the area, that has the responsibility of advising the governmental agency "with respect to the operations of the center, which committee shall be composed of individuals who reside in the center's catchment area, who are representative of the residents of the area as to employment, age, sex, place of residence, and other demographic characteristics, and at least one-half of whom are not providers of health care" (Public Law 94-63, Section 201 [c] [1] [B]). While some advisory boards, for various reasons, may actually wield considerable power and authority if they are set up to function as pseudo-governing bodies, the governing board retains final responsibility for CMHC operation.

Depending upon circumstances, an advisory board may be weak, ineffectual, and mostly window-dressing; on the other hand, it can provide important and meaningful advisory functions to help the board.

In addition, every CMHC is specifically required to establish a professional advisory board or committee "to advise the governing board in establishing policies governing medical and other services provided by such staff on behalf of the center" (Public Law 94-63, Section 201 [d]). A professional advisory board makes recommendations. It advises and may exert a great deal of influence in policy determinations of the governing board. This advisory board, since it is composed of professional staff with a wide background of clinical and programmatic experience, is in an excellent position to provide valuable input concerning needed changes in CMHC services or service delivery and ways to improve quality of services offered to the community.

Board Member: What about the relationship of the executive director to these various advisory boards?

Executive Director: In most cases, the relationship is similar to the executive director's relationship to the governing board. Staff assistance is provided to these advisory boards to the extent necessary for them to do an effective job in the areas of responsibility assigned by the governing board. The executive director may participate in the activities of these advisory boards to a greater or lesser extent, however, depending upon local options. These advisory boards usually report directly to the governing board.

Board Member: You talked about the governing board setting policy for CMHC operations and described this as perhaps the most important function of the governing board. What are other reasons a governing board needs to exist?

Executive Director: There are many other reasons a CMHC governing board is necessary and important. Let me mention a few of these. As in the case of policy determination, each of these additional areas requires joint efforts of both board members and the executive director. These are shared responsibilities, and both the executive director and his/her staff and board members work toward common goals. The board members, however, have the decided advantage of being community volunteers interested only in what is best for the community.

The governing board needs fully to accept its responsibility in developing the necessary financial resources to make adequate CMHC services possible. At the local level, board members can have tremendous influence in generating the necessary local funding from city and county government, United Way, school board, and other local financial resources. They are in an excellent position to contact local foundations that may be able to contribute to various worthwhile projects.

The board's ability to help generate and maintain local funding can mean the difference between a successful and an unsuccessful CMHC. As you know, these local funds form the basis for the entire financial structure of the CMHC. They have the magic potential of being able to draw down state and local dollars. The ratio of local money to state and/or federal money may vary from 1:1 to as high as 1:10; that is, for every dollar of local financial support, the CMHC may be able to draw down from one to ten dollars in support from other sources. Therefore, an extremely important responsibility for the governing board and the executive director is the preservation of the funding base for the CMHC. Without a solid local funding base, it is not possible to engage in meaningful planning for future services. The executive director is responsible for preparing a realistic budget proposal and identifying local funds necessary to maintain or improve CMHC services. After evaluating and approving the budgetary recommendations of the executive director, the governing board has the responsibility of working hand-in-hand with the executive director and his/her staff to effectively present these budgetary needs to local government. The role of the governing board then becomes one of advocacy. The governing board, due to the fact that it is composed of individuals who are "broadly representative" of the community, is in the best position to speak to the mental health needs of the community in a manner that local governmental officials can best understand and appreciate.

Board Member: The board members may then assume responsibility for making the formal budget presentation to local funding groups—or at least a large portion of that responsibility.

Executive Director: I personally feel that members of the governing board should "carry the ball" to a large extent in instances where local political decisions may greatly influence the future of the CMHC. Budgetary decisions influence the very survival of a CMHC, and the governing board needs to give high priority to constructive ways of influencing these decisions. A central issue in the future survival of CMHCs is the problem of securing more stable funding so that realistic long-term program planning can take place (Sharfstein & Wolfe, 1978; Weiner, Way, Sharfstein, & Bass, 1979). Protection or maintenance of the CMHC's funding base is a role of primary importance for both the executive director and the board. The roles to be played by the executive director and by members of the governing board in funding matters require careful review so that each is clearly aware of what is expected in the political-budgetary arena.

Board Member: I have served on other boards where the executive director assumes full responsibility for budgetary presentations and "carries the ball." That is, while the executive director is accountable to the governing board and acts under the board's general guidance, he assumes the major responsibility for obtaining funds. You are suggesting a quite different emphasis.

Executive Director: Yes. I am at least suggesting that careful study be given to what would be the most effective approach to local government. This may vary from community to community. The ultimate goal needs to be kept clearly in mind. It is the goal of adequate financing for an extremely important service to the community. How can that best be achieved? Members of the governing board may be able to be quite persuasive in the local political arena due to factors such as reputation, high credibility, successful business experience, and political ties. The governing board should look carefully at how their role and the role of the executive director can be best defined in their particular community in order to achieve the goal of obtaining the local financial support necessary to operate the CMHC.

Board Member: I can see that participation of the governing board could help ensure to the governing bodies that there is responsible, local control of the CMHC's activities—that the money is being responsibly spent and accounted for, and that services are needed and are evaluated by local citizens. The assurance of local control seems to be an important, implicit message that could be communicated by such advocacy of the governing board.

Executive Director: Yes. The interaction of the executive director with the local community can build an image of the CMHC as being a truly "professional" organization. The interaction of the governing board with the community can further enhance the image of the CMHC as an organization that is locally controlled by responsible, cost-conscious citizens who are volunteering their personal time toward improving health resources in the community.

Let me touch on another related area of importance and one that involves a close working relationship between the executive director and the board.

Both the executive director and the governing board have the challenge of developing a positive image of the CMHC to people in the community. Both have the job of making CMHC services not only visible, but "acceptable." There is without doubt, for many people, a stigma attached to the type of services provided by a CMHC. Members of the CMHC's governing board and advisory board can make an extremely important contribution through being able to articulate the CMHC's goals and objectives to the community, by being an effective advocate for adequate and stable local financial support, and by interpreting CMHC services in a positive manner. This public relations role of the governing and advisory boards, if it is to be effective, obviously presumes that board members are kept well-informed and have received the inservice training necessary to prepare them to speak knowledgeably in the community. I am certainly talking in favor of an active, participative board, although I am well aware that some boards do not choose this path and instead rely heavily upon an executive staff who make most decisions and pretty well run the show (Steckler & Herzog, 1979).

Board Member: How does our CMHC go about preparing new board members for this type of community liaison work?

Executive Director: In two or three ways. Both myself and other members of the staff meet with new board members to educate them about the CMHC and its services. A workshop is provided that includes a historical review of the CMHC movement, current state and federal legislation affecting CMHC operations, the organizational and financial set-up of the CMHC, and an explanation of the board committee system. We try to provide a broad perspective of all issues that the CMHC faces now and will face in the future and give them some idea of how they fit into the work of the CMHC. They are encouraged to attend state and national meetings that deal with CMHC issues and concerns. Each board committee has a staff member assigned to it, and this person is able to provide additional technical information to members of the committee throughout the year. Each monthly meeting of the governing board begins with a 20-30 minute educational "special program" that is prepared and presented by staff. These "special programs" are a built-in, continuing education mechanism for the board members and cover, over a period of time, all important aspects of CMHC operations, including an explanation of all CMHC services, the manner in which the CMHC relates to other agencies, and a review of administration.

Board Member: Members of the governing board, in your view, should assume considerable responsibility not only for the internal operations of the CMHC but also external relationships to the community.

Executive Director: I believe so, and in addition to the relationship of the governing board to the local community, there is also an important relationship to other outside groups.

Board Member: Such as to the state mental health authority?

Executive Director: Yes, certainly to the state. In addition, our CMHC is accountable to the National Institute of Mental Health, National Institute of Alcohol and Alcohol Abuse, National Institute on Drug Abuse, Law Enforcement Assistance Administration, the Department of Education, and several other funding sources. Each of these groups influences the nature and extent of services we provide to the community. Each group is responsive to specific federal legislation and promulgates rules and regulations that guide the services provided by the CMHC. Years ago when CMHCs were in their early development, it was commonplace for the executive director to have almost exclusive contact with these external funding sources. That is no longer the case. Governing boards must have a fair knowledge of each of these agencies that regularly review the CMHC, and increasing attention is given in these reviews to the extent of board knowledge and participation and appropriate board functions. Board members are viewed as being able to represent accurately the needs of the community. Because they are supposed to be representative of the community at large, it is their responsibility to ensure that the services needed by the community are developed. It is also their responsibility to evaluate how effective these services are and also to concern themselves with the cost-effectiveness of these services. The executive director has the job of providing the staff skills necessary to assist the board in answering such important questions as these: what services are needed? what population groups are most in need of which services? are the services reasonably accessible and acceptable so that they will be well-utilized by the people who need them? are services cost-effective? are the needs of all age groups and diagnostic groups being adequately considered? how can we most effectively communicate these needs to the community so that services can be adequately funded and implemented? This type of continuing evaluation is essential.

These and many other management questions must be constantly reviewed and dealt with. It is the executive director's job to help the board find meaningful answers.

Board Member: As a new board member, I must admit I am a bit unnerved by the many expectations you seem to have of a board member. It appears to me that an effective board member would have to become an expert in many areas. How realistic is this expectation?

Executive Director: You touched upon a very important topic. That is, what are the expectations an executive director may have of a board and, conversely, what are the expectations that boards often have of the chief administrator of the CMHC.

Board Member: I think that is something we need to talk about because, as a new board member, I am beginning to feel a bit overburdened before I even start my work on the board.

Executive Director: The areas of responsibility I've mentioned are numerous, but each one is important to the successful operation of the CMHC. I can well understand how you might feel "overburdened" at the start when you look at the entire picture. You can take some comfort, however, in knowing three things: (1) You will be given a great deal of assistance in gaining the knowledge you need. I am available to you and the other board members, and it is my job to keep you informed. Other CMHC staff will also be of assistance. There is a continuing program of inservice education. A great deal is learned at committee meetings. (2) You don't have to learn it all in a short time. You will gain a great deal of knowledge about CMHC operations and how you can be of assistance in the first few months you serve on the board, and a year or so down the line, you will be even better prepared to contribute your special skills. (3) The volunteer work in which you will be involved will be tremendously challenging, interesting, and fulfilling. There is no getting around it—it is quite a responsible undertaking, but your contribution will bring many personal rewards.

Board Member: That's reassuring. I am interested, and I am quite willing to give a reasonable amount of my time to help wherever I can.

Executive Director: That's all that's really expected.

Board Member: I was wondering also what type of personal expectations you may have of the board.

Executive Director: The "ideal" relationship between the executive director and a CMHC board would certainly be one of mutual trust and respect. My expectation is that we will both work toward that end. If I am to implement both board policies and CMHC services effectively, I must have the support of the board. The board has the right to expect me to manage the CMHC in a responsible manner. I have the expectation that the board will support my efforts to do what needs to be done in all areas of management and service delivery. I don't mean a rubber-stamp approval, but rather evidence of support for my actions as the chief administrator with the understanding that I am always accountable to the board. This means, of course, that board members do not become involved in the day-to-day operations of the CMHC. That's my job. Thus they should respect the need to go through the proper channels if they wish to suggest modifications in CMHC operations.

I would like for the board to understand that while I represent the board—and thus management—I am also perceived as an advocate for client and staff needs and concerns. Therefore, I feel I must try to articulate the points of view of both "labor" and "management" when issues are being considered by the board. The bottom line, of course, is that I represent the board, and it is my job to implement board decisions. If I find I cannot in good conscience do that, then I should find another job. With this understood, however, I would expect the board to permit and encourage a fair representation of both "labor" and "management" views in the hope that whenever these viewpoints diverged, reasonable accommodations could be made and the decisions that resulted would strengthen rather than weaken the CMHC and its service potential.

Board Member: From your experience working with this board, and perhaps other boards, what do you think are some of the reverse expectations—that is, the expectations the board has of you?

Executive Director: I think the board expects me—or whoever may occupy this position—to keep them well-informed and to keep them out of trouble. This means that I must keep current with federal, state, and local requirements for CMHC operations, legal requirements, and all legislation relevant to community mental health services. The board has the right to expect me to take seriously my need for continued professional growth in the area of improving management and administrative skills. They expect me to place a very high priority on ensuring competent fiscal management procedures and to explore all avenues to make CMHC services more cost-effective. They also have a right to expect me to explore avenues to develop new funding sources, stabilize existing funding sources, and increase the CMHC's financial self-sufficiency in any way possible (Morrison, 1977a). They expect me to maintain visibility in the community so that I have many opportunities to explain the goals and objectives of the CMHC and build community support. They expect me to recruit and maintain competent and skilled staff, to take the evaluation of our services seriously, and to try to improve quality of services.

    Board Member: There are a number of mutual expectations.

    Executive Director: There really are. The board can help the executive director develop his or her capabilities, and the executive director can help maximize the individual talents, skills, and leadership potential of the board. The basic ingredients for a constructive relationship between board and director is that of mutual trust and teamwork.

    Board Member: I am ready to go to work.

    Executive Director: Then let's get started!

REFERENCES

Buntz, C. Gregory. Developing human service administrators: The educational challenge. Administration in Mental Health, Spring 1977, 4, 42-51.

Citizens Participation Program, National Institute of Mental Health. Orientation manual for citizen boards of federally funded community mental health centers. Department of Health, Education and Welfare Publication # (ADM) 78-759. Washington, D.C.: Superintendent of Documents, U.S. Government Printing Office, 1979.

Feldman, Saul (Ed.). The administration of mental health services. Springfield, Ill.: Charles C. Thomas, 1973.

Hinkle, Andrew, and Burns, Mark. The clinician-executive: A review. Administration in Mental Health, Fall 1978, 6, 3-21.

Howell, Jon P. The characteristics of administrators and the effectiveness of community mental health centers. Administration in Mental Health, Spring 1976, 3, 125-132.

Howell, Stuart P. Training for citizen governance in community mental health: A proposed model. Administration in Mental Health, Spring 1979, 6, 240-250.

Mazade, Noel A. Future issues in mental health administration: A report. Administration in Mental Health, Winter 1978, 6, 154-160.

Morrison, Lanny J. Barriers to self-sufficiency for mental health centers. Hospital and Community Psychiatry, March 1977, 28, 185-191. (a)

Morrison, Lanny J. Legislative change is not enough for self-sufficiency. Presented at the National Conference on Self-Sufficiency for Community Mental Health Centers, Louisville, Kentucky, September 8-9, 1977. (b)

Public Law 94-63, Title III: Community Mental Health Centers Amendments of 1975.

Price, Wolfgang S., Associates. Manual on governance and policy planning for board members. Silver Springs, Md.: Wolfgang S. Price Associates, 1977.

Robins, Arthur J., & Blackburn, Cheryl. Governing boards in mental health: Roles and training needs. Administration in Mental Health, 1974, 2, 37-45.

Sharfstein, Steven S., & Wolfe, John C. The community mental health centers program: Expectations and realities. Hospital and Community Psychiatry, January 1978, 29, 46-49.

Steckler, Allan B., & Herzog, William T. How to keep your mandated citizen board out of your hair and off your back: A guide for executive directors. American Journal of Public Health, August 1979, 69, 809-812.

Weiner, Risa S., Woy, J. R., Sharfstein, Steven S., & Bass, Rosalyn D. Community mental health centers and the "seed money" concept: Effects of terminating federal funds. Community Mental Health Journal, Summer 1979, 15, 129-138.

6

VOLUNTEERS IN MENTAL HEALTH SETTINGS
Marsha Matson Silverman

An important part of any mental health organization, volunteers can be grouped into two basic types, the service deliverers and the community representatives. This chapter describes the range of activities each group performs in a variety of mental health settings. Special attention is given to the background and role of the community representative volunteer whose function is usually that of an advisory/governing board member. Also considered are reasons for using volunteers, tasks performed, volunteer characteristics, and impact of the experience on clients and volunteers themselves. The chapter concludes with a discussion of seven important factors contributing to a successful volunteer program: volunteer needs assessment and planning, recruitment, selection, task assignment, orientation and training, on-the-job factors, and termination.

DEFINITION

The volunteer is an individual whose entry into, performance at, and exit from a mental health organization are matters of choice rather than financial remuneration or legal coercion. This definition encompasses persons whose motivations are often identified with volunteerism, such as serving the community and helping disadvantaged people. It also includes those wishing to earn favored status for job promotion, try out a new experience, receive college credit, or secure a permanent position.

Volunteerism is characterized by its secondary importance to the individual. Compared to job and family obligations, it is a low priority activity occupying leisure time and surplus resources

(Begalla, 1976). Involvement is often time-limited, with a narrow
range of objectives, and more often than not lies outside one's area
of education or occupation. In other words, volunteerism is an avo-
cational behavior occurring relatively infrequently.

WHAT DO VOLUNTEERS DO?

Volunteers at mental health agencies can be categorized into
two groups, the community representatives and the service deliverers. They perform three kinds of prevention activities. The first
group, the community representatives, embody community values
and link an agency's programs to the needs of its service population.
They perform as its advisory or governing board and monitor its
performance. Community representatives are typically concerned
with the primary prevention activities of mental health planning,
community organization, agency accountability, and organizational
policy making.

The second basic group is the service deliverers, who are
sought for their skills in primary, secondary, and tertiary prevention. In primary prevention, these volunteers form problem-solving
groups on such topics as nutrition, employment, housing, and race
relations. Acquainting the community with the agency's programs
is also an important function, while other primary prevention projects involve presentations to civic groups on mental illness, consultation in specific areas in which volunteers have been trained,
and organization of self-improvement groups.

Service delivery volunteers have only recently undertaken
such secondary prevention roles as cotherapists in family therapy,
counselors on crisis hotlines, conveners of self-help groups, and
directors of psychodrama. These activities are almost always conducted in concert with a supervising professional. Individuals from
many walks of life—even former inpatients, who have been regarded
as a valuable resource for treating current inpatients—can function
in a direct service role.

Tertiarty prevention activities are the traditional bailiwick of
the service delivery volunteer. The more common duties of staff
assistant or part-time secretary have been supplemented by newer
roles as helpers of parents of drug abusing teenagers, "cultural experts" who interpret unique aspects of the service population for
staff, and companions to isolated persons. Other responsibilities
may include friendship for ex-inpatients, recreation, and home
visits.

THE SPECIAL CASE OF THE VOLUNTEER
AS COMMUNITY REPRESENTATIVE

Volunteerism boasts a long history in mental health, usually in tasks confined to staff aide, fund raising, and community goodwill. As members of boards of trustees, middle- and upper-class citizens were recruited to generate charitable contributions and to lend legitimacy to an agency. In the last three decades, however, the community mental health movement has advocated expanded control over service delivery by consumers and residents. These two groups were often composed of lower-class whites and minorities, who had rarely acted as advisors to or governors of mental health organizations. They frequently had no previous knowledge of mental health or organizational management. Amendments to the federal CMHC Act of 1963 have required formal citizen participation in federally funded community mental health centers (CMHCs). This focus has spread to many mental health settings where community representative volunteers occupy visible and sometimes controversial positions.

The importance of the community representative volunteer lay not in his/her capacity to augment services or raise money but rather in (1) the ability of the volunteer by virtue of residence, sex, age, race, or income to be the political embodiment of a segment of the community, and (2) the ability of the mental health agency to be accountable to that volunteer as one of the community's representatives. Issues of organizational control, community power, and institutional change increasingly challenged professional autonomy and, on occasion, placed staff in conflict with other social service agencies.

Another source of conflict arose from misunderstandings over the skill/representative function of indigenous volunteers. The unique role of each volunteer group was confused and often remains so today. Service delivery volunteers residing in the community should not be considered representative of its values although characteristics shared by volunteers and clients can enhance their relationship. However, the proportion of volunteers with mental health training on advisory/governing boards should be smaller than the proportion of residents with no background in mental health in order to allow community representativeness to prevail.

Another facet of the debate over citizen participation was the political climate of the 1960s and early 1970s. Part of the protest of that time was lodged against the insensitivity and inefficiency of big government. Through a number of domestic programs including community mental health centers, the federal government experimented with returning responsibility for solutions of social problems to the local level.

A neglected aspect of the representative function is that volunteers in public decision-making positions have long been part of U.S. political tradition. Citizen volunteers have been active on local planning, school, and zoning boards. The federal government, too, had encouraged voluntary action as early as 1914 in the form of 4-H Clubs.

Thus, four separate patterns coalesced to define a special group of volunteers as community representatives in mental health agencies. First, U.S. tradition had incorporated volunteers into public policy-making positions. Second, the federal government attempted to channel the energies of the social action movements of the 1960s and 1970s into local organizational structures, the CMHC program being one. Third, acceptance of volunteers in mental health settings was longstanding. And, fourth, the community mental health movement gave a distinctive emphasis to citizen involvement as a means of agency accountability to its service population. Currently, the extent of citizen control depends on legal requirements and the willingness of the staff to share power with board members. Since 1963 citizen boards at federally funded CMHCs have moved from an advisory role to governance as mandated by the 1975 Amendments.

WHAT IS THE DIFFERENCE BETWEEN VOLUNTEERS, NONPROFESSIONALS, PARAPROFESSIONALS, AND PROFESSIONALS?

A volunteer can be a nonprofessional, paraprofessional, or professional. The professional holds an academic degree—such as a Ph.D., M.D., M.S.W., or R.N.—in a mental health related field. Persons who have not been educated in traditional postbaccalaureate or professional training programs are alternately referred to as nonprofessionals or paraprofessionals. The distinction between professional and nonprofessional volunteer is quite important when constituting a citizen board. Currently, governing boards of federally funded CMHCs must be comprised of a majority of volunteer nonprofessionals, the remainder coming from the ranks of volunteer "providers." Providers include such professional groups as planners, physicians, employees of social service agencies, and hospital administrators.

WHY USE VOLUNTEERS?

The most common reason for using volunteers has been to compensate for inadequate staffing. McGee (1974) states: "The real professional crisis worker has emerged in the form of the volunteer, whose availability has only begun to be tapped and whose devotion and dedication to the needs of fellow human beings are not constrained by time honored roles and artificial status distinctions" (p. 112).

Volunteers assist staff in a variety of ways. They can help the center coordinate community services for clients. One study of all the rape crisis centers in the United States found that the number of interorganizational contacts was directly related to the number of volunteers on staff (O'Sullivan, 1977). The volunteer also helps clients directly. A volunteer who possesses a common attribute such as race can contribute a special sensitivity to the cultural under-pinnings of mental disorders. In the same way, a volunteer who has previously experienced a mental disorder may serve as a model of recovery.

Nicoletti and Flater-Benz (1974) describe an innovative pro-gram at one CMHC serving 65,000 persons. Thirty-one volunteers taught behavioral approaches to family and alcoholism groups, dem-onstrated anxiety management through deep breathing, and formed a relaxation/diet group. In addition, they established groups for wives of policemen and for welfare mothers, and delivered community lec-tures. They not only wrote articles on mental illness and the CMHC for the local newspaper, but also presented editorials on radio and TV.

HOW MUCH DO MENTAL HEALTH AGENCIES USE VOLUNTEERS?

It has been estimated that in 1974, 107 million Americans held membership in some voluntary organization, and that 70 million had actively volunteered that year (Smith & Baldwin, 1974). The vast majority of these persons were involved in school groups, trade unions, fraternal organizations, and sports clubs. Only a small pro-portion, less than 4 percent, were active in service-oriented organi-zations. It is unknown how many volunteers participated in mental health settings.

Data on volunteers at all 410 CMHCs operating in 1973 indicate that 7 percent of their staff persons were regularly scheduled volun-teers (NIMH, 1974). However, only 1 percent of total scheduled staff hours were attributed to volunteers. Volunteer hours as a per-cent of staff hours ranged from none to a high of 28 percent. Three settings described in the mental health literature are notable in their use of volunteers. One urban CMHC engaged 50 volunteers who donated approximately 240 hours weekly in group interview sessions (Sata, 1974), while a psychiatric unit of a children's hospital aver-aged 90 volunteers giving 1,900 hours of service a month (Siepke et al., 1977). Crisis intervention centers tend to use many volunteers as staff. By 1973, there were 1,000 hotlines in the United States, with 50-100 volunteers on a given line (Carothers & Inslee, 1974).

A recent examination of federally funded CMHCs found that utilization of volunteers was the most poorly implemented of all CMHC goals (M. Silverman, 1978). Over 50 percent of the 410 centers scored in the "ineffective" category. CMHCs tended to use volunteers when one or more conditions existed: the CMHC was located in an urban catchment area, the state mental health department was weak relative to the state health department, the CMHC did not possess a poverty designation, and the state political environment was considered hostile to community mental health. It was speculated that adverse governmental influence coupled with a politically antagonistic atmosphere prompted the CMHCs to turn to the community in the form of volunteers for support.

No figures exist that directly compare volunteer time devoted to service versus representation. Nevertheless, some data can be gleaned from different sources. Length of service of crisis intervention volunteers in Tennessee varied from 6.9 months on a community-sponsored hotline to 29.6 months on those run by churches (Engs, 1973). Volunteers for school-sponsored hotlines averaged 9.17 months of service. In contrast, board members at 19 mental health centers located in a metropolitan area served an average of 2.5 years (Silverman, in press).

WHO VOLUNTEERS?

Volunteers in a wide variety of organizations tend to possess what could best be described as integrated personalities (Howarth, 1976). Contrary to a popular belief that disturbed people are attracted to volunteer service with the mentally disadvantaged, many examples of volunteers' personality adjustment can be found in the literature. Direct service volunteers display less conflict and variability in their personality than do nonvolunteers (Horn, 1973). These same volunteers also express a greater affinity for close interpersonal relationships and hold a larger number of community-centered values. Elderly volunteers in senior citizen centers have a wide scope of social interests, express interest in senior citizen activity, and believe in their capacity to serve others (Monk & Cryns, 1974). When volunteers at a suicide center were compared to suicide attempters, they were found to have greater emotional stability, less fantasy about suicide, almost no suicide attempts, and were less likely to consider suicide as a justifiable problem-solving option

(Weis & Seiden, 1974). Advisory/governing board members reported a high degree of purpose in life and good family adjustment (Russem, 1976).

In terms of demographic characteristics, volunteers in general are more likely to be white, male, and middle-aged, with a higher level of education, income, and social class (Cutler, 1976; Hyman & Wright, 1971). Mental health board members tend to match this profile (Silverman, 1979a). However, over half of the 74 volunteers at five crisis intervention services in Tennessee were nonprofessional women over 30 (Engs, 1973).

Volunteers have typically volunteered more than once. Their motivations are of two fundamental kinds: helping others or helping themselves. The latter classification includes such motivations as improving social skills, choosing an education or career field, and feeling personally useful. People who volunteer for the purpose of helping others remain longer—as much as twice as long—as those participating for self-growth or experience (Engs & Kirk, 1974).

WHAT IS THE IMPACT OF VOLUNTEERING ON CLIENTS AND VOLUNTEERS?

Certainly the strongest case based on research findings for volunteerism can be made in terms of the benefits accruing to the volunteers themselves. Degree and direction of change in volunteers varies according to the intensity of the experience. "High risk" volunteers, those who work with the mentally disordered for at least six months acquire greater self-insight, self-assurance, and tolerance than do those who volunteer for less than six months (Smith & Baldwin, 1974).

Much less is known about the impact of volunteers on patients. Housewives have helped reduce recidivism in a poor risk population of schizophrenic women (Katkin et al., 1971), while higher levels of empathy, warmth, and genuineness in hotline counselors were associated with callers' greater self-exploration and lowered anxiety and depression scores (Knickerbocker, 1972). Empirical evidence of the long-term effectiveness of volunteers does not exist.

SEVEN STEPS TO AN EFFECTIVE VOLUNTEER PROGRAM

There are several important factors contributing to a successful volunteer experience. They are (1) assessment of agency need for volunteers and planning for their use, (2) recruitment, (3) selection, (4) task assignment, (5) orientation and training, (6) on-the-job factors, and (7) termination. These "steps" are discussed in the order in which they should be implemented by the agency.

1. Volunteer needs assessment and planning. All staff should be asked if they can use a volunteer, what the volunteer will do, who will be responsible for supervision, and what objectives they wish to achieve. Once this survey is completed, planning for volunteer use becomes simpler and more rational.

It is important at the outset to delegate the person(s) responsible for the coordination of volunteers. This person will recruit, select, and train volunteers. As the planner of volunteer activities, the coordinator will work with staff to specify types of needed activities and gear these priorities to recruitment and training strategies. The coordinator also acts as a liaison between the staff and volunteers.

2. Recruitment. An important element in recruitment is to match desired volunteer characteristics to the volunteer task. To illustrate, a hypothetical community mental health center has determined that it needs volunteers for three common volunteer functions. A first group of volunteers would provide counseling on a crisis intervention hotline. A second group would constitute a citizen governing board. The third group would operate a self-help prevention program—in this case, one in which volunteer parents would act as teachers of communication skills to families with problem children. For the three projects chosen by the hypothetical CMHC, volunteers with widely divergent attributes would be needed. For example, the most effective hotline workers score highly on openness, self-acceptance, flexibility, and altruism (Sakowitz & Hirschman, 1975; Natali, 1974). They also exhibit moderate levels of independence, nonconformity, and rejection of authoritarian attitudes (Werner, 1976).

An excellent mode for locating this type of individual is through a mass appeal campaign, employing radio and TV spots, newspaper articles, and lectures to community groups. An extensive advertising campaign not only attracts a large pool of applicants but also publicizes the activities of the center. A compelling reason for using a mass appeal campaign is its time-limited nature, since the time between recruitment and task performance need only be a few months (McGee, 1971).

Volunteers for board membership have requirements different from those for hotline counselors. Since board members will, on occasion, meet with community decision makers, they should either have or be able to learn appropriate negotiation and leadership skills. The most likely candidates are probably already known to various community organizations, and for this reason, consulting with them results in nominations of interested persons. One author has stressed the importance of recruiting influential community people who, through their affiliations, represent a large number of residents (Rabiner, 1972). At that author's CMHC, over 700 organizations were consulted at 50 meetings in order to constitute a community-based board. A less extensive canvas combined with a mass appeal campaign described above can produce an array of attractive candidates for board membership. However, it should be cautioned that using nomination as a sole recruiting technique tends to garner individuals whose first loyalty lies with another organization or whose tenure is shortened by commitments elsewhere.

The only criterion for the third group of volunteers, the parent self-help group, is sharing the condition, that is, being a parent. In describing one such group, Beier et al. (1971) suggest that empathy and an ability to listen are the most important qualities of such a volunteer. Other personality or demographic characteristics appear to be less important in effective leadership of a self-help group. Candidates can be located by eliciting the cooperation of local schools and social service agencies. Letters explaining the program to parents and asking for volunteers can be sent home with the children from schools, day care centers, and organized recreational activities.

Recruitment literature should emphasize opportunities for helping others and self-improvement. Mothers with preschool children, for instance, volunteer as a form of human capital maintenance in that they tend to participate to keep or learn skills for later use in the job market (Mueller, 1975). Recruitment materials for the parent self-help group can, thus, profitably emphasize developing communication skills as well as improving family interaction.

Special attention should be paid to the temporal constraints of potential volunteers. Many persons who would otherwise volunteer cannot do so during daytime working hours. Recruitment messages should note that boards meet in the evening, a crisis hotline operates around the clock, and parent self-help groups are offered at different times of the day.

3. Selection. Screening devices are available to aid the judgment of the selector. Paper and pencil tests have helped to accept and reject hotline candidates. The MMPI is the most well-known (Evans, 1977), but the Barrett-Lennard Relationship Inventory (Mullins, 1973), the Human Empathy Scale, and the Whithorn-Betz A-B Therapist Scale (Jamison & Johnson, 1975) were also useful in selecting volunteers. No matter what device is employed, some selection procedure should be used, for self-selection tends to result in poorly adjusted volunteers (McClure et al., 1973).

Selection of board members is often achieved under legal constraints, when, for example, a certain percentage must represent community residents while the remainder are comprised of providers. This is usually accomplished by obtaining a demographic representation of the service population; in this case residence, age, ethnicity, sex, or consumer experience become selection criteria. A second consideration is the desirability of volunteer participation in other community organizations or activities. His or her current activity enables the volunteer to represent a larger constituency than the unaffiliated individual and to act as an agency connection to the community power structure. Community representative volunteers can be selected by administrative staff, community organizations, or community-wide election. While election is difficult to implement, it offers greater volunteer representativeness and independence than do the first two methods.

4. Task assignment. If a number of different jobs are available to the volunteer, professional sensitivity in matching volunteers to clients and tasks becomes paramount. The first priority is using volunteers in ways that are personally rewarding to them. Similar age and interests have been found to improve the likelihood of a successful volunteer-client relationship.

In lieu of staff assignment, another avenue is for volunteers to choose their own jobs. This works well when the tasks are all related to a common goal, such as resocialization or rehabilitation. Since the selection process has already produced volunteers whose qualities are appropriate to a goal, it is assumed that whichever task is selected will be adequately performed.

5. Training/Orientation. Orientation acquaints volunteers with staff and jobs. In one individual or group session, it provides the volunteer with an introduction to the workings of the center. Its purpose is to address the nature of the task and its value to the center as a whole.

Training differs from orientation in that it is a planned sequence of courses combining didactic and experiential materials necessary for successful volunteer performance. Didactic materials include lectures, readings, and discussions, while experiential materials "teach through doing." Role-playing, awareness exercises, simulated crisis calls, and practice lectures for the parent self-help group are all experiential techniques.

Before turning to the content and format of training, the question of whether volunteers really need training should be addressed. The weight of evidence overwhelmingly confirms the value of training to service volunteers' improved opinion of themselves (Callahan, 1976), improved therapeutic skills (Sakowitz & Hirschman, 1975), greater communication effectiveness (Nicoletti & Flater, 1975), and preparedness for performing their duties (Minor & Thompson, 1975). Training for board members elevates their level of knowledge of board and center functioning (Silverman, 1979b).

Findings from a smaller number of studies on the effect of volunteer training on improved functioning of clients or target system have been contradictory. While the training of volunteer teacher assistants did improve the academic achievement in educable mentally retarded children (Powers, 1974), it has not been demonstrated that volunteer counseling behaviors resulting from training were associated with client change (Tyler et al., 1978). Nor has it been shown that volunteers consistently apply training in actual counseling situations. On the other hand, board members have attributed changes in board and center operations to their training (Silverman, 1979b).

It should be noted here that board training programs must be provided by a training organization independent of the agency. Its autonomy ensures the objectivity of the information and allows the board members to prepare for their governing responsibilities without regard for staff preferences.

6. On-the-job factors. The effectiveness of a volunteer program depends on the volunteers, clients, staff, and organization. Certainly a most important volunteer quality is dependability; warmth, genuineness, and empathy are also vital for direct service volunteers. For board members, length of membership on the board contributes to all-around board accomplishment (Meyers et al., 1974). Client interest and understanding of the volunteer's role also enhance the experience.

Volunteers should receive consistent supervision combined with positive feedback. Regularly scheduled supervision provides needed role clarity and helps to place realistic limits on involvement with clients. It also gives continuous feedback on whether the volunteer has an acceptable quantity of work. A system for recognition is a means of rewarding volunteers, who, after all, work without pay.

Certain organizational factors have been associated with greater accomplishment of boards. Such seemingly minor items as permanent office space and getting needed secretarial and technical help contribute to board achievement. Staff must understand that certain organizational limitations are characteristic of citizen boards. Their decisions often take longer to make because scheduling and attending meetings is more difficult for volunteers than staff. Diversity of backgrounds and problems with the technical language of mental health also restrict their decision-making ability.

7. Termination. Volunteerism is essentially a short-term, leisure time activity, ranking below work and home obligations for

most people. One can realistically expect volunteers to terminate when other responsibilities supersede, or when their learning or helping needs have been satisfied. Since volunteers have a history of volunteerism, other projects may catch their interest and they will leave to pursue them.

To counteract volunteer attrition, the agency can place a time limit on the duration of a program, or it can build in routine replacement. For example, the parent self-help group can continuously recruit new parent trainers as they "graduate" from the program and express a desire to remain in some capacity. Boards can replenish their membership through their contacts in the community. Hotline volunteers can be asked their motivations during the selection process, so that those wishing to help others can be given preference; they tend to stay on much longer than those who join for self-improvement.

SUMMARY

Voluntary activity in a mental health organization is a matter of choice rather than financial remuneration or legal coercion. It is an infrequent behavior, commanding less time than family and employment responsibilities. Volunteers at mental health agencies are either service deliverers or community representatives; both have long histories of involvement in mental health settings. Community representatives are usually board members, while service volunteers are engaged in a variety of primary, secondary, and tertiary prevention activities. Service volunteers are professionals, paraprofessionals, and nonprofessionals, while community representatives should come only from the latter two categories.

Typical volunteers are described as well-adjusted; they tend to be white, male, and middle-aged, with a higher level of education, income, and social class. They participate to help others or to improve their own skills and knowledge. The greatest impact of the volunteer experience is on the personality of the volunteer. Little is known about the effect of volunteer activity on clients or target systems.

Seven "steps" to an effective volunteer program are described. It is suggested that an assessment of agency need for volunteers makes subsequent planning for their use more rational. An important element in recruitment is matching desired volunteer characteristics to the volunteer task. This process requires determining which qualities are most effective in certain roles and keying recruitment strategies to those qualities. An intuitive feeling about a candidate's suitability can be assisted by various objective tests;

unique board member requirements, however, necessitate recruitment strategies of nomination or election. Tasks can either be assigned to or chosen by the volunteer. While training has been shown
to be a vital component in a successful volunteer program, volunteer
dependability, regular staff supervision, client interest, and organizational assistance also contribute to its success. Finally, an
agency can counteract volunteer attrition by placing a time limit on
a particular project or by building in routine replacement procedures.

REFERENCES

Begalla, M. A. The comparison of the performance and achievement value of work, volunteer, and homemaking behaviors of
supervisory male and female employees, non-supervisory female
employees, and female volunteer workers. Doctoral dissertation, The University of Tennessee, 1976.

Beier, E., Robinson, P., & Micheletti, G. Susanville: A community
helps itself in mobilization of community resources for self help
in mental health. Journal of Consulting and Clinical Psychology,
1971, 36, 142-150.

Callahan, J. The effects of two training procedures on volunteers
in corrections. Doctoral dissertation, Boston University School
of Education, 1976.

Carothers, J., & Inslee, L. Level of empathetic understanding offered by volunteer telephone services. Journal of Counseling
Psychology, 1974, 2, 274-276.

Cutler, S. Age differences in voluntary association membership.
Social Forces, 1976, 55, 43-58.

Engs, R. The personality traits and health knowledge of crisis intervention volunteers in the state of Tennessee. Doctoral dissertation, The University of Tennessee, 1973.

Engs, R., & Kirk, R. The characteristics of volunteers in crisis
intervention centers. Public Health Reports, 1974, 89, 459-464.

Evans, D. Use of the MMPI to predict effective hotline workers.
Journal of Clinical Psychology, 1977, 33, 1113-1114.

Horn, J. Personality characteristics of direct service volunteers. Doctoral dissertation, United States International University, 1973.

Howarth, E. Personality characteristics of volunteers. Psychological Reports, 1976, 38, 853-854.

Hyman, H., & Wright, C. Trends in voluntary association membership of American adults: Replication based on a secondary analysis of national sample surveys. American Sociological Review, 1971, 36, 191-206.

Jamison, R., & Johnson, J. Empathy and therapeutic orientation in paid and volunteer crisis phone workers, professional therapists, and undergraduate college students. Journal of Community Psychology, 1975, 3, 269-274.

Katkin, S., Ginsburg, M., Rifkin, M., & Scott, J. Effectiveness of female volunteers in the treatment of outpatients. Journal of Counseling Psychology, 1971, 18, 97-100.

Knickerbocker, D. Lay volunteer and professional trainee therapeutic functioning and outcomes in a suicide and crisis intervention service. Doctoral dissertation, The University of Florida, 1972.

McClure, J., Wetzel, T., Flanagan, M., McCake, M., & Murphy, G. Volunteers in a suicide prevention service. Journal of Community Psychology, 1973, 4, 397-398.

McGee, R. Selection and training of nonprofessionals and volunteers. In J. Zusman & D. Davidson (Eds.), Organizing the Community to Prevent Suicide. Springfield, Ill.: Charles C. Thomas, 1971, 37-42.

McGee, R. Crisis intervention in the community. Baltimore, Md.: University Park Press, 1974.

Meyers, W., Dorwart, R., Hutcheson, B., & Decker, D. Organizational and attitudinal correlates of citizen board accomplishment in mental health and retardation. Community Mental Health Journal, 1974, 10, 192-197.

Minor, K., & Thompson, P. Development and evaluation of a training program for volunteers working in day treatment. Hospital and Community Psychiatry, 1975, 26, 154-156.

Monk, A., & Cryns, A. Predictors of voluntaristic intent among the aged: An area study. Gerontologist, 1974, 14, 425-429.

Mueller, M. Economic determinants of volunteer work by women. Signs, 1975, 1, 325-338.

Mullins, R. Evaluation and prediction of success of volunteer counselors. Doctoral dissertation, The University of Oklahoma, 1973.

Natali, R. An investigation of the personality characteristics of volunteer and nonvolunteer counselor trainees as they related to personal growth, group participation and counselor effectiveness. Doctoral dissertation, University of Pittsburgh, 1974.

National Institute of Mental Health (NIMH). Unpublished data from the 1974 Inventory of Community Mental Health Centers.

Nicoletti, N., & Flater-Benz, L. Volunteers in a community mental health agency. Personnel and Guidance Journal, 1974, 53, 281-284.

Nicoletti, J., & Flater, L. A community-oriented program for training and using volunteers. Community Mental Health Journal, 1975, 11, 58-63.

O'Sullivan, E. Interorganizational cooperation: How effective for grass-roots organization? Group and Organizational Studies, 1977, 2, 347-358.

Powers, L. The effectiveness of volunteer college student helpers in improving the social and academic behaviors in educable mentally retarded children. Doctoral dissertation, University of Oregon, 1974.

Rabiner, C. Organizing a community advisory board for a mental health center. Hospital and Community Psychiatry, 1972, 23, 118-121.

Russem, P. Differences in the meaning in life and quality of intrafamily relationships of four selected groups of volunteers. Doctoral dissertation, Boston College, 1976.

Sakowitz, M., & Hirschman, R. Self-ideal congruency and therapeutic skill development in nonpaid paraprofessionals. Journal of Community Psychology, 1975, 3, 275-280.

Sata, L. Group methods: The volunteer and the paraprofessional. International Journal of Group Psychotherapy, 1974, 24, 400-408.

Siepke, B., Crawton, L., Schutman, J., & Kandara, C. The volunteer program in the psychiatric division of a children's hospital. Hospital and Community Psychiatry, 1977, 28, 697-699.

Silverman, M. Factors associated with effective implementation of the Community Mental Health Centers Act of 1963. Doctoral dissertation, Northern Illinois University, 1978.

Silverman, W. H. Some aspects of advisory board functioning in a large urban area. Journal of Social Service Research, in press.

Silverman, W. H. A state-wide assessment of mental health advisory/governing board training needs. Unpublished manuscript, University of Illinois Medical Center, 1979. (a)

Silverman, W. H. Self-designed training for mental health advisory/governing boards. Unpublished manuscript, University of Illinois Medical Center, 1979. (b)

Smith, D., & Baldwin, B. Voluntary associations and volunteering in the United States. In D. Smith (Ed.), Voluntary Action Research 1974. Lexington, Mass.: Lexington Books, 1974.

Tyler, M., Kalafat, J., Boroto, D., & Hartman, J. A brief assessment technique for paraprofessional helpers. Journal of Community Psychology, 1978, 6, 53-59.

Weis, S., & Seiden, R. Rescuers and the rescued: A study of suicide prevention center volunteers and clients by means of a death questionnaire. Life-Threatening Behavior, 1974, 4, 118-130.

Werner, R. Personality characteristics of citizen volunteers in relation to their level of human relations skill. Doctoral dissertation, Boston College, 1976.

II

FUNDING

No topic in community mental health is more controversial or misunderstood than funding. With the continuing reduction in government financing for public services, there is greater competition for limited money and stricter accountability for spending. Executive directors pressure boards to seek multisource funding, and boards look with a sharper eye at the ways hard earned dollars are spent.

The purpose of this section is to demystify the processes of obtaining and spending money for mental health services. From the chapter on Congressional procedures that create mental health programs and appropriate funds through chapters detailing alternative financial sources, boards and directors will be able to form rational policies and strategies in the funding area.

Cavarocchi gives an account of the federal authorization and appropriation process with special attention to mental health programs. He summarizes the structural components in Congress responsible for working on a mental health bill and notes appropriate junctures where interested citizens may have an impact. He takes the reader through a timetable of events starting with the introduction of a bill and ending with its passage into public law. Then another series of events, called the budget process, begins, in which the President and Congress decide upon an appropriation for the law.

A major portion of funding for mental health service is provided by government. Elpers reviews federal, state, and local government sources and weighs methods for securing financing. There is a section specifically devoted to board roles in funding. Elpers warns that obtaining dollars should never be an end in itself, but rather a means toward fulfilling the goals of the CMHC.

The most neglected source of mental health funding is private philanthropy. Silber states that the survival of many CMHCs may depend upon tapping this resource. He pinpoints individual gifts, foundation grants, deferred gifts, and corporate gifts and grants as potential contributors to special projects or long-range budgeting.

Grassroots fund raising has had a colorful and successful history in charitable activities, but it has been neglected as a source of revenue for CMHCs. Beckett notes that grassroots activities not only raise money, but they also strengthen the morale of the board and make the center more visible to the community. Beckett offers advice for choosing and carrying out successful efforts.

Securing funding does not necessarily lead to effective programming. Finances must be efficiently managed and related to performance. Rydman notes that this requires three sets of information. A service information system incorporates data on utilization and performance. A client outcome information system uses data on individuals and programs to monitor productivity. A cost information system explains how data are generated on unit-of-care and add-on costs. These information systems aid in recording resource consumption and services productivity. A decision-making schema is presented for use of the data in cost-effective allocation of funds.

7

THE AUTHORIZATION AND APPROPRIATION PROCESS AND MENTAL HEALTH FUNDING
Nicholas G. Cavarocchi

The purpose of this chapter is to describe the Congressional process by which public funds are appropriated to support government programs such as community mental health centers (CMHCs). In order to understand the appropriation process, it is necessary to know how these programs are created, extended, or changed, and how the level of funding is formulated. To this end, the chapter is divided into sections that describe the organization of Congress; the legislative process by which programs are authorized; the budget process by which the executive branch (the President and his agencies) formulates a budget and allocates limited resources to thousands of federal programs; the work of Congressional budget committees; and the appropriation process. Emphasized are those points at which public input is most effective.

THE STRUCTURE OF CONGRESS

Juxtaposed between individual members of Congress and the assemblage of the entire House or Senate, committees were created by Congress as an intermediate level where most of the detailed work occurs. The committees are where the most intensive consideration is given to the legislative and budgetary proposals and, most important, where citizens are given their opportunity to be heard.

In health policy, the House of Representatives and the Senate each have three main committees with jurisdiction over the creation or funding of health programs. In the House of Representatives, the principal committee responsible for legislation authorizing (creating)

97

health programs is the Committee on Interstate and Foreign Commerce. This Committee, like most of the committees in both houses, divides its work among subcommittees. Its Subcommittee on Health and the Environment performs the intensive work on health legislation and has jurisdiction over the programs of the U.S. Public Health Service, such as the National Institute of Mental Health (NIMH), the National Institute on Drug Abuse, and the food and drug laws. It also has jurisdiction over the CMHC, Medicaid, and the Maternal and Child Health Programs.

The second committee in the House of Representatives concerned with health programs is the Ways and Means Committee through its Subcommittee on Health. The full Ways and Means Committee has jurisdiction over tax laws. Its Health Subcommittee reviews health programs involving special taxes such as Medicare and most National Health Insurance proposals. Some of these proposals incorporate coverage for mental health care. As one might expect, there is considerable overlap between the work of this Subcommittee and the Subcommittee on Health and the Environment. For example, when the Hospital Cost Containment bill, which was designed to reduce hospital spending and to save money for the Medicare and Medicaid programs, was introduced in the House, it was referred to both Committees and each reported a bill.

The third committee of the House of Representatives involved in health programs is the Appropriation Committee through its Subcommittee on Labor and HEW. This Committee does not have the authority to create programs, but it does provide the funds necessary to operate them, and its control over the purse strings makes its work every bit as important as the work of the committees that authorize the programs.

In the Senate the corresponding committees have slightly different but clearer jurisdictional boundaries. The Committee on Labor and Human Resources is responsible for the programs of the U.S. Public Health Service, such as CMHCs, but lacks jurisdiction over Medicaid.

In contrast to the House, the Senate Finance Committee has jurisdiction over both programmatic and revenue aspects of all legislation relating to taxation. This gives the Committee exclusive responsibility for the Social Security Act, which authorizes the Medicare, Medicaid, and Maternal and Child Health Programs. Payments for some mental health services are allowed in these programs. Since most National Health Insurance proposals, in which mental health care may be covered, involve a tax credit or deduction of some sort, the Finance Committee has jurisdiction over those bills in the Senate. Although the Committee has a Health Subcommittee, most of its work is done in full committee. (This is different from the usual procedure, in which a subcommittee makes recommendations to the full committee for further consideration and action.)

The third Senate Committee concerned with health policy is the Senate Appropriation Committee through its Subcommittee on Labor-HEW Appropriation. This Subcommittee has the same jurisdiction and power as its counterpart in the House.

THE LEGISLATIVE AUTHORIZATION PROCESS

This section will trace the path that authorization bills follow from the time they are introduced until they become public law. Congress deals with two basic types of legislation in the health area: Authorization bills, which create, extend, or change programs; and Appropriations bills, which provide the money to carry out the programs. This distinction created a persuasive argument for Congress' successful override of President Gerald Ford's veto of the 1975 CMHC Amendments. Ford claimed that the bill was too expensive, but supporters argued that it was an authorization rather than an appropriations measure. They maintained that the Appropriations Committees could properly reduce the bill's authorization levels at a later date.

An Authorization bill defines the need for a program (or its modification), establishes the scope and nature of federal involvement, assigns the program to a specific department of the federal government, and identifies the amount of money that can be spent on it. An authorization bill can create an entitlement for benefits that requires the government to pay valid claims, or it may create a discretionary process that leaves the annual funding up to the budget and appropriation process.

A recent example of an authorization bill is the Mental Health Systems Act sent to Congress by President Carter on May 15, 1979. This legislation would reform the nation's mental health delivery system by giving monies to states for community-based services for the chronically mentally ill, by allowing CMHCs to tailor their services to selected populations rather than to all groups as had been required, and by encouraging integration of general and mental health care services. The President asked for a $99.1 million authorization, of which $30 million would come from reductions in existing mental health programs.

The enactment (signing into law by the President) of an authorizing bill other than an entitlement program does not guarantee that the program will be funded at all. This will be discussed in greater detail later in this chapter.

There are various sources of legislation. Some bills are developed by a Senator or a Representative because of a perceived need or because his constituents have come to him with their complaints or recommendations. In this case, the more information a constituent can bring to a meeting with the Senator or Representative, and especially the specifics of what should be done, the better the chance of getting a favorable response. If draft bill language can be provided, the chances for success are even higher.

Another source of legislation is the "Administration," that is to say, the President and the executive agencies. President John F. Kennedy was the originator of CMHC legislation in 1963. Administration proposals are usually drafted in bill form by agency lawyers and submitted to Congress for introduction. Since the President cannot introduce a bill, this is usually done for him by a senior member of the House or Senate. Many times, the words "by request" will appear next to the sponsor's name, indicating that the sponsor was asked by the Administration to introduce the bill and that the sponsor does not personally support the proposal.

Yet another source is existing legislation that is due to expire and must be extended in order for a given program to continue to operate. Most health programs, such as community mental health centers, have a specific time limit and must be renewed every three years.

After the bill has been introduced, it is referred to a committee by the Parliamentarian, recorded by the Journal Clerk, assigned a number, and sent to the printer. Once bills are printed, copies are available to the public from the House and Senate Document Rooms. Upon receiving a bill referred to it, the committee turns it over to the appropriate subcommittee. This is done by the Chairman of the full committee or—as is most often the case—by his Committee Clerk.

The next important step in the process is the holding of hearings by the subcommittee. Such hearings on a bill, depending on how important or controversial it is, may involve only one witness and last only a few hours, or may extend for days and weeks. The principal supporter of the bill is usually the first witness to testify. If the bill is an administration health bill, then someone from HEW, almost always the Secretary, will be the first to testify.

A Secretary does not always testify in favor of a bill. When the Senate Labor and Public Welfare Subcommittee on Health held a one-day hearing in 1973 on a bill to continue funding for CMHCs, HEW Secretary Casper Weinberger testified that he wanted to phase out the program. He argued unsuccessfully that the program had been intended by Congress as a demonstration project and that it had fulfilled that purpose.

Following the leadoff witness, the subcommittee will hear from individuals who can demonstrate the need for legislation or who generally support the bill. Next the subcommittee will hear from those people who object to the bill or who wish to propose changes in the bill. In the interest of time, most subcommittees try to have witnesses testify in "panel" of up to six people with similar concerns or interest. Also, this allows the witnesses to comment on each other's statements.

Upon announcing the date for a hearing, the subcommittee will accept requests from interested individuals to testify, and all possible witnesses are accommodated on a first-come-first-served basis. Occasionally, a subcommittee will hold hearings on a "by invitation only" basis. In this case, the subcommittee staff selects the witnesses, and only those individuals testify. Typically, CMHC bills attract individuals representing such groups as the National Association for Mental Health, the National Council of Community Mental Health Centers, the American Academy of Child Psychiatry, the National Association of Social Workers, the National Committee Against Mental Illness, the American Psychological Association, and the American Psychiatric Association.

Once the hearings are completed, the next step in the process is referred to as "subcommittee mark-up" of the bill. This simply means that the entire subcommittee will consider the bill section by section (and sometimes line by line) and will amend (add or delete) the master copy of the bill. This part of the process is important because none of the subsequent steps will go into this level of detail on the bill. During the mark-up the subcommittee will use the information received during the hearings but will also use information obtained from the General Accounting Office, the Congressional Budget Office, the Office of Management and Budget (OMB), and the federal agency to which the program will be assigned.

Prior to the announced mark-up—often there is little advance notice of mark-up sessions—those persons interested in the legislation should meet with the subcommittee members or their staff to reinforce their concerns or support for the bill. Private publishing firms and interest groups such as those mentioned above send out newsletters following the progress of legislation through Congress. Members or subscribers can then time their communications and are often urged to do so by the interest groups. A short summary of their views can be left with the member or the staff. This summary will often be used during the mark-up session.

Upon the completion of the subcommittee mark-up and approval by the subcommittee (only a simple majority is needed to approve), the bill is forwarded to the full committee for consideration. The full committee usually deals with two situations. The first is when committee members who are not on the subcommittee wish to offer an amendment to the bill. Usually subcommittee members are expected to have offered their amendments during the first consideration of the bill. However, a subcommittee member may announce at subcommittee mark-up that he/she intends to offer an amendment at the full committee level, where he/she believes there will be stronger support for the amendment.

Prior to the mark-up on Carter's Mental Health Systems Act, three members of the Senate Labor and Human Resources Health Subcommittee met to resolve their differences. Senator Richard Schweiker had prepared amendments on follow-up for chronic patients in community settings, and Chairman Edward Kennedy met with Schweiker and Senator Jacob Javits to devise a bill to gain subcommittee and full committee acceptance.

The second situation is when the subcommittee is unable to resolve a controversial issue, and thus it is carried forward to the full committee. The format most often used at full committee is to consider amendments by major section or title, rather than line by line.

At the completion of the mark-up, the full committee votes on whether to order the bill reported to the full Senate or House. If an affirmative vote is taken, then an official version of the bill with all the amendments approved by both the subcommittee and the full committee is prepared along with a report. The bill and the report are sent to the chamber, constituting the actual "reporting" of the bill.

The report describes the purpose and scope of the bill and the reasons for its recommended approval. Usually, a section-by-section analysis is set forth in detail, explaining precisely what each section is intended to accomplish.

The report is perhaps the most valuable single element of the legislative history of the law. It is used by the courts, executive departments and agencies, and the public as a source of information about the purpose and meaning of the law. The report, like the bill, is assigned a number at the time it is filed and is printed and subsequently available in the House and Senate Document Rooms. Along with many other federal documents, it is forwarded to federal depositories, many of which are large libraries scattered throughout the country. The Committee Report prepared for House consideration of the 1973 CMHC Amendments is a document rich in detail on CMHC history, funding, administration, important facts, and issues of interest to Congress. Even a lengthy bibliography is attached.

The writing of a report is another point in the process where an interest group may be able to influence the direction of a program. The group may wish to indicate a strong preference to the responsible agency that a specific aspect of the program be given top priority or be funded in a certain way. On the other hand, the group may wish to insert clarifying language about a specific section of the bill in order to avoid future conflict with the agency.

When the bill is reported out of committee, the next step is to establish the time and ground rules for Floor debate. In the House of Representatives, the Rules Committee determines the amount of time allowed for debate on a bill, what amendments (if any) will be in order, the amount of time each amendment will be debated, and who controls the time during debate. Generally, the chairman of the committee that has favorably reported the bill appears before the Rules Committee accompanied by the bill's sponsor and one or more members of the committee in support of his request for a resolution for its immediate consideration.

After the Rules Committee has reported a rule on a bill, the House leadership must schedule the bill. Floor action may be delayed for weeks, especially if the bill is controversial, while the leadership determines whether it has the votes to get a bill passed.

The rules of procedure in the Senate differ to a large extent from those in the House. First, the Senate does not have a Rules Committee. The scheduling procedure is performed by the majority leader in the Senate, and debate can be limited by "unanimous consent agreements" that set the rules for debate. A typical agreement would be "two hours of debate equally divided between the majority and the minority, with 30 minutes for amendments." Another major difference between House and Senate floor procedures is the existence of unlimited debate in the Senate. This is the tactic known as "filibustering" and is usually employed by Senators opposed to a bill who intend to prevent or defeat the action to schedule the measure for debate. Filibustering has never been employed against CMHC legislation.

Once the bill is scheduled for floor action, debate usually begins with a statement by the chairman of the subcommittee or committee that reported the bill, followed by a statement from the ranking minority member. These two members, called "managers" of the bill, yield to others who want to make statements. After the general debate, amendments are called up, discussed, and voted on individually. For example, S66, an omnibus health services bill containing the 1975 CMHC Amendments, was in itself not a subject of debate during Senate floor action. However, a controversial amendment to S66 eliminating federal funding of abortions was tabled after a heated floor debate.

Even during floor action, an interest group can have input in the process by communicating to the Congress via telegram or letter that it supports a particular amendment. When all the amendments have been acted on, the final step is a vote either to approve or reject the bill. It is also in order prior to this final vote for a motion to recommit the bill to the committee, either to kill it or to provide instructions to re-report the bill with a particular section added or deleted.

Just such a recommittal attempt was made by Representative Samuel Devine on the House version of S66, the omnibus health services bill containing the 1975 CMHC Amendments. Devine maintained that the bill should be split into separate bills for individual program consideration and vote. The House voted 9-352 to reject his motion.

The last step in the floor debate process occurs when an official copy of the bill is prepared, customarily referred to as "engrossed," with all the changes approved in the floor debate. This document is signed by the presiding officer and transmitted with considerable ceremony to the other body. If the House acted first, then the bill will be handcarried to the Senate.

Since the House and Senate separately consider and amend bills, and since only a single document can be sent to the President for his consideration, there is a mechanism called the "Joint Committee of Conference" that is used to work out the differences in the two bills. A new conference committee is created for each bill. When it completes its work, it goes out of existence.

When House and Senate reauthorization bills for the CMHC program did not match in 1978, it was thought that they would be sent to a conference committee for compromising. The final version was worked out by staff and members of the House Commerce Committee and the Senate Human Resources Committee when it became obvious that the 95th Congress was about to adjourn without action.

The Conference Committee is allowed to discuss only issues in dispute between the House and Senate. However, there are times when either the House or Senate has substituted its bill for that passed by the other, and in fact it can be said that the entire legislation is subject to revision and compromise. Under these circumstances, it is not unheard of for the Conference Committee to write a completely new bill that does not resemble either of the bills passed by the two bodies.

When the Conference Committee reaches a compromise and thereby has completed its work, a "conference report" is prepared that explains the legislative agreements that were reached. The report is accompanied by a "statement of the managers," which sets out the House position, the Senate position, and the compromise for each section of the bill. The Conference Report is then considered by both the House and Senate, and if approved, the bill, after some Congressional formalities of printing and signing, is finally sent to the President.

A conference committee was held to resolve differences in the funding levels of the House and Senate approved versions of the 1975 omnibus health services legislation, of which the CMHC Amendments were a part. The committee cut authorizations for almost every program in an attempt to head off an expected veto by President Ford. Both houses adopted the conference report by voice vote without debate.

The President now has three choices. First, he can sign the bill, and it immediately becomes public law. Second, he can refuse to sign the bill: if Congress is still in session, the bill automatically becomes law after ten days. However, if Congress had adjourned (for example, at the end of its second session) before the ten days are up, the bill does not become law. This is known as a "pocket veto." President Ford pocket vetoed a bill authorizing funding for the CMHC program after the 93rd Congress adjourned in 1974. Third, the President can veto the bill. In this case he is required by the Constitution to send the bill back to Congress along with his reasons for rejecting it.

Upon receiving the bill, the Congress can attempt to override the veto. This can be difficult because an override requires the approval of two thirds of the members voting in each of the House and Senate. If the override vote is successful, then the bill immediately becomes law. If the override fails, then the Congress must start over again at the subcommittee level. President Ford vetoed S66, the omnibus health services bill, on July 26, 1975. Within hours, the Senate overrode the veto by a 67-15 vote, and the House followed on July 29 by a 384-43 voice vote.

THE BUDGET PROCESS

Assuming the President signs the bill that permits creation of a program, the next step is for the President to determine how much money he wishes to spend on the program and to include that amount in his budget. The actual formulation of the President's budget starts about 19 months before the fiscal year in which the funds become available for expenditure. The current government fiscal year is October 1 through September 30. Thus, using Fiscal Year 1981 as an example (October 1, 1980 through September 30, 1981), the budget process for this fiscal year started in March of 1979. As one can imagine, it is very difficult to predict what the economic conditions will be 19 months hence, and more important, what the mood of the Congress and the people will be when the fiscal year starts.

The federal budget process can be divided into three phases. Phase I covers the period from March through June and is the period during which the budget policy is developed. During this phase the President's Office of Management and Budget (OMB) (1) develops economic assumptions; (2) obtains forecasts of international and domestic situations; and (3) prepares fiscal projections in coordination with the Treasury Department and the Council of Economic Advisers. Upon completion of the forecasting aspects of the budget process, the OMB issues guidelines to the various departments, such as the Department of HEW, which in turn passes these guidelines down to agencies such as NIMH. Once the agencies receive these guidelines, they begin to review their current operations, their program objectives, and future plans in relation to the upcoming annual budget. This is a point where interested groups can and should work with the agency to express their views regarding the level of funding needed for an existing program or for a new program never before funded.

After the agency has completed its internal review, it submits its requirements through the department, which reviews the material and may modify it prior to submitting preliminary estimates to the OMB. The OMB compiles the estimates received from the departments and compares the total estimated expenditures with the Treasury Department's estimate of revenues. Once this step is completed, OMB develops recommendations for the President on fiscal policy, program issues, and budget levels. By the end of June, OMB conveys the President's decisions to the department heads, including budgetary planning targets for individual agencies.

In July, Phase II begins. During this phase, the agencies prepare their budgets based on the target figures issued by the OMB. At this point, OMB may issue one figure for all health programs within HEW, or it may issue an estimate for research, one for manpower, one for services, and another for prevention. The HEW Secretary then allocates an amount to the NIMH, an amount to the Alcohol, Drug Abuse and Mental Health Administration (ADAMHA), and so on. Each agency, such as ADAMHA, will further allocate the budget dollars among its programs. This is another point at which interest groups should be working closely with agency personnel such as the ADAMHA administrator, the Assistant Secretary for Health, and the HEW Secretary.

By the end of September, the departments forward their budgets to OMB. This is Phase III—OMB final review and presidential decisions. During this phase, OMB analyzes the budgets received from the departments and holds hearings with agency representatives on budget, program, and management issues. Also, during this period, OMB reexamines its economic assumptions and fiscal policies developed in March. In light of its revised forecast, OMB prepares budget recommendations for the President. By mid-November, the agencies are notified of the President's decisions.

Generally, the agencies are given an opportunity to appeal the President's decisions, and they often are successful in getting additional money for their programs. During November, interest groups can meet with key OMB staff to impress upon them the need for adequate support of a particular program, and in doing so will be reinforcing the budget request of the agency.

In mid-December, OMB once again reviews its economic assumptions and finetunes the President's budget. By December 31, the budget numbers and the President's budget message are completed, sent to the printer, and officially submitted to Congress 15 days after it convenes.

The process of formulating the President's budget is often overlooked by interest groups. Admittedly, it is a closed process (as opposed to the open congressional affair with its hearings), but it is equally important. In fact, I believe it to be more important because, if the President's budget contains adequate funding for your program, you avoid a fight at the Congressional level for the few dollars that Congress might be able to add to the budget and still get the bill through the House and Senate. The names of the key persons in OMB are available at public libraries in directories of federal government employees. More often than not, they are willing to meet with interest groups in order to learn how the programs are actually working at the local level.

THE CONGRESSIONAL BUDGET COMMITTEES

The budget committees are recent arrivals to the Congressional process. The Budget and Impoundment Control Act of 1974 created the budget committees in a sweeping and complex piece of legislation. Traditionally, Congress would each year take the President's budget, chop it up into many small pieces, and distribute it among many committees and subcommittees. Each committee or subcommittee would work on its own piece with little or no regard for the impact that its changes might have on the total budget. It is safe to say that only a few within the Congress were aware of the emerging totals.

Under the requirements of the Budget and Impoundment Act of 1974, the budget committees establish, for each fiscal year, levels of total spending, revenue, and national debt. The intent is to give Congress a means by which it can set national fiscal and economic policy through a comprehensive and unified approach to the budget.

The new congressional budget process sets the following timetable:

Deadline	Activity
November 10*	President submits current services budget.
January 18†	President submits budget to Congress.
March 15	All congressional committees report on their reaction to the President's budget, along with their recommendations.
April 1±	Congressional Budget Office reports to House and Senate Budget Committees.
April 15	House and Senate Budget Committees report out first budget resolution.
May 15	All committees must report on authorizing legislation requiring an expenditure of funds in the upcoming fiscal year. Congress completes action on first budget resolution.
Labor Day plus 7 days	Congress completes action on all spending bills.
September 15	Congress completes action on second budget resolution.
September 25	Congress completes action on reconciling the spending bills with the budget resolution.
October 1	Fiscal year begins.

With this chronological information as background, we can proceed with the details of the process.

When the House and Senate officially receive the President's budget, it is immediately referred to the Budget Committees and the Appropriation Committees, and they concurrently begin to analyze and interpret the document. In February, the Budget Committees hold hearings in preparation to draft the first concurrent budget resolution. Witnesses are usually invited by the Committee and may include the OMB Director, Secretary of the Treasury, Chairman of the Council of Economic Advisors, leading economists, and

---

*The current services budget is a new concept in the budgetary process. Basically it requires the President to show what it will cost to maintain the current year's level of government services in the upcoming fiscal year.

†Or 15 days after Congress convenes.

±The Congressional Budget Office was created by the Budget and Impoundment Control Act of 1974 as an analytical and informational arm of the Budget Committees.

experts on particular issues such as defense, health, and transportation.

Around March 15, after other committees of the Congress have submitted their views and estimates for the upcoming fiscal year, the Budget Committee begins to draft its first budget resolution and usually attempts to complete its work by the end of the first week in April. The budget resolution does not address itself to specific amounts of money for given programs such as mental health research. Rather it addresses itself to major functions of the government, such as defense, transportation, and health.

The first budget resolution must be adopted by the House and Senate by May 15. (By this date, the two bodies will have resolved any differences in a Joint Conference Committee.) This first resolution merely establishes revenue and expenditure boundaries within which the other committees of the Congress attempt to stay.

In September, after the authorization and appropriation bills have been acted on, the Budget Committees prepare a second budget resolution that sets a specific ceiling for expenditures and places a floor under revenues. This resolution must be reconciled with the appropriation, authorization, and revenue bills acted on over the summer months. Once the reconciliation process has been completed—and it must be completed before Congress can adjourn—any subsequent bill that exceeds the expenditure ceiling or breaches the revenue floor is subject to a point of order, preventing the bill from being considered by the full House or Senate.

The budget resolution is not sent to the President for his signature, and it is not a law. It receives the designation of "Concurrent Resolution" because it simply expresses the sense of the Congress concerning fiscal and economic policy. But the rules of the House and Senate require the committees to comply with budget resolutions, which are therefore of great importance and affect every unit of Congress.

THE APPROPRIATION COMMITTEES

The Appropriation Committees approach the budget differently from the Budget Committees. The Appropriation Committees look closely at individual programs and activities, such as mental health research, mental health manpower, community mental health centers, drug abuse, and alcoholism services.

The Committees require each program within that agency to justify its need for funds in the upcoming fiscal year: how it is spending its money in the current fiscal year, and what it accomplished with the money it spent in the previous fiscal year. They

examine how well the program is carrying out the intent of the law
that created it and how efficiently its money, manpower, and equipment are being managed. A tremendous amount of detail is submitted by the agencies. For example, the U.S. Public Health Service submits four volumes totaling more than 1,000 pages.

The Appropriation Committee begins its process early in February by holding a special overview hearing on the budget with the
OMB Director, the Secretary of the Treasury, and the Chairman of
the Council of Economic Advisors. Subsequently, each of the 13
subcommittees begins detailed hearings with the departments under
its jurisdiction by first inviting the departmental secretary to testify.
It then invites the agency heads to testify, and sometimes also program directors such as the NIMH Director or the Director of the
National Institute of Arthritis, Metabolism and Digestive Diseases.

Approximately two months are devoted to hearing testimony
from the Administration witnesses in support of the President's budget, and an additional two weeks is devoted to taking testimony from
the general public. In the case of the Subcommittee on Appropriation for the Departments of Labor and HEW, as many as 200 witnesses appear before the subcommittee, and practically all of them
request additional money for a specific program.

During the first two weeks of May, the subcommittees mark-up
their section of the President's budget, using the budget resolution
as a guide. This is usually done in an open session, that is, with
the public sitting in the room, and usually amounts to the Chairman
presenting his recommendations on a line-by-line basis. Each of his
recommendations is either accepted or amended by the members of
the subcommittee.

The mark-up takes approximately a full day to complete, and
unless one has a copy of the President's budget, it is extremely difficult to follow the committee actions. Prior to the official mark-up,
considerable negotiation takes place between the Chairman and individual members, and between the committee staff and the staffs of
the individual members. By the time the public mark-up takes place,
a substantial percentage of the work has been done, and only the
highly controversial items remain.

In addition to testifying, citizens should work closely with the
subcommittee members and staff in the two weeks preceding the
mark-up, in order to assist them in formulating their recommendations for the budget. The staff and the members need supplemental
information, usually in one or two pages—instead of volumes that
no one has time to read—explaining program accomplishments, how
the program helps people, and how additional money will be spent.

Once the mark-up is completed, the subcommittee staff prepares an appropriation bill and a report that explains the subcom-

mittee's action. The report is often a vehicle used by the members to instruct the agencies to undertake a certain activity or to give special emphasis to an area of research. Interest groups should not overlook this report as a means of advancing their program objectives.

The next step is for the subcommittee to present its bill, which is still not assigned a number at this point in the process, to the full committee. The full committee usually completes action on the bill in half a day, and few, if any, changes are made to the bill and report. The bill is reported, assigned a number, and subsequently scheduled for floor debate. The appropriation bill and the accompanying report are available in the Document Room within 24 hours after the bill has been introduced.

Floor debate and action on an appropriation bill can last from a few hours to several days. The Labor-HEW bill usually takes in excess of ten legislative hours to complete, depending on the number of amendments to be offered on the bill.

Interest groups can have money added to the appropriation bill by working closely with a member of Congress. During floor consideration of the Fiscal Year 1975 appropriation bill, Congressman Silvio Conte of Massachusetts offered an amendment to add money for the community mental health centers. Earlier that morning, all 435 members of the House of Representatives were inundated with telegrams from their constituents back home urging them to support the Conte amendment. It was obvious that the mental health community had reached an agreement with Mr. Conte to offer the amendment and then, with perfect timing, unleashed an avalanche of telegrams in support of the amendment. Members were walking down the aisle of the House Chamber with telegrams in their hands, asking the staff for more information on the Conte amendment and asking the Chairman of the subcommittee if he planned to oppose the amendment. Most members urged the Chairman to accept the amendment because of the substantial constituent interest. The amendment was adopted overwhelmingly.

The House of Representatives always acts first on appropriation bills, and therefore as soon as the House completes its work on the bill, the comparable Senate subcommittee schedules a mark-up. The bill then moves to full committee and the Senate floor, basically following the same process as in the House of Representatives. A separate bill is written, as is a separate report containing directives and emphasis on areas of special interest to the Senate. The instructions in the House and Senate reports are often conflicting, and the agencies must find creative ways to respond to the directives.

As with the authorizing legislation, a Joint Conference Committee is created to resolve the differences between the House and

Senate appropriation bills. The work of the Joint Conference Committee is restricted to resolving the differences in the two bills. It cannot reopen an item that was agreed to by the full House and Senate. Here again, as in the authorization process, when the Joint Conference Committee completes its work, a conference report and a statement of managers is prepared that explains the agreements. The conference report is then considered by both the House and Senate, and if approved, the bill is finally sent to the President.

Once again, the President has the same choices he has in the authorization process. He can sign the bill, in which case it immediately becomes law. Or he can refuse to sign the bill. If the Congress is in session, the bill automatically becomes law after ten days. If the Congress adjourns before the ten days have passed (as might happen, for instance, at the end of a session) the bill does not become law. This is known as a pocket veto. Finally, the President can veto the bill. If he does so, the Congress can attempt to override the veto. This override requires approval of two-thirds of the members voting in the House and Senate.

But even if the appropriation bill is enacted, the agency does not immediately get the money. Authority to actually spend the money must come to the program from the Treasury Department, through the OMB. The OMB may decide with the President's approval to withhold funds from the program. President Richard Nixon impounded monies for CMHCs authorized to begin operations. After losing a law suit filed against him by the centers, he released the monies. Impoundment of these and other programs' funding as a means of control over appropriations led to the passage of the Budget and Impoundment Act of 1974.

This then brings us to that part of the process created by the Act dealing with recessions and deferrals. If the President decides that Congress appropriated too much money for a program, he can ask that it be rescinded. If Congress rejects the request, the President must make the money available to the program.

In 1975, President Ford asked that $14.2 million for construction and renovation of CMHCs be rescinded. The House agreed, but the Senate disapproved. The money was not rescinded. The other option available to the President is to inform Congress of his intent to defer the expenditure of funds until some later date in the year. Here again, if Congress rejects the proposal, the funds must be immediately available for expenditure.

We are now at the end of a long and complex process that has taken many months, and involved numerous actors. In order for an interest group to surmount this process, it must be tenacious, patient, and, at all times, on top of the legislative process.

REFERENCES AND SUGGESTED READINGS

Fenno, R. The power of the purse: Appropriations politics in Congress. Boston: Little, Brown, 1966.

Kirst, M. W. Government without passing laws. Chapel Hill: University of North Carolina Press, 1969.

Wildavsky, A. The politics of the budgeting process. Boston: Little, Brown, 1974.

8

FUNDING THROUGH
GOVERNMENT SOURCES
J. R. Elpers

Without a solid funding base, it is difficult for any mental health agency to carry out its function. Since the various levels of government provide a major part of the funding for mental health services, topics in this chapter address survival issues in our service effort. I will first present a brief history of the role of government in mental health care, then turn to a description of governmental sources of funding. The last three sections deal with nongovernmental sources, securing public monies, and the role of board members in funding.

HISTORY OF GOVERNMENTAL RESPONSIBILITY

Over the centuries, the mentally ill have been widely recognized as a dependent population, and their care has been placed either with religious or governmental institutions. The mode of service has ranged from remote asylums to active community care programs.

Modern systems of treatment are generally traced back to the eighteenth century. Philippe Pinel (1745-1826) is usually credited with freeing patients from chains in the institutions he supervised in Paris, France, the Asylums of Bicêtre and La Salpêtriere. William Tuke (1732-1822) and Benjamin Rush (1745-1813) led similar reform movements in England and the United States, respectively. These movements gave impetus to the further emergence of the "moral" treatments of the nineteenth century in which a great deal of optimism, perhaps an excessive amount, was held regarding the treatability of the mentally ill. It was during this period that

Dorothea Dix (1820-1877), a retired school teacher, led the crusade
for better care from state to state. Her efforts resulted in the acceptance of responsibility for the mentally ill by state legislatures
and the establishment of state "asylums." These asylums were initially designed to provide humane treatment; and in fact, being
small and well-staffed, they had considerable success in returning
patients to the community. However, because of increased service
demands and limited fiscal resources, a new system of large state
institutions evolved in which many components were no better than
the Asylums of Bicêtre and La Salpêtriere. As more people were
institutionalized and stayed for longer periods of time due to the
lack of appropriate treatment, the burden on state governments became overwhelming. By the mid-1950s well over half of all the hospital beds in the entire country were psychiatric beds located primarily in state institutions.

By the mid-twentieth century, the scene was set for a redis-
covery of moral treatment, although this time it was called community mental health. Leaders in mental health care reached a general consensus that the huge state institutions could not themselves
be improved because the cost would be prohibitive. Under the aegis
of the community mental health movement, local services were offered as alternatives to state institutions. However, since the state
was the major provider for the treatment of the chronically emotionally disabled, other governmental jurisdictions were unwilling
to assume significant fiscal responsibility. For example, when the
federal government established Medicaid, it avoided paying for patient care in state hospitals by limiting benefits to outpatient care
and to treatment in psychiatric wings of general hospitals. When
the first federal community mental health center (CMHC) program
was instituted in 1963, many recognized that the federal government
would never have adequate resources to assume a significant level
of support for state facilities. Thus, the decision was made to fund
a new model on a pilot basis. The declining grant structure of the
CMHCs was devised to allow the federal government to experiment
with a new pattern of care while utilizing minimal federal resources.

SOURCES OF GOVERNMENT FUNDING

This review of the various sources of governmental funding
is undertaken in general terms because a great deal of variability
exists from state to state regarding fiscal responsibilities.

Federal Funding

Federal per capita expenditures for mental health care are small when compared to state expenditures. Primary sources of federal money are grants from the National Institute for Mental Health (NIMH), especially service funds for CMHCs, and patient care reimbursements through Medicaid and Medicare. CMHC legislation continues to be modified, particularly in the range of mandated services, organizational structure, and reporting requirements. Because funds are awarded on the basis of competitive applications and there are more fundable grants approved than money to support them, grant-writing skills and effective program defense are essential for applicants. Funding priorities are given to poverty areas, which also receive a higher level of federal participation in the operating costs of the centers.

Since federal grants are awarded on the basis of catchment areas and priorities defined in each state's CMHC plan, each community should work with the appropriate state agency to assure that the definitions are appropriate. Each grant application is reviewed by the local Health Systems Agency and, in most cases, by the state Health Systems Agency. In addition, the state agency for CMHCs must review and comment on the proposal. Detailed reviews of the application are generally conducted in the regional offices of the federal Department of Health and Human Services, with final approval or deferral coming after review by the national review committee of NIMH.

Among the many types of CMHC grants are those for planning, initiating new programs, and special categories. Because many of these categories will be revised with new legislation, there is no need for a review here. Staff at the regional offices of the U.S. Department of Health and Human Services are generally eager and able to give the latest on grant information to both CMHC boards and personnel. A close and cordial working relationship with this staff is highly recommended.

Medicaid is a major source of funding for most public mental health programs. Medicaid is a complex program that constitutes a joint undertaking by the federal government and the individual states to finance health care for the poor. Funding is based upon a formula that varies according to the state's resources. The federal government agrees, within certain limits, to match the state's contributions for most types of health care to eligible persons. Eligibility is determined by the patient's income and whether he/she is receiving other forms of governmental assistance. Both the covered services and the eligible population vary from state to state. A CMHC board is able, therefore, to influence state legislators and administrators to strive for the broadest possible coverage for mental health services and the most reasonably inclusive eligibility standards.

Since Medicaid is a medical program, there are many CMHC services not covered. Services usually considered "social" rather than "medical" are case management, social model residential care programs, activities centers, and consultative services. One of the problems of Medicaid funding is that it frequently forces a CMHC to bias its programs toward medical treatment rather than social rehabilitation. This problem presents a major policy issue because it is often difficult to decide at what point one should stop tailoring programs to meet Medicaid regulations in order to preserve the relevance of programs to the community.

For centers that serve a large number of older persons, Medicare can become a significant portion of patient revenues. Medicare eligibility is far more universal for older persons throughout the country, and covered services are uniform. Since definitions and coverages are limited, Medicare patient fees are only a small part of the average CMHC's revenues.

Many programs funded under CMHC legislation are not eligible for reimbursement under Medicaid and Medicare. Consequently, the executive director must choose judiciously which programs he/ she attempts to fund via the grant mechanism, in contrast to which programs to fund via reimbursement under the major third-party payment systems. Maximization of revenues will be achieved through matching the revenue source to a program plan rather than arbitrarily distorting programs to meet funding requirements.

Among the number of other federal government funding sources that are not mainstream but should be considered are Housing and Urban Development (HUD) funds for residential care facilities, Farmers' Home Administration (FMHA) grants to small communities for special projects, such as apartments for the "disabled," Community Development Block Grants, and Title XX monies. These last named funds vary among the states and are dependent on a state plan similar to that of Medicaid. They can be a major source of funding for social services designed to avoid institutionalization and to move the client toward social and economic independence.

State Funding

As noted previously, funds for the treatment of the mentally ill are most readily available through state government. States presently have a large investment in their care, and in a majority of the states, this is primarily in state hospital services. Most states now have some mechanism to fund local mental health services.

Local services are expected to be cost effective, from the perspective of state government, by reducing the utilization of state hospitals. On occasion, state funding is directly tied to this reduction.

Unfortunately, over the years the community mental health movement has been sold to legislators on the basis that it will reap great savings in state hospital costs. As state hospital populations decline, legislators tend to lose sight of the fact that the patients who formerly were in hospitals still require help, even though they now reside in the community. Savings from hospitals revert to the general fund, rather than becoming available to local programs.

There are many factors that influence both the cost and the speed of instituting local services for ex-inpatients. These include the availability of residential care settings, the capacity to attract the necessary staff, required training time, and the complexity of negotiating contracts. Reduction of state hospital utilization is not a goal, but only a secondary effect of good community mental health. Hospital admissions should be reduced only if patients have better community alternatives.

Local Funding

The availability of local governmental funds is highly variable throughout the country. In some states, local funds are mandated as matching formulas to state funds. Occasionally, states legislate a special taxing authority to enable local governments to fund their own programs. Frequently, the mental health program is competing with other community priorities for local funds. With this in mind, it is wise to choose a program for local funding that has broad appeal or is readily visible and closely linked with other community services. Typically, one finds that local funding sources are most responsive to unique community needs.

In recent years, many local governments have used federal revenue sharing funds to provide human services. These funds are generally considered one-time funds with limited commitments for the future. Local agencies should keep in mind that revenue sharing was created through the aggregation of funds from federal categorical aid programs, including human services programs, into block grants. Its history presents a strong argument for the inclusion of human services in revenue sharing projects.

Funding from local government is often the least stable source of revenue because priorities change frequently. Income is closely related to the local economy. Also, it is difficult for any human service program to compete with the needs of police, fire, and other essential municipal services.

Governmental Priorities

To understand the full range of governmental funding for mental health services, both quantitative and qualitative comparisons are in order. We can see from the data in Table 8.1 that the bulk of funding comes from state government. Nationally, there is more interest in how NIMH utilizes its resources, not because of the amount of money it distributes, but because it exerts a leadership role through seed money and pilot projects. NIMH is a trend setter to whom we look for future directions in funding.

TABLE 8.1

Direct Support of Mental Health Programs
by NIMH, New York, and California

	Support	Population*	Per Capita Support
NIMH			
Research	$145,250,000	216,332,000(US)	$0.67
Training	90,354,000	"	0.42
Services	297,943,000	"	1.38
Program support	35,000,000	"	0.16
Total	$568,547,000	216,332,000(US)	$2.63
New York (state and local support)			
State hospitals	$422,200,000	17,924,000	$23.56
Community programs	198,800,000	"	11.09
Total	$621,000,000	17,924,000	$34.65
California (state and local support)			
State hospitals	$130,558,000	21,896,000	$ 5.96
Community programs	300,556,000	"	13.73
Total	$431,114,000	21,896,000	$19.69

*July 1, 1977 population estimates.
Source: U.S. Bureau of the Census.

The quantitative differences in the various funding sources suggest different agenda at different governmental levels. From the federal government there is start-up money and funding for special projects via the grant route. Medicaid and Medicare provide a major portion of our most stable long-term funding. State governments, on the other hand, are fundamentally concerned with mainstream services to the chronically and severely ill. These are the services that will reduce their obligation to fund state institutions. Therefore, state governments are unlikely to look favorably upon other services, particularly prevention. Finally, local governments are more interested in programs that meet the needs of highly visible populations. These include programs for children, particularly those who are abandoned and neglected, minority populations, and those services with which the general population can easily identify.

NONGOVERNMENTAL FUNDING SOURCES

A brief word on nongovernmental funding sources is needed in order to assess the relative importance of governmental funding to the mental health care system. Conceptually, we can break down our funding needs into one-time projects and ongoing support. One-time projects include such items as the acquisition of new facilities, remodeling of old ones, and special purchases of expensive fixed assets or equipment. Such expenditures are ideal targets for special fund-raising projects because the product is highly visible to potential donors.

Philanthropic sources of money, discussed elsewhere in this book, can be used both for one-time projects and for ongoing support. However, philanthropic support requires large endowment funds, multiple bequests, and aggressive pursuit of foundations and special donors. Many smaller agencies do not have the capacity to gather a significant part of their operating expenditures from philanthropy, but some do obtain a portion from community-wide combined giving drives, such as United Way or Community Chest. These organizations tend to be stable and traditional. Although it is difficult for a new agency to obtain a portion of the distribution, once it has become a recipient, it can expect to remain so. Agencies undertaking these large charitable drives do, in fact, assume a quasi-governmental role in that they distribute money based on a broad community input and they attempt to protect the public good in much the same way as do public officials.

The major advantage of funds from philanthropy or combined giving agencies is that they are not usually tied directly to specific types of programs or services. They are more flexible in their use than governmental or fee-for-service sources.

A portion of revenues for any mental health agency should be patient fees. They may come from the patients themselves, from government programs such as Medicaid or Medicare, or from insurance payments. The mix of these types of fees varies according to the population served. Poor communities will depend primarily upon Medicare and Medicaid, while blue-collar communities can expect greater contributions from large group insurance. More affluent communities will gain a larger portion of revenues from patient fees. Vigorous collection of fees is important because most governmental funding programs require the agency to secure all such fees possible before it spends governmental funds, and the fees help to compensate for declining monies for human services.

SECURING FUNDING

Knowing which agency at any given level of government should fund your mental health program in no way guarantees they will do so. Obtaining public funds involves more than turning in grant applications, program proposals, or bills for patient services. It is necessary that the director, staff, and board agree about the type, range, and focus of its services. Only after they reach a clear understanding of the mission can they begin to secure these monies. Each center should first undertake an advocacy role with local elected officials, state legislators, the governor, and their Congressmen and Senators to assure that programs are properly defined and budgeted at the appropriate governmental level. Programs with common needs can join together in broad coalitions, such as the National Council of Community Mental Health Centers, to lobby for legislation. In larger metropolitan areas, an alliance of competing agencies may be necessary to assure the support of local officials for adequate mental health appropriations. Otherwise, the mental health agencies can be reduced to squabbling among themselves for a very small pot of available monies.

In order to accomplish legislative goals, board members and executive staff must have a thorough knowledge of current legislation. The key is to direct attention to the proper committees or executives at the proper time, particularly when decisions are due to be made, and to present a simple, concise argument. Legislators respond to people, not statistics. When we are forced to present statistics, we generally have lost the cause, and when we are asked for them, the legislators are seeking a reason to reject our proposals. Politicians are reluctant to turn down persons in need when those persons, their friends, relatives, and other concerned citizens are willing to stand up for the agency.

When funds are being sought, board members and the executive staff must clearly delineate what part each can play best. For example, board members can attract the attention of the political leadership of the community; the executive director can then provide the necessary information to them. It is the board and its extension through community liaison groups that can mobilize community support for the agency. For the director and staff to attempt to do so appears self-serving. They are at a disadvantage when defending the agency's programs if they lack the strong, consistent, and informed support of their board and constituency groups.

BOARD ROLES

There are many different types of boards for community mental health programs: some are operating boards, others are advisory, and others are governmental in nature, that is, appointed by public bodies. Board members may be elected from the community or selected from among the community leadership. The type and character of boards should be determined by the needs of the population served by the host agency. Thus, agencies that depend primarily on philanthropic sources will tend to have boards made up of persons who have access to philanthropic monies, or in some cases, individuals who themselves can afford to donate to the agency. Boards of governmental entities tend to be selected from the community at large, and also have contacts in the political sector. Federally funded CMHC boards are required to be representative of the community and are composed of interested citizens and consumers. Because each type of board will have different resources and skills available to it, it can utilize its membership to assure the adequate and appropriate funding of its agency. It is the responsibility of the board membership to assess their own capabilities and duties and the needs of their centers.

Close collaboration with the executive director and administrative staff is essential. Many functions can be undertaken by board members that would seem self-serving if carried out by the director or staff. Among these functions are advocacy before governmental funding authorities such as state legislatures, local commissions, boards of supervisors, and other political authorities. Another function boards assume is leadership in articulating agency requirements to the public, either through the media or to planning bodies and public coordinating agencies. A properly selected and constituted board can and should present itself as being primarily concerned with the representation of the needs of the people served by the agency. Thus, for a board to assume an effective advocacy role, each member should know about the goals, priorities, and methods of the agency. He/she must feel personally responsible for the quantity and quality of services provided and should have a sincere interest in its clientele. We are, in summary, speaking of the necessity for dedicated and committed board membership.

The board's responsibility in evaluating the various sources of governmental funds goes beyond speaking for the agency in the political arena. It should accept funds only under such conditions that the goals of the agency can continue to be met. No agency should prostitute itself by assuming unwanted or inappropriate responsibilities or by carrying out its functions in an unacceptable manner in order to obtain funding.

Board members must carefully evaluate the strings attached to various sources of money. Nearly all governmental agencies function with objectives defined by law to guarantee that specific types of service are provided. These laws assure that their own mission or function is carried out, although the mission may appear narrow when viewed in the perspective of the total gamut of human service needs. It may help to view each funding source as a special interest agency more concerned with its own survival than the needs of the local population for particular services. With this understanding, each request for funding can be assessed to assure that your agency's goal will not be harmed if you accede to the demands of the funding source. The vast majority of conditions imposed by funding services are for good and reasonable purposes. They assure that the recipient carries out the duties for which it is receiving money and that there is accurate reporting of activities. Vigilance must be maintained to assure that the various reporting requirements, accounting practices, or other such strictures of one funding source do not destroy the ability of the agency to integrate its support with that of others.

SUMMARY

In this chapter, I have attempted to give a general review of the various funding sources and an orientation for board members to the particular interest of those sources: namely, the federal government's interest in innovative, trend setting programs, state government's interest in reducing the population in institutions providing services to the chronically ill, and local government's tendency to fund programs of special interest or unique value to the community. This review has necessarily been general since every state and community has special needs and opportunities to obtain funding for mental health services. The role and responsibilities of board

members vis-à-vis agency staff have been discussed with emphasis
on the board's responsibility to interface with the political sector
as well as protect the goals and policies of the agency from undue
distortion by the various funding resources. Finally, it must be
emphasized that every board has a unique and fundamental role to
play in guaranteeing the fiscal survivability of its agency. This
role must be carefully delineated and effectively carried out if the
service goals of the agency are to be successfully attained.

9

PRIVATE PHILANTHROPHY:
AN OPPORTUNITY FOR BOARD INITIATIVE
IN SUPPORT OF
MENTAL HEALTH PROGRAMS
Stanley C. Silber

In a rural community in the southwestern United States, a community mental health center (CMHC) is operating a thriving food processing business. Consisting of hothouses, a sorting factory, and a canning plant, the business was started for the purpose of assisting clients who had serious problems in returning to meaningful functioning. The project grew out of determined board action under the leadership of the president, who convinced the local Chamber of Commerce to donate $30,000 to purchase a program site. An agricultural agency and a vocational agency also helped to fund it as a result of the Chamber's participation. The combination of public and private community support were the critical elements that led to several incremental grants totaling well over $200,000 given by a national foundation over a three-year period.

This type of board initiative and many others have been successful for several reasons. These include (1) an increasing awareness of the critical nature of funding problems facing community mental health programs today; (2) shrinking federal, state, and local tax sources and increasing operating costs; (3) knowledge that national health insurance will not cover all service needs and, indeed, may not become a reality for many years; and (4) the need for strong community initiative and action to sustain an ever-increasing demand for service.

When these boards faced the question of what could be done at this time, their choice was to return to one source of funding that has been neglected in recent years—private philanthropy. This free and unencumbered dollar is used today as a catalyst for combining a multiplicity of other public and private sources to accomplish service goals required by the community. The private philanthropy dollar is no longer a major source of support for health, education, and welfare services; it is still, however, significant as a creative supplement to both public and private dollars for research, training, evaluation, and special innovative projects. Such projects in the long run are needed to revolutionize our care systems. It also can pay for preventive programs that are our greatest hope for reducing the incidence of mental illness. Furthermore, private funds generated at the state or local level can add a healthy measure of local influence on program development.

Despite current inflationary pressures, private philanthropy continues to be a growing business. Historically, government has granted privileges to private citizens in exchange for their commitment to the public interest. It encourages philanthropy today through the overall tax structure. During 1978, the last year for which complete figures are available, philanthropic giving reached $39.56 billion, up almost 145 percent since 1968. This was a 9.4 percent increase over the previous year when the rate of inflation was 9 percent. It is estimated that $43 billion from all sources was raised in 1979, and the estimate for 1990 is $80 billion. These projections are based on a fairly reliable rule that philanthropic donations consistently approximate 1.9 percent of the gross national product.

These philanthropic funds come from four principal sources: individuals, foundations, bequests and deferred gifts, and corporations. Individual gifts have consistently made up more than three fourths of the annual total; during 1978 they amounted to $32.8 billion or almost 83 percent of the total. In the same year, foundations increased their charitable giving by 7.5 percent to a total of $2.16 billion. A sizable part of the increase can be attributed to the reduction from 4 percent to 2 percent of excise taxes that foundations have paid to the government since 1969. Bequests produced $2.6 billion in 1978; this does not include the billion-dollar bequest of the late John MacArthur for the establishment of two foundations. However, the $2.6 billion figure represents 13 percent less than the amount bequeathed to philanthropic organizations in 1977. The picture of corporate giving is much brighter. The $2 billion given to charitable causes by U.S. businesses in 1978 is the largest increase in the history of corporate giving, up 17.6 percent from the $1.7 billion given in 1977.

The scope of philanthropic giving has great significance for local communities in that the story of the southwestern community already mentioned could be repeated in various forms by other boards throughout the country. Many sources at both state and local levels can be tapped if an organized approach to seeking funds is taken. To develop philanthropic support for a program, a board should first look at the potential of the four major sources of support.

The remainder of this chapter examines these sources in detail and cites examples of creative board action in obtaining them.

INDIVIDUAL GIFTS

Individual giving has been and continues to be a promising source of income. Contributed in the form of cash, securities, appreciated property, and goods in kind, these gifts can often be used for capital and operating costs and are designated for either special projects or general purposes. They are acquired from persons directly or through professional business, civic, social, labor, and service organizations. Complete information about developing an individual gifts program is available from the American Association of Fund Raising Counsel, Inc., 500 Fifth Avenue, New York, New York 10036, or from the Fund Raising Institute, Plymouth Meeting, Pennsylvania 19462.

Once the individual contributor has decided to support a program, the tax incentives provided under the Internal Revenue Service Code help to determine the size of the gift. Cash gifts can be deducted at full-face value up to 50 percent of the donor's adjusted gross income, and they may be averaged over five years. Gifts of appreciated property may be deducted at their full market value up to 30 percent of the donor's adjusted gross income, and the donor does not have to pay capital gains tax on the appreciation. For example, if a man gives a mental health center some land that he bought for $6,000 but which now has a market value of $50,000, he is entitled to a $50,000 deduction and he pays no capital gains tax on the appreciation of $44,000. Complexity of the tax law requires expert legal counsel on all large gifts of appreciated property in order to determine tax consequences.

It is more important to understand the individual giver and his/her motives for giving than the form of the gift. We might choose to see the giver as being strongly motivated by tax incentives provided by the federal law, and indeed, this is often true. However, service organizations are able to raise money partly because people believe in what they do. People are motivated to give for a variety of reasons. Many give out of a sense of personal identification with the cause or the services, and they will support it because they or their relatives have been helped by it. Many donors, such as wealthy individuals who support a variety of causes, give because they respect another person's opinion of a cause; they may be influenced by a board member who cannot individually give large sums but may persuade those who can. Many clubs and organizations support specific programs, and some clubs have even been formed for philanthropic reasons. Some individuals give significant sums to alleviate a social problem of concern to the community because they hold strong convictions that a community should solve its own problems and maintain control of its programs.

Many others enjoy giving for the satisfaction they receive. All they need is some understanding of the relationship between the activities they support and the effects those activities have on them: all individual giving is ultimately done for personal reasons. Perhaps those in the mental health field who traditionally have given help are reluctant to ask for it. The giver feels the same sense of well-being in helping us with our critical problems as we do in helping those who come to us in crisis. Both situations require the open communication of needs.

One urban CMHC located in a mid-Atlantic state offers an illustration of how a board began its individual gift program. The community had experienced a rapid growth in population, and the center concomitantly experienced increased service demands for its drug and alcoholism program. The critical need was for an adequate treatment facility that could relate to the shifting service population. While staffing needs were met through federal grants, the space problem was addressed in a unique fashion. The board formed a separate receiving corporation for the purpose of acquiring properties. Initial funding came from the contributions of some affluent board members, their business associates, and friends. The nonprofit holding company was able to acquire an adequate facility for a minimal down payment. The mortgage was paid through the rent allowance available to the CMHC through a federal grant. When the population began to shift to another part of the county, an additional facility was purchased and financed in the same manner. The first facility was sold at a profit, and the corporation remained in a position to purchase additional properties as service needs changed.

In another case, an individual board member undertook a project that grew out of his own special skills. A West Coast building contractor was concerned with family violence and child abuse. In order to develop programs to address this community problem, he built a "showplace house" by garnering the support of labor unions, women's groups, government, and suppliers. He did this with the assistance of other board members and sold the house at a substantial profit, thus enabling the CMHC to begin its new programs.

It is important to view individual gifts as an ongoing source of support for ongoing programs. A laissez-faire approach to seeking individual gifts will, by and large, result in limited amounts of money given on a one-time basis. Properly organized, individual giving can become a springboard for all other endeavors to obtain private philanthropic support. It is the single most important source of dollars as well as a promoter of wider community participation.

It is axiomatic that individual giving requires both programmatic and financial commitment by members of the board. From
that point forward, a rule of thumb for successful fund raising has
three parts. First, 70 percent of total giving in a campaign should
be provided by 10 percent or fewer of the contributors. Second,
the size of the first 10 to 25 gifts solicited and received often determines success or failure in reaching a goal. Finally, all giving
is highly personal and should be solicited on a personal basis. A
good text that explains the mechanics of fund raising is Harold J.
Seymour's Designs for Fund Raising—Principles, Patterns, Techniques.

Operating business enterprises such as thrift shops and annual
book sales are another form of individual philanthropy that has produced significant sums of money for worthy causes. Mental health
facilities might do well to adopt such devices. These enterprises
are generally organized by relatively affluent women and attract
support from influential people in the community. They require
little time from professionals because they are usually run entirely
by volunteers.

Although individual giving has increased over the years, the
major limitation of this category has been the increase in the number of persons taking the standard deduction for income tax purposes. Some legislative activity in Congress at this time calls for
allowing taxpayers to take the standard deduction while itemizing
charitable contributions. In 1979, the Fisher–Conable Bill was introduced in the House and the Packwood–Moynihan Bill in the Senate;
both bills attempted to change the tax law, including those parts affecting charitable contributions.

FOUNDATION GRANTS

There are over 22,000 foundations in the United States, and
they are another important source of income for mental health programs. A foundation is a philanthropic nongovernment organization
with a principal fund derived from gifts or bequests from its founder.
Its operation and purpose as defined by the Internal Revenue Code is
to receive and grant funds for the advancement of human welfare.
The larger foundations have wide-ranging interests and generally
try to improve the quality of life by supporting new and experimental programs.

Foundations hold approximately $32.4 billion in assets. Their
grants of $2.6 billion in 1978 almost doubled the amount given at the
beginning of the decade. Twenty percent of the grants were to
health, and 15 percent of those health dollars were for mental health
exclusively. Interestingly, many state mental health departments

have set up private foundations to enable them to develop research, training, and special projects that could not otherwise be funded under state law.

There are five principal types of foundations: general purpose, special purpose, corporate, community, and family. General purpose foundations number approximately 350, and account for more than half the grants and two thirds of the assets of the foundations. Among them are Ford, Danforth, Johnson, and Rockefeller Foundations. They have professional management, distinguished boards, and specific policies, procedures, and areas of interest.

Special purpose foundations hold some 10 percent of all foundations assets. Although each generally supports a specific project, grants can be made for broader programs in health, education, and welfare. These may include special educational projects for population groups such as American Indians, and treatment of specific handicaps or medical conditions, such as cancer and heart diseases.

Corporate foundations number 2,000 and hold 6 percent of foundation assets. They are funded by annual corporate appropriations, generally no more than 1 percent of net profits. Among the fastest growing group of foundations, they have varied interests and good potential for providing support for mental health programs. Furthermore, they have the advantage of being locally based, so that support for local programs that are in the interest of both community and corporation can be more easily developed.

Community foundations serve a specific geographic area. In 1978 they gave an estimated $87 million in grants, and their assets were more than $1.3 billion. Presently, there are 230 such foundations in the nation, and although these foundations have not increased appreciably in number, their assets have grown. Current developments in tax law have increased interest in the role of the community foundation. As a community entity, it supports essential community services and research, and holds both special purpose and general purpose funds. As a public charity, its assets are attained through contributions of cash, securities, and properties given either directly or through bequests that offer tax advantages to the contributor.

Some CMHCs are interested in helping to create community foundations as a mechanism for philanthropic grants. It should be noted, however, that they are intended to serve a variety of local concerns rather than any specific one. Guidelines for setting up such a community foundation are contained in a two-volume publication entitled Handbook for Community Foundations. This excellent guide may be obtained by writing to the Council on Foundations, 1828 L Street, N.W., Suite 1201, Washington, D.C. 20026. The price is $40.00. Another helpful publication, Community Foundations: Their

Structure and Use in Tax Planning by Norman A. Sugarman, may be
obtained as a reprint from Prentice-Hall, Englewood Cliffs, New
Jersey.

The largest group of foundations, numbering an estimated
120,000, is family foundations. Their funds derive annually from
an individual or family, and grants are made to organizations in
which the founders have a personal interest. Because there are so
many of them located throughout the country, they are accessible to
many mental health programs and represent a prime source of potential support.

Changes brought about by the 1969 Tax Reform Act and subsequent amendments made family foundations an especially important
source of funding. For the first time in the history of philanthropy,
the 1969 Act levied an excise tax on the investment of income of all
private foundations. Combined with legal restrictions on the use and
management of the principal fund, this tax makes it fiscally prohibitive for some of the smaller family foundations to remain in operation. The only way they can liquidate without severe tax penalties
is to turn their assets over to a community or public foundation or
to a tax-exempt nonprofit or government group, classified in the Internal Revenue Code as 501(c) organizations.

It is important to remember in approaching a foundation that
its funds are generally limited, that it has the expectation of concrete evidence of community support, and that it prefers the program to be self-supporting within three years. The best means of
obtaining foundation funds is by studying the policies of the foundations, their particular program emphasis, and their required application procedures. The Seventh Edition of the Foundation Directory
(1979) is available in many libraries and lists by state almost 3,100
foundations whose assets are at least $1 million and whose annual
grants total $100,000 or more. The Directory and the National Data
Book, which lists 22,152 foundations by address, IRS number, and
other identifying information, are published by the Foundation Center, 888 Seventh Avenue, New York, New York 10019. The Center
has repositories in New York, Washington, and San Francisco that
contain IRS information returns detailing the assets and activities
of foundations located by state or region. There are also 73 regional cooperative collections that provide basic information on
foundations by state or region. The list of locations may be obtained by writing to the Foundation Center in New York.

Procedures vary among the foundations on how grant applications should be prepared. Specifications can be obtained by writing
to the foundation directly. A more detailed, regularly updated analysis of 400 to 500 foundations can be obtained from the Foundation
Center in its Foundation Center Profiles publication.

For mental health programs, foundation sources should be realistically viewed as a limited resource. Development of these grants, nevertheless, should be an integral part of a multiple source funding plan. An example of this kind of fund raising can be seen in the activity of the board and executive director of a center in the Midwest. Eight years ago, they began visiting the founder of a family foundation, describing their work and purpose to him. The first visit resulted in a $2,000 grant. As the years progressed, grants increased to $15,000 per annum. Upon the death of the founder, the family awarded a grant of $150,000 to the center for the purpose of developing a facility to house clinical services, administrative offices, and a halfway house for returnees from the state hospital. This $150,000 was utilized to secure a 30-year, $3 million loan at 5 percent interest under a special government guaranteed loan program. The mortgage on the facility will be paid vis-à-vis the grant rental allowance for the specific programs being offered. Additional income would then be forthcoming from third-party payments, grants, and other public and private resource sources. Needless to say, this was an intelligent, farsighted, and innovative approach to multiplying private resources.

DEFERRED GIFTS

Deferred giving is the third major source of philanthropic funding, representing 6.6 percent of all giving in 1978. Gifts of this kind range from simple bequests to highly technical trusts and annuities. Because annuities and trusts provide lifetime income to the donor, one leading tax attorney has described them as "the donor's giving away the tree and retaining the fruit for life." Over the years this type of support has been most aggressively pursued by universities and religious and cultural organizations; more recently, a significant number of health and welfare agencies have joined in. Legal details about deferred gifts are contained in the Philanthropy Tax Institute Manual of Deferred Giving, available by writing to Tax-wise Giving, 13 Arcadia Road, Old Greenwich, Connecticut 06870.

Before the tax reform legislation of 1969, the most prevalent form of deferred giving was the classic charitable trust. The donor gave appreciated property or securities to a tax-exempt organization, but received all the earnings for life. The principal went to the organization upon the death of the donor or of his/her designated heirs. He/she could add funds to the trust at any time and receive a charitable deduction immediately, thereby avoiding short- and long-term capital gains taxes, estate taxes, and gift taxes, while at the same time lowering the rate of taxable income.

Although this kind of trust no longer generates a charitable deduction under recent legislation that closed many loopholes in the game of tax avoidance, other forms of trusts and annuities retain most of the benefits of classic charitable trusts. These forms include charitable remainder unitrusts, annuity trusts, pooled income funds, and gift annuities. Under a charitable remainder unitrust, the donor receives a fixed percentage of the trust income as prescribed by law, regardless of the value of the principal fund. Under a charitable annuity trust the donor receives a fixed annual sum for life regardless of the trust left to the institution.

Pooled income funds allow multiple donors to contribute fixed amounts to a trust maintained by an institution; each donor receives a share of the earnings of the pooled funds. A gift annuity involves both the transfer of securities and property to the charitable organization, in return for which the donor receives a tax deduction and a specified life income. Obviously, all these deferred giving plans are geared to the well-established and older citizens in the community. As a result of their donations, they reap numerous tax benefits, and upon their death a sizable amount of money goes to their recipient organizations.

An organization that receives deferred gifts must, in effect, operate an investment program that requires the services of a professional fund development director, a business manager, and an investment policy committee. For mental health programs, the committee accrues the advantage of involving trust officers, attorneys, insurance men, prominent physicians, businessmen, and other influential community figures, along with their goodwill and personal interest in the program. While it is not feasible to employ a professional development director, it might be advantageous to use the services of investment bankers along with the committee.

Establishment of a pooled income fund is the most significant means of obtaining deferred gifts for a medium-sized mental health program or for a group of mental health programs working collaboratively. A less ambitious approach is to develop a bequest committee that actively interprets the program to potential donors and to those who help draw up wills.

Life insurance offers another significant potential for deferred giving. For example, anyone who designates a mental health program as the beneficiary of a paid-up policy can deduct the amount of the policy's replacement value, irrespective of his/her age or physical condition, up to 50 percent of adjusted gross income. For unpaid policies, the tax deduction is slightly above the cash surrender value, and all future premium payments are tax deductible. Another potential source of gifts is term insurance given as a fringe benefit to corporate executives. The law interprets all such insurance over $50,000 as income to the executive. If he/she designates a charitable organization as beneficiary for the amount over $50,000, he/she can claim a deduction for the premiums even though they are paid by his/her company.

Bequests programs sometimes result from a successful program of seeking individual gifts, such as a campaign to raise capital funds. A colleague of mine reported that after completion of a fund campaign for a CMHC, he began to receive about two calls a week from attorneys asking for the legal name of the organization so that it could be included in a will. Two years later, the first bequest, totaling $75,000, was received. He then started a formal bequest program by organizing a volunteer committee of leading citizens.

The bequest due to the death of the foundation president cited in the previous section is the more typical activity leading toward sizable gifts. However, another CMHC in the Midwest discovered that, although a bank was holding a trust the proceeds of which were to be used for the care of the mentally ill, it had never disbursed those proceeds. The bank had, in fact, turned down a number of bona fide requests. Because of the size of the trust, several mental health facilities in the area took the case to court and won. As a result, all the mental health programs serving people from that area are receiving funds from the trust. The center that initiated the suit has been able to underwrite all of its inpatient care for indigent patients.

CORPORATE GIFTS AND GRANTS

The fourth principal source of support is corporations. They give charitable contributions totaling more than $250 million annually, in addition to the $2 billion they gave in 1978 through their foundations and granting mechanisms. Under the tax law, they are able to contribute to programs that qualify as legitimate business expenses, a definition that includes programs attacking community problems. Some observers estimate that corporations give as much as $1 billion annually in this way. With more than one and a half million corporations filing tax returns listing charitable contributions, and with the proximity of these organizations to mental health facilities, they can be a major source of philanthropic support.

Since the beginning of modern philanthropy, and particularly in the last 25 years, larger corporations have emphasized the importance of management personnel's involvement in community philanthropy. These executives provide sophisticated volunteer manpower to generate donations. Financial support by a corporation frequently spells the difference between the success and failure of service programs.

An interesting approach to obtaining corporate gifts was developed by an executive and board president in a southwestern community. The president was an official of a large oil company headquartered in a medium-sized community. He proposed a plan aimed at developing corporate support on a short-term basis to solve a number of problems being experienced by the CMHC. One major problem was the loss of a psychiatrist, whose replacement required higher remuneration than might be expected in a large urban center. The executive and board president recruited for board membership three additional officials of the oil company—namely, the head of the Equal Employment Office, the Chief of the Accounting and Management Service, and the vice president of International Trade. As a team, this group discussed the center's needs and services to the community with the corporation's president. They were able to obtain a $75,000 grant over a three-year period to pay for psychiatric services. At the conclusion of this period, they demonstrated as per agreement the ability of the center through sound management to meet the cost of professional services. The success of this action led in turn to additional contracts with the corporation for services they would have purchased from the outside.

Another center in the Midwest operates a number of contracts with major manufacturing firms located in their service area. They train company supervisory personnel to deal with absenteeism of employees with emotional problems, principally alcoholism. As a result of the contractual services, the center has received over $40,000 annually from the corporate foundations.

Trends in patterns of sources of support for CMHCs, as reported in the Alcohol, Drug Abuse and Mental Health National Data Book published in December 1979, indicate that public tax sources of funding from all sources have declined from 80 percent to 65.7 percent between 1969 and 1976. It would appear that this trend will continue owing to the state of the economy and the current "tax revolt." During this same period, private funding in federally supported CMHCs remained constant at 3 to 4 percent. With the passage of Propositions 4 and 13 in California and similar referenda in other states, it would seem that financing is becoming the most critical issue for CMHCs and their boards. What is needed is the development of new financing models of multiple funding with a configuration of public, private, and third-party resources. The catalyst for these new patterns of funding can well be the philanthropic dollar. "Philanthropy . . . is most certainly not a substitute for government, but a creative supplement that provides new options or different options . . . that would not have otherwise existed" (Silber, 1973). Beginning a search for philanthropic sources requires the services of a professional director of financial development with highly specialized knowledge and skills in working with boards.

He/she has to be given appropriate authority as a member of the administrative team, which includes the administrator, the program director, and the business manager, to assist in carrying out this task.

Operations in many centers do not warrant hiring a professional funding director. However, it may be feasible for several smaller centers to hire a single director to develop their philanthropic programs collaboratively. Another possibility is for state mental health authorities to employ a financial management consultant to work as part of a group composed of members of the department's public relations and research staff. My experience indicates that a professional funding director can raise at least five to ten times the cost of his/her salary and overhead within a two-year period.

In the final analysis, private philanthropic funding can amount to as much as 10 percent of the overall budget of many CMHC programs and provide dollars more consistently than the public tax dollar. Board members must bear in mind that it is not so much the dollars as the ideas that translate into funding, which in turn supports the programs. There are many dollars that may be gained from private philanthropic sources. Of equal importance are the spin-off benefits. Philanthropy is a strong force for unifying the community and building a constituency for mental health programs because it demonstrates community support and credibility. Philanthropy also gives feedback to local and state taxing bodies. Besides relieving them of additional expenditures, it provides a public platform that, in the short run, holds the tax base and, in the long run, may increase it by developing a constituency of local support.

Many programs throughout the country have never received federal tax support and have utilized private philanthropy in innovative ways. One that comes to mind is located in a western state. Through the help of board members' contributions, favorable financing was obtained from a local bank to purchase rental property. This property produced enough income to support the center's retirement program for its employees. With the combination of federal housing dollars and private funds, another center developed services and housing for the deinstitutionalized mentally ill. We might well learn from these experiences and those of centers that have continued to operate at the termination of their federally funded period. The survival of many programs in today's economic climate may well depend on the initiatives supplied by board members, and private philanthropy can contribute significantly to the success of their efforts.

SUGGESTED READINGS

Books and Pamphlets

Dickinson, Frank G. Philanthropy and public policy. New York: National Bureau of Economic Research, 1962.

Fortune double 500 directory of the largest U.S. industrial corporations and the 50 largest commercial-banking, life-insurance, diversified-financing, retailing, transportation and utility companies. New York, 1978.

Foundation directory, The. (7th Edition). New York: Russell Sage Foundation, 1979.

Nielsen, Waldemar A. The big foundations. New York: Columbia University Press, A Twentieth Century Fund study, 1972.

Seymour, H. J. Designs for fund raising—Principles, patterns, techniques. New York: McGraw-Hill, 1966.

Silber, Stanley C. Foundation support for mental health and related services. Department of Health, Education and Welfare Publication # (NIH) 74-658. Washington, D.C.: U.S. Government Printing Office, 1974.

Silber, Stanley C. Multiple source funding and management of community mental health facilities. Department of Health, Education and Welfare Publication # (ADM) 74-66. Washington, D.C.: U.S. Government Printing Office, 1973.

Sugarman, Norman A. Community foundations: Their structure and use in tax planning. Englewood Cliffs, N.J.: Prentice-Hall, 1972.

Periodicals

Aid to Education Programs of Some Leading Business Firms. Council for Financial Aid to Education, 6 East 45th Street, New York, N.Y. 10017.

The Bulletin. American Association of Fund Raising Counsel, 500 Fifth Avenue, New York, N.Y. 10017.

College Development. Gonser and Gerber, 105 West Madison Street, Chicago, Ill. 60602.

The Foundation News. Foundation Library Center, 1001 Connecticut Avenue, N.W., Washington, D.C. 20036.

Giving, USA. Annual Yearbook on Philanthropy, American Association of Fundraising Counsel, Inc., 500 Fifth Avenue, New York, N.Y. 10036.

Philanthropic Digest. John Price Jones Company, 30 East 42nd Street, New York, N.Y. 10017.

Philanthropy Today. John Price Jones Company, 30 East 42nd Street, New York, N.Y. 10017.

Voluntary Support of Education. Council for Financial Aid to Education, 6 East 45th Street, New York, N.Y. 10017.

10

GRASS ROOTS FUND RAISING
Jane Beckett

Grass roots fund raising is an activity carried out by volunteers in order to generate money from their own communities for special charitable projects or ongoing community programs. Activities range from knocking on doors, to bake sales and bowling tournaments, to elaborate carnivals and banquets.

Mental health governing and advisory board members are volunteer activists. Should they be involved in grass roots fund raising? What types of events are most successful? Are there techniques that guarantee success? These questions form the basis of many discussions I have had with board members. The answers we have found can help any board decide when, why, and how to undertake grass roots fund raising as part of its function.

The role that advisory and governing boards of mental health agencies play in the funding process has changed greatly since the days when mental health services were considered a "plus" for the community or as a gift from the well-to-do to the poor. The overwhelming bulk of funding for both routine and experimental programs offered by mental health clinics is now derived from client fees, third-party payments, taxes, and grants. This shift reflects the fact that mental health care has moved from the periphery to the center of the public agenda. Now that it is seen as necessary and valuable to society as a whole, mental health care can make claims on the mainstream economy in the form of taxes, insurance, and corporate giving that marginal and special interest activities cannot make.

For many boards, this has meant that raising money has moved from personal contacts with individuals and appeals to the community to more indirect methods. When their power entails choosing staff directors, approving budgets, and other "hands on" responsibilities, boards can use the excellence and efficiency of the services they provide to solicit public and private monies and to increase their clientele. When, as is the case with many advisory boards of publicly funded agencies, their responsibilities are of a more informal nature, they can lobby, provide community outreach and visibility, and qualify their agencies for government or corporate funding by their mere existence. In their role as individual citizens or as representatives of constituencies, board members can also participate in the political decision making that determines governmental and foundation giving.

Most board members are aware that their major money producing role has undergone this transformation from direct to indirect. Does the transformation mean, then, that grass roots fund raising has no value for governing and advisory boards? Not at all. While Americans in general favor public support of community-based mental health services, grass roots fund raising is, nevertheless, still a unique and powerful tool both for maximizing an agency's income and for achieving other goals. Before describing such techniques, however, I want to explain why locally based projects can bring added benefits to a board and its mental health center.

1. Visibility, public relations, and outreach. Clients and their families may be the only persons in a community who know about the services you provide unless you create opportunities to tell the community at large. Grass roots fund raising events provide such opportunities. These events give boards a chance to describe the variety of center services and to interact with individuals whose donations, ticket purchases, or direct help may be needed. They may result in press coverage, thereby presenting an opportunity to show the community that your board is active and imaginative. They publicize the needs of the center to a broad array of citizens and institutions. All in all, they deepen your roots in your community.

2. Legitimation and positive feedback. One major reason why community mental health agencies have boards is to ensure that the services currently offered are needed by and acceptable to the community. By representing various groups who provide, use, or care about those services, board members are a sort of fail-safe system. They weed out irrelevant services and initiate those that are needed. For example, imagine that one of an agency's goals is to provide assistance to young persons with drug problems. If its services are aimed at older teens, but the age group presenting the most serious problem is junior high school youngsters, it may well be that board members through their personal and institutional contacts will be the first to realize the lack of fit between the services offered and those actually needed.

In this context, successful money raising serves as a visible sign to the center and to outsiders that the community wants the services the agency is providing. When a board conducts a raffle, for example, and sells 1,000 raffle tickets, those tickets can be interpreted as 1,000 messages that say "I approve of what you're doing."

3. Extra Income. A mental health agency that is both visible and legitimized through grass roots financial support is far more attractive to foundation executives, corporate donation officers, and government agencies. The various forms of matching grants earmarked specifically for those agencies that can raise money from their communities are evidence of this attractiveness. Any grant proposal stands a better chance of approval if the submitter can demonstrate board initiative and local support. A grant proposal, for instance, might request funding for a program leader and two field workers for an outreach to the home-bound program, with two additional field workers to be paid through grass-roots events. The benefit to the granting organization is threefold: a relatively modest grant will result in a relatively larger program; the overall size of the grant will be smaller than if five salaries are requested; and there is solid proof of the grantee agency's commitment to the program, as well as of the community's support for the agency.

4. Independent Income. What do you do when you want to offer a program but cannot get funding for it? If you have community-generated income, you have options that are not otherwise available to you. You may, for instance, be able to use those monies to hire the staff to deliver the services. Or you may use grass-roots-generated money to do a needs assessment or feasibility study to persuade a grantor such as the U.S. Department of Health and Human Services or the Ford Foundation to fund the service. The few hundred dollars you raise on a square dance may not be enough to set up a counseling program for abusive parents, but it will be enough to let you conduct a survey of numbers and types of reported and presumed cases of child abuse in your area, based on records of social agencies, law enforcement agencies, schools, and pediatric clinics and hospitals. The survey, in turn, may well convince a large donor to fund your counseling program.

Taking a different tack, you may initiate a campaign for a specific project. For instance, you might want to sponsor a Walk-A-Thon for a drop-in center for those newly discharged from institutions. This will get some money to deliver that service as well as help you demonstrate to a grantor that it should take over the continued funding of the program since the community has demonstrated support for the center through its participation in a Walk-A-Thon.

5.   Board Development.   Grass roots fund raising can have
several beneficial effects in terms of strengthening a board.   An
active local program can be a factor in recruiting valuable individuals for board membership.   The energy and commitment that it requires will discourage lazy but title-hungry people from seeking or
accepting board membership.   Also, the real doers in any community do not just accept any invitation to be on a board.   They want
evidence that the organization they are joining is also made up of
doers.   A good local money-generating program is one of the best
indicators there is.   Imagine that you are trying to choose between
membership on an agency board whose members appear to do little
besides listen to long staff reports and approve them, and membership on a board that conducts an active program that raises significant amounts of money, attracts even more from funding sources,
and provides outreach into its community.   Which would you choose?

It is common for boards to have difficulty exercising leadership vis-à-vis directors and staff.   Successful fund raising can dramatically increase the likelihood that a lay board's opinions and decisions will be considered.   Moreover, within the board, individual
members can also promote their own credibility with more powerful
members when they demonstrate effectiveness in generating money.

I hope that this discussion of the reasons why grass roots fund
raising should be done, even by boards whose agencies receive most
of their funds from other sources, illustrates its usefulness.   It is
a vehicle for many organizational gains, as well as a source of operating funds.

CHOOSING AND CARRYING OUT A GRASS
ROOTS FUND RAISING EVENT

In this section, I will discuss the mechanics of choosing and
carrying out a grass roots fund raising event.   After a few general
comments, I will limit myself to issues that arise directly out of
the special nature of governing and advisory boards of mental health
agencies.

The question that most board members ask is, "What types of
events are most profitable?"   By this they mean what types give the
highest return compared to the time investment and risk involved.
There is no graph or chart that can answer this question for every
group, but there are a few guidelines that generally hold true.

1.   Fund raisers that are actually methods of asking for
medium-to-large donations, or that involve sales of expensive items,
give the highest return per person-hour of work.   Ad books and art
auctions are good examples of this.

2. Fund raisers that demand a high degree of skill on the part of the workers are more profitable. A board member can raise $300 or more in an hour on the phone selling tickets to a $50 a place dinner, if he/she is aggressive, outgoing, and has the necessary contacts.

Unfortunately, not every board is in a position to jump into fund raising by planning a $20,000 ad book or a dinner/dance at the Waldorf Astoria. The challenge is to choose the event that has the lowest overhead and also calls on the skills your current members possess. The bottom line is that your board members should never be putting so much time into a low-yield event that they could contribute more by working at regular jobs and donating their wages.

A special characteristic of most mental health boards that limits their ability to conduct local events is their relatively small size. Unlike larger organizations, such as the PTA, these boards cannot send scores of people out to sell raffle tickets, collect old newspapers, or solicit contributions through program book sales. They must, therefore, either create auxiliary volunteer organizations ("Friends of the Maple Street Clinic") or they must select functions that can be accomplished with a small work force.

Another constraint is that the public is aware that the agency's operations are for the most part underwritten by outside sources. Consequently, individuals may be reluctant to make donations or purchase tickets to expensive events unless the agency has a distinct and well-presented plan for using the money to sponsor a special project. The exception to this rule is that very small donations or purchases such as raffle tickets are a matter of personal liking for the solicitor/salesperson and not of demonstrable need for the money.

On the other hand, several other characteristics of mental health agency boards are definite assets in local fund raising. Chief among these is that board members usually have close ties to other community institutions, such as churches, civic associations, schools, and fraternal orders. Through these other organizations, members will have been exposed to or even conducted local money-raising projects. Thus, they may be familiar with what types of events are popular with the community and will know what resources are available. I have met board members who through their activities with their churches, the Rotary, or the Scouts, were experienced in conducting Ice Capades benefits, rummage sales, annual dinners, gold outings, and literally dozens of other types of benefit events.

Another asset is that the potential market for any board project is everyone in the community. Although there may be many people for whom community-based mental health care is not a priority, there are also few people who actually oppose the concept.

Because of this very wide potential appeal, boards could conduct the same sort of door-to-door solicitation campaigns as do the Heart Fund and the Cancer Society (small donations received from a very high proportion of the households in the target community) if they have the kind of sophisticated public relations programs those charities possess. Even without sophisticated "PR," door-knocking by a group of well-trained, well-informed volunteers is a real possibility.

The following suggestions are a few of the other types of projects that the workforce and market characteristics suggest. First, for a board that will be conducting the project on its own without a sizable auxiliary, there are many seasonal food specialty events that are traditional in most communities: fish fry, pancake breakfast, spaghetti dinner, sugar party, clambake, or ice cream social. These are feasible particularly if local churches, youth service agencies, and the like will help sell tickets or even buy blocks of them. Auctions, house tours, lectures by visiting VIPs in the mental health field—any event where the tickets will "sell themselves" if preceded by good publicity—are good possibilities too. Raffles can be successful even for a relatively small group if a way is devised to have the bulk of the tickets sold by local merchants. And, of course, a car wash or plant sale conducted by board members and their families can raise a respectable amount of money and provide seed money and experience for larger events. A relatively small group can also sponsor a Walk-A-Thon or Bike-A-Thon, since people who are not joiners will often make a sizable commitment of time and energy on a once-a-year basis. For example, the Chicago Chapter of the National Organization for Women sponsors an annual Walk-A-Thon in which well over half of the walkers are nonmembers.

With the assistance of an auxiliary group, a board can move into events where a large number of workers is necessary: carnivals, fashion shows, catered dinners, and theater benefits. Most raffles depend on a large number of chance sellers, and the profit of almost any event rises in direct proportion to the number of people who are selling tickets. Compare, for example, the amount of money raised by a ten-girl Scout Troop on its cookie drive with the amount raised by a 30-girl troop.

Whether or not a board can succeed in recruiting volunteers depends partly on the history of the agency. If it started out as a charitable organization, the community may well have the expectation that its talents are needed for annual cleanup and maintenance work or for auxiliary services to clients such as emergency shelter, food, and clothing. If this is the case, an existing core of volunteers, be it formal or informal, can be recruited.

If, on the other hand, the agency has always been funded by third-party payments and federal monies, the recruitment of volunteers to help with grass roots fund raising will be more difficult. It will depend chiefly on the board members' ability to recruit their own acquaintances through enthusiasm and persuasion and also on the attractiveness and "fun quotient" of the planned event. To some extent volunteers can be brought into the organizational money raising function by first asking them to do something simple, familiar, and enjoyable, such as baking a cake, chaperoning a teen dance, or refereeing a sports event. In the course of this easy task, the potential volunteer can be told in more detail about the services the agency offers; he/she can learn to enjoy working with the group and can develop some attachment to the agency. The next time around, such volunteers can be asked to do something more taxing.

What other types of events might you do? Consult your local newspapers, especially the women's pages, for an overview of ideas that other organizations are using. Visit any medium-size or large library for books on fund raising for charitable organizations. And don't forget that supermarket magazines such as Women's Day and Family Circle often report on interesting ideas both in feature articles and in their regular columns and Letters to the Editor.

Finally, you will want to consider the probable dollar return per person/hour that can be expected for your group. The range is very wide. Consider that ten people could each spend ten hours on planning a rummage sale. Depending on the effectiveness of their "PR," the number of personal contacts each person has, the value of the goods donated, the weather on the day of the sale, the effectiveness of the pricing, traffic in the vicinity of the sale, and the skills of the salespeople, the sale could make between $100 and $10,000. The dollar return could, therefore, be anywhere between $1 and $100 per hour.

Once a board has chosen a fund raising project that is appropriate to its capacities and attractive to its community, how can the members maximize the profit on the event? Four considerations to keep in mind are suggested below.

1. <u>Gathering information.</u> Consult people you know who have directed similar events. Attend some events to take notes. If possible, offer to help with another organization's version of the same event before starting your own.

2. <u>Breaking down the task.</u> This means analyzing it in three ways:

    a. Money. Prepare a budget.

    b. Time. Prepare a time line describing which tasks will be accomplished in the weeks before the event, and the deadline for each task. Note how many tickets will be sold during each week if tickets are involved.

      c. Task. Assign workers to committees on arrangements, publicity, program, ticket sales, and any other necessary jobs.

    3. <u>Assigning responsibility</u>. Place a specified person in charge of each task/committee. Scheduling regular meetings for committee members to report to their chairs and for the chairs to report to an overall coordinator guards against falling behind on assignments.

    4. <u>Paying attention to morale and motivation</u>. Like many other challenging activities, fund raising is enjoyable if people feel adequately prepared for it. If you and your fellow board members/auxiliary volunteers feel uncomfortable asking for money, do some role playing. Write a script, use the buddy system, celebrate when you've sold two thirds of your ticket goal. Choose events in which you will have fun working and select a coordinator whom you all like and respect. Serve refreshments at your working meetings. Generating financial support is gratifying if people are rewarded and recognized for their effort. Make sure the board president personally thanks every person or organization that helps make your event a success.

    These ideas barely suggest the range of factors that are important in grass roots fund raising. The novice group must above all read widely, talk to others, capitalize on its own experience, and expect to improve with practice.

    I hope that this outline has demonstrated how such events can help boards meet their organizational and financial goals. In order to illustrate the kind of event that can give a board this sort of boost, I will describe a project of a mental health board with which I'm familiar.

    The project was a raffle. The members of the board designed a Bicentennial quilt on which each 12" x 12" square depicted a scene or event from the history of the community. Each board member then worked her square in patchwork and embroidery, and the quilt was pieced together. When it was completed, the board arranged to have the quilt hang for one week in the lobby of each bank and savings and loan association in the catchment area served by their center. During the week, a board member would display the quilt during heavy banking hours, lecture on it, explain the services offered by the mental health center, and sell chances to win the quilt in a drawing. During the slow hours, the banks and S&Ls agreed to allow their tellers to sell the chances, partly out of community spirit and partly because the quilt itself generated a fair amount of foot traffic for them.

At the same time, of course, board members were also sell-ing chances to all their friends, acquaintances, and other contacts. Imagine how difficult it would be to refuse to buy a chance from one of the people who had helped make the quilt! At the end of the sev-eral week display period, the winning ticket was drawn. The board had collected over $10,000, all of it profit. Thus, the board had created a fund raiser that capitalized on the talents of the members, their contacts with community institutions, the wide appeal of the services provided at their mental health center, the community's longstanding interest in its regional history, the current popularity of handcrafted items, and the celebration of the Bicentennial.

We can't hit a winning combination every time, but the poten-tial is clearly there. The thing to remember is that money-making projects are not like mathematical formulas that will produce the same results for each group that uses them. They are more like recipes for Grandma's old-fashioned stew: the exactness of the measurements, the quality of the ingredients, the skill of the cook, and the tastes of the people who eat the product all help determine the outcome.

SUGGESTED READINGS

The best source for boards who are just beginning in grass roots fund raising or who are focusing on small- to medium-sized events is Flanegan, Joan. The Grass-Roots Fund Raising Book, Chicago: Swallow Press, 1977. In fact, this is really the only book that both covers the field in a clear and up-to-date way and is also aimed at volunteers rather than professionals.

If you do contemplate using a professional, or if your chair becomes very skilled and you decide to try some big-time events, you should read a book aimed at professionals, such as Warner, Irving R. The Art of Fund Raising, New York: Harper and Row, 1975.

11

USING SERVICE, CLIENT OUTCOME, AND COST INFORMATION SYSTEMS FOR DECISION MAKING
Robert J. Rydman

INTRODUCTION

Because of rapidly rising health care costs, the price tag for mental health care has taken on greater visibility to legislators, funding agencies, third-party payers, and the public. At the same time, adequate financing and quality of community-based mental health services remains a major concern to local boards and agency administrators. As sources of funding diminish and the supply of money becomes tighter, public and private funders increasingly inquire about the most effective services at the most reasonable price. Presently, few boards or administrators are prepared to answer that question. In the near future, administrators and boards will be required to demonstrate efficient use of fiscal resources. For many agencies, this will mean becoming familiar with and installing improved financial management and program evaluation techniques.

TODAY'S PROBLEM

Although the technology exists to compare mental health programs on the basis of cost effectiveness, boards do not make routine use of it. Part of the difficulty is that board members are volunteers, and they rely on information gathered and supplied by their administrators. Agency administrators are often unfamiliar with cost effectiveness techniques and may downgrade the importance of collecting information critical to rational policy making. Consequently, many agencies are managed solely by budgets and client data generated to satisfy external funders since compliance with their informational requirements is a necessary condition for continued funding. Not only is this situation insufficient for effective management, but it compounds the difficult tasks of boards. Inadequate, irrelevant, or unretrievable information reduces each board's ability to be responsible to its constituency. Boards must have their own information system in order to fulfill an advisory or governing role.

This chapter seeks to explain features of an information system that will enable a mental health board to account for the effectiveness and cost of its services. The materials presented here are based on the work of other authors (Carter & Newman, 1976; and Sorenson & Phipps, 1975). I will, however, attempt to convey it in a way meaningful to board members.

THE BASIC COMPONENTS OF AN INFORMATION SYSTEM

It is important that boards subscribe to fundamental principles of accountability. First, a community mental health board should be an advocate for and responsive to its constituents, and second, a board is responsible for its agency's services and costs. Put another way, the identification and justification of what services public and private dollars buy at your center makes your board answerable to the community.

To exercise accountability, a primary decision-making arena for boards is programming. Programming refers to questions about what types of services work best for what kinds of clients and at what cost. Programming also refers to delivery aspects of an agency's services such as availability, awareness of consumers and other agencies, extensiveness, appropriateness, and accessibility. In order to formulate program policy, three information systems are necessary. These will be explained in the remainder of this chapter. They are:

1. a Service Information System;
2. a Client Outcome Information System; and
3. a Cost Information System.

Using these systems, a board's programming decisions will influence methods, scheduling, and utilization of treatment. It must be noted that carrying out board policy on programming is the responsibility of the agency administrator. The role of the board is to empower its administrators not only to set up the systems and gather information but to implement its program decisions. The agency administrator is the instrument of the board. For the administrator, empowerment does not necessarily mean more money to solve problems, but rather greater freedom to improve the organization.

THE SERVICE INFORMATION SYSTEM

A service information system is a monitoring procedure that examines selected service elements and provides an overview of the mental health organization's responsiveness to the community. Elements of such a system include services utilization and certain performance measures such as appropriateness, accessibility, availability, acceptability, extensiveness, and community awareness. More specifically, utilization data enable a board to determine which segments of the community are using services. Continuous monitoring of client problems and their levels of severity reveal the most common types of problems seen at the agency and the direction of clients' mental health status while in treatment. Appropriateness measures such as length in treatment and planned versus actual client progress establish and maintain standards for service usage and continuity of care. Extensiveness measures detailing the amount and type of services offered by all community agencies indicate whether service gaps or duplications exist. These extensiveness measures suggest the point at which referral networks or cooperative programs with outside agencies should be developed. Acceptability measures such as consumer satisfaction with various aspects of agency services provide additional insight about present and future client willingness to support existing agency efforts. All the utilization and performance measures mentioned here have expanded utility for planning and programming decisions and will be discussed in greater detail in the four subsections to follow.

How to Determine Who Is Being Served

Certain population characteristics (demographics) such as age, sex, race, ethnicity, economic status, and family organization, are associated with various types of mental health problems (Beech, Fiester, & Silverman, 1976). Community demographics can provide useful information for planning mental health services and can be obtained from U.S. Census data. Comparing community demographics with the same set of demographics for center clients can provide the board with an assessment of the extent to which various segments of the community are served. Underserved and unserved populations targeted by this comparison may indicate a lack of community awareness, inaccessibility, or inappropriate services. If even more detailed client information, such as geographic location, previous hospitalization, and initial observed level of social functioning, is obtained from the agency's case records, it can also be of great value to the board in planning, evaluating, and assessing the need for specialized services and identifying targets for public relations campaigns.

How to Determine Clients' Problems and Progress

Boards should be able to understand consumer problems in the context of both the individual and the community. Mental health agencies have a variety of ways to express severity of consumer problems on scales of observable levels of social functioning. These scales vary in their descriptiveness from vague (5-point scale) to specific (9-point scale). Regardless of increments of scale, client status is usually assessed along five dimensions: physical health, personal self-care, education/vocation performance, emotional/stress tolerance, and social interaction (see Carter & Newman, 1976). Figure 11.1 illustrates how a five-point scale from 1 (extreme dysfunction) to 5 ("normal" functioning) is used to organize services around individual client needs.

Upon a client's admission to the agency, service providers assign a level from dysfunctional to functional that most accurately describes the client's personal and social status. This assessment, or "demand," allows providers to develop a treatment plan. Ratings are periodically completed for all subsequent contacts throughout the client's treatment career. Thus, changes in level of functioning permit a measurable record of client status in terms of progress, maintenance, or regression from beginning through the termination of treatment. Scores become an integral part of the service information system by "quantifying" and "operationalizing" demand (need) for and outcome (results) of social services. (For further information on outcome measurement, see Hargreaves and Attkisson, 1978).

How to Determine Service Appropriateness
and Continuity

A service information system should reveal whether clients are receiving appropriate and continuous treatment. Appropriate treatment occurs when clients receive the correct amount and type of service for their particular problem. Indicators (such as average

FIGURE 11.1

Community Services Provided for Varying Levels of Client Functioning

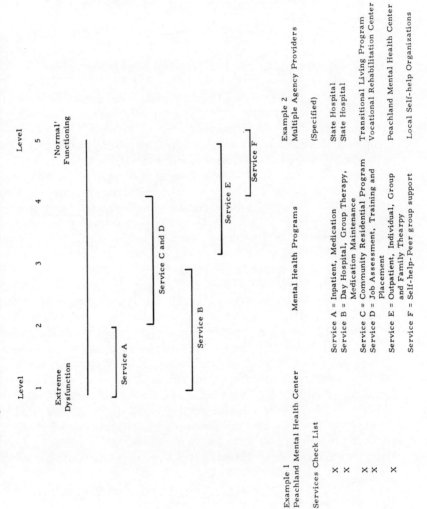

Level   Level

1   2   3   4   5

Extreme   'Normal'
Dysfunction   Functioning

Service A

Service B

Service C and D

Service E

Service F

	Example 1	Example 2
	Peachland Mental Health Center	Multiple Agency Providers
	Services Check List	(Specified)
Service A = Inpatient, Medication	X	State Hospital
Service B = Day Hospital, Group Therapy, Medication Maintenance	X	State Hospital
Service C = Community Residential Program	X	Transitional Living Program
Service D = Job Assessment, Training and Placement	X	Vocational Rehabilitation Center
Service E = Outpatient, Individual, Group and Family Thearpy	X	Peachland Mental Health Center
Service F = Self-help- Peer group support		Local Self-help Organizations

Mental Health Programs

length in treatment, planned time versus actual time spent in treatment, and planned progress versus actual progress for their problem) provide a measure of appropriateness and a check on the fit between diagnosis and treatment. Continuous treatment means that the agency responds to multiple and changing needs of consumers, thereby preventing consumers from getting lost in the system.

A board should be able to display its agency's services in terms of consumer problems on an ordered social functioning scale. In Figure 11.1, Example 1, we see that Peachland Mental Health Center provides comprehensive and continuous services for all levels of social functioning. This figure also reveals that clients at certain levels of functioning may receive multiple services or "service mixes." Individual client records should contain a ledger on all services received. As we will see in the later section on the cost information system, individual client ledgers are necessary in determining the amount of effort (services) and cost (expenses) that contribute toward improving clients' mental health (level of functioning).

How to Map Referral Networks and Develop
Interagency Programs

When a single agency cannot provide services for all its potential consumers within the community, referrals are made. Boards should be familiar with their own services and those of nearby agencies. Extensiveness measures indicate how many types of problems and populations an agency's services are designed to treat. A listing of types of services offered by community agencies not only can prevent service gaps or duplication, but can also aid in planning and coordination among sister agencies.

Let us look at the services provided by Peachland Mental Health Center in Figure 11.1, Example 1. In many communities these services are provided by different agencies at various locations (Figure 11.1, Example 2). For illustrative purposes, let us say you are on the board of Peachland Mental Health Center. Imagine Peachland Mental Health Center as only the outpatient clinic that provides three basic services: individual, group, and family therapy (Service E). These are designed for all populations at levels 3, 4, and 5. A state hospital nearby provides inpatient and day hospital services (Services A and B) for all populations at Levels 1, 2, and 3. Community apartment residences and supportive therapy (Services C) for Levels 2, 3, and 4 are provided by a transitional living program. A vocational rehabilitation center provides job skills training (Service D) for Levels 2, 3, and 4. Local self-help organizations provide peer group support (Service F) for Levels 4 and 5.

With this information, an array of social services within a
community can be displayed on a matrix check list to determine:
(1) where your agency fits in the scheme of available services within
the geographic area; (2) which services are accessible in terms of
location, costs, and severity of problem; (3) where agencies are
currently referring consumers; (4) to what other groups or organizations your agency could be referring consumers; and (5) how your
agency could better use outside support services. Additionally,
boards should be familiar with existing formal interagency agreements for purchase of care contracts, program evaluation, and
provider-referral responsibility. It would also be helpful to know
the cost and effectiveness of outside services and interagency programs since referral networks and interagency programs influence
the cost and effectiveness of programs delivered by your agency.

A service information system is a constant search and monitoring process. A mental health agency is rarely an isolated service: a single agency must allow for interdependent relations with
others. Profound changes can occur in overall community mental
health care as your agency or nearby agencies add, modify, or drop
programs.

THE CLIENT OUTCOME INFORMATION SYSTEM

Outcome measurement provides another set of data regarding
strengths and weaknesses in a system of mental health service delivery. Outcomes are essentially a primary product output indicator.
In industry, product output refers to the quantity of tangible goods
produced within a given time. With mental health services, such
output is less easily measured. Customarily, desired product output refers to amount of client progress or outcome of service consumption over time. This is expressed here in nonmonetary terms
using the social functioning skill mentioned earlier. In this section,
we will discuss simple client outcome measurement, namely, how
individual clients respond to certain services. Program outcomes,
which are aggregate client outcomes for numerous individuals participating in a particular treatment approach, will also be discussed.
Both sets of measurements collected routinely are a useful part of
an integrated management information system.

What Client Outcomes Tell You

Service programs should have treatment plans with time-
sequenced goals and objectives that directly relate to improvement

in a client's level of functioning. These treatment plans should be reviewed weekly, monthly, or quarterly to determine and record the amount of planned services actually provided and the direction and degree of client progress. This information should be immediately retrievable not only for clinical management purposes but for overall program evaluation.

By continually tracking an individual client's level of functioning while in treatment, we can construct a picture of change for groups of clients within any service program for any given period of time. This picture is actually a matrix of <u>client outcomes</u> over specified time periods.

Each matrix in Figure 11.2 illustrates how individual client outcomes can be displayed for one given treatment program. This figure represents 30 client outcomes for two demographically similar groups of clients receiving 90 days of treatment in different service programs. Assessments based on a five-point scale (1 = extreme dysfunctioning, 5 = normal functioning) are made for all clients at the beginning and end of the time period to be measured. An initial assessment rating of 2 would place the client in the 2, 2 diagonal cell; a 90-day outcome rating of 4 would move the client into the 2, 4 cell, an improvement of two levels. Client status over time is determined by following the cell location directly to the left margin for initial rating or assessment. Assessment ratings reveal the existing condition at the start of the time period. By following the cell location directly to the upper margin we obtain an evaluative rating. Evaluative ratings reflect client status resulting from a course of treatment. The difference between the two ratings represents outcome over time. To illustrate program outcomes over time, the matrices can display inside each cell multiple numbers of client outcomes and overall costs of services. (Determination of cost is discussed in a subsequent section entitled "The Cost Information System.") The cells above the diagonal represent improvement. The cells on the diagonal represent no change or maintained status, and the cells below the diagonal represent regression while in treatment.

Client outcome tabulations for each service program are detailed below each matrix. The client group for matrix 1 program has a net level improvement of 14 levels. Net levels are calculated by multiplying the number of clients within each cell by the increment of improvement (+) or regression (-), using zero increment for clients in no-change categories, and totaling all positive and negative outputs. For the client group in matrix 2, we see a net improvement of nine levels. These net levels of change represent a measure of <u>program outcome</u> and in this case show Services C and D represented by matrix 1 to be superior to Service E in matrix 2.

FIGURE 11.2

Comparison of Client Outcomes in Two Mental Health Programs

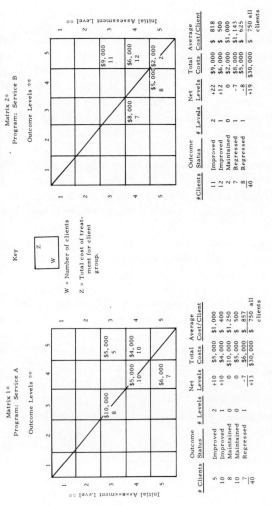

Key

W = Number of clients.
Z = Total cost of treatment for client group.

Matrix 1*
Program: Service A

# Clients	Outcome Status	# Levels	Net Levels	Total Costs	Average Cost/Client
5	Improved	2	+10	$5,000	$1,000
10	Improved	1	+10	$4,000	$400
8	Maintained	0	0	$10,000	$1,250
10	Maintained	0	0	$5,000	$500
7	Regressed	1	-7	$6,000	$857
40			+13	$30,000	$750 all clients

COST PER NET LEVEL OF IMPROVEMENT $30,000/13 = $2,307.69

Matrix 2*
Program: Service B

#Clients	Outcome Status	# Levels	Net Levels	Total Costs	Average Cost/Client
11	Improved	2	+22	$9,000	$818
12	Improved	1	+12	$6,000	$500
2	Maintained	0	0	$2,000	$1,000
7	Regressed	1	-7	$8,000	$1,143
8	Regressed	1	-8	$5,000	$625
40			+19	$30,000	$750 all clients

COST PER NET LEVEL OF IMPROVEMENT $30,000/19 = $1,578.95

* N = 40 Adult clients, age 18-45. Time period = 60 days
** Based on 5 point scale when 1 = Extreme dysfunctioning, 5 = Normal functioning.

Source: Adapted from D. E. Carter and F. L. Newman, A client oriented system of mental health service delivery and program management: A workbook and guide. Department of Health, Education and Welfare Publication # (ADM) 76-307. Washington, D.C.: U.S. Government Printing Office, 1976.

A number of factors can be compared and measured using the program outcome criterion. Because Figure 11.2 illustrates a comparison of two discrete service technologies on demographically similar populations, its information is useful in determining the relative effectiveness of one treatment approach compared to another. Thus it is possible to compare alternate treatment approaches within one agency or between two or more agencies. Outcome comparisons can also be made to determine if similar service programs have equal impact on dissimilar client populations, for example, prior hospitalization versus no prior hospitalization, adults versus adolescents, or Blacks versus Hispanics versus Whites. Poor outcome totals for certain client populations indicate the need for more specialized or different treatment approaches, and funds could be better directed to them.

Additional outcome comparisons can be made to determine manpower strengths and weaknesses by using similar client groups and treatment technologies and then comparing different service providers such as psychiatrists, psychologists, social workers, and paraprofessional mental health workers. These data may be used for decisions on personnel competencies and could influence hiring practices, staff assignments, supervision time, training, and expenditures for each of the employees (Wynne, 1979).

Limitations of Client Outcome Information

A board must weigh the significance of using net levels of improvement as an indication of program success or failure when formulating policy. One consideration is that while social functioning scales demonstrate ordered change in client mental health status, they do not indicate distances between levels. For example, it may require greater time and effort for clients to move from Levels 2 and 3 than from Levels 4 and 5. It may also require huge efforts just to maintain a client at a given level using a particular service technology. This raises questions about comparing program outcomes on client groups that have unequal numbers of individuals at initial assessment levels. By aggregating groups of clients with equal or closely equal numbers at initial assessment levels, the problem of achieving a meaningful program comparison in this regard can be reduced. Boards can set acceptable limits for expenditures of time and effort on clients with certain initial assessment ratings by observing outcomes for a variety of treatment programs through time. To determine the best program design, outcome comparisons can be made between similar client groups experiencing different treatment methods, and vice versa. Track records for individual staff providing similar services for similar client groups can also be compared to evaluate staff competency. To set valid limits on program outcomes, boards may wish to match their internal program comparisons with similar programs provided by outside agencies.

Another consideration is that any service "producing" a given outcome cannot be viewed as having a causal impact on client functioning. One can only assume that mental health services contribute to the direction of a given client's mental health status. Even this statement can be accepted only when one observes improved mental health status on the part of one population in treatment and little or no improvement by a similar population without that treatment. For many mental health centers this comparison is not practical. Monitoring the mental health status of clients in treatment gives the best available information for evaluating program effectiveness, but findings must not be interpreted as proof that the program actually caused client change.

Validity checks should be performed on the ratings each provider gives to his/her clients. A validity check is accomplished by selecting individual cases to be rated by independent providers or by having agency staff rate each other's ongoing cases anonymously. The provider's rating is considered reliable if two or more raters agree with it. A rating is also considered valid if multiple raters share a consensus on whether the provider ratings match external behavioral criteria from other rating procedures (see Carter & Newman, 1976).

Finally, indicators of program effectiveness via outcome measurement are important but insufficient data for allocating resources among various services. Boards cannot dismiss the element of the cost of "effective" services. Figure 11.2 shows that Services C and D had greater impact on clients than Service E. Providing Services C and D would seem to be the obvious programming choice; however, we do not know the difference in cost. This unknown factor is so important that it can negate a choice between programs. Just as client outcome (output) data are necessary for setting acceptable performance standards, program cost data are needed to measure resource consumption (input). Although client outcomes are necessary for program evaluation purposes and can be studied independently of cost analysis, it is only when the two are combined in a cost outcome evaluation between two or more programs that cost effectiveness can be determined.

THE COST INFORMATION SYSTEM

Obtaining cost information is not only a necessary step in policy formulation, but it is a basic management tool. Cost finding is an accounting procedure yielding the cost of a unit, usually an hour, of mental health care; it is the dollar value of this unit that determines fees for services. The amount of fees an agency collects reveals which programs are self-supporting and which require a subsidy. Unit costs are also used for negotiating third-party payments, purchase of care contracts, and grants to support direct service programs.

Board members need not concern themselves with the machinery of cost finding, such as models of expense allocations producing unit costs (see Sorenson & Phipps, 1975), since detailed cost finding is a subject for bookkeepers and accountants. However, because of its impact on resource allocation decisions, the cost of professional activities contributing to unit-of-care costs should be known.

Computing Unit Costs

The mental health industry is labor intensive. Generally speaking, 80 to 85 percent of operating expenses are for professional salaries. Professional time spent in a therapy hour is the foundation of unit-of-care cost. Professionals are paid at different rates, so unit-of-care costs depend on who is providing direct services. Unlike most industries, differentiated remunerations for line staff in mental health organizations are related more to discipline and formal training background than to job function, performance, or degree of specialization. It is not unusual for the management-trained executive administrator to be paid less than the staff psychiatrist.

Highest to lowest paid direct service workers usually are psychiatrists, psychologists, social workers (or master's degree equivalents), baccalaureate mental health workers, and nondegree paraprofessionals. Their hourly direct service rates can be calculated by obtaining a weekly rate (annual salary divided by weeks worked) and dividing it by hours of direct service worked per week.

Other "organizational" costs are built into direct service unit costs. For example, not all professional time is spent in direct services. Professionals spend varying amounts of time on administration and supervision. Nondirect staff activities are treated either as overhead or add-on costs because they directly serve the organization rather than the client.

Add-on Costs

Tracking the amount and content of professional time is necessary for calculating unit costs. Supervisory add-on costs are determined by assessing professional time in supervision—the number of hours multiplied by the supervisor's hourly rate—to obtain a lump sum figure. For purposes of illustration, let us assume that the supervisory cost figure is $3,800. The direct service hours of supervisees, say 1,040 hours, is divided into supervisory costs, $3,800, to obtain the add-on cost to supervisee hourly rates: $3,800 divided by 1,040 hours = $3.65/hour. Supervisors' hourly rates are not subject to these add-on costs. This procedure is called a "step-down cost allocation," and it is used in order to arrive at adjusted rates for supervisees' consumption of staff time. It may also be applied in trainer-trainee and consultant-consultee relationships.

Boards can monitor supervisory, training, and part-time consultation costs since excess activity may seriously inflate unit-of-care costs. For example, line staff in mental health organizations may hold lengthy supervisory meetings to discuss diagnostics, treatment plans, budgets, or evaluations. Some alternative management actions that may reduce nondirect costs include reassigning staff, hiring more highly trained personnel, or investing in continuing education programs, any of which could ultimately lead to less consumption of staff time in nondirect activities.

Overhead Costs

Personnel time costs for nondirect organizational activity, such as administration, community consultation, prevention programs, and communications, may be determined for each staff and totaled to obtain a lump sum overhead figure. Let us assume this cost is $8,695.00. There are additional categories of overhead cost that usually include salaries of support service personnel (say $13,560) and rent, maintenance, utilities, communications, travel, supplies, and equipment (say $20,000). Expenditures in all these categories are treated as overhead that influences the magnitude of unit costs. The items mentioned here total $42,255. A direct allocation of these expenses is made by dividing the total direct-service staff hours, say 1,580, by 42,255. This procedure allows us to obtain total hourly organizational overhead costs, which in this example are $26.74/hour. This figure is added to all adjusted and nonadjusted personnel hourly rates or unit costs.

Using Cost Outcome Information

As mentioned earlier, individual client records should contain a ledger of all services rendered. A ledger, such as that shown in Figure 11.3, identifies time-sequenced client status, service type,

FIGURE 11.3

Client Ledger

Name _____

Address _____

ID # _____

Telephone _____

Date	Level of function	Service program	Provider	Units Rec'd	Unit cost	Total cost	Balance 1* amount able to charge client	Balance 2 Amount payable by 3rd party reimbursement or subsidy
6/10/80	3	E	1(MD)	2	49.82	99.64	40.00	59.64
6/15/80	3	E	2(Ph.D.)	2	45.99	91.98	40.00	51.98
7/01/80	4	E	1(MD)	1	49.82	49.82	20.00	29.82
7/15/80	5	E	3(MSW)	3	40.03	120.09	60.00	60.09
Total cost for 6 week, 4 visit episode of care						361.53	160.00	201.53

*Balance 1 based on ability to pay $20.00/hour.

Source: Adapted from D. E. Carter and F. L. Newman, A client oriented system of mental health service delivery and program management: A workbook and guide. Department of Health, Education and Welfare Publication # (ADM) 76-307. Washington, D.C.: U.S. Government Printing Office, 1976.

number of units consumed, the service provider, unit cost, total cost, and charges to specified sources. With this information we can follow client outcome and cost through time.

Through the select aggregation of client ledgers, measures of cost and outcome can be obtained for groups of clients in various service programs. Figure 11.4 illustrates costs and outcomes for two programs. Each cell contains the number of clients with a particular pre/post assessment of level of functioning and the total cost of their 60-day treatment. Below each matrix are the data derived from using this approach.

Given that both these programs serve similar clients in terms of previous hospitalizations or demographics, Program B proves to be more cost effective. Although total program dollars expended and average costs per client served are the same, Program B demonstrates greater output in terms of net levels of improvement. Program B is not only more effective but is also less costly in producing these net levels of improvement. Overall cost efficiency values are computed by dividing net levels of improvement by the total cost of the program. Using these cost/outcome comparison criteria, Program B would be the superior choice in deciding resource allocations.

DECISION RULES IN SELECTING PROGRAMS FOR RESOURCE ALLOCATION

The logic of cost-effective decision making among service programs is based on maximizing client progress per fixed cost and minimizing cost per net level of improvement.

Boards must make judgments in cases of extremes. Additional information is needed when considering a program that is most effective and most costly. Selection in this case may be prohibitive due to lack of available funds. If adequate financing of one program requires service cutbacks in another, adverse repercussions from citizens or agency staff may be too much to risk. Where a program is least effective and least costly, boards must consider standards of impact and quality. A program may be inexpensive but of unjustifiable productivity.

SUMMARY

Cost effectiveness is basic to a system of accountability for local mental health care. The essence of a cost-effectiveness investigation is a simple value comparison among various service

FIGURE 11.4

Comparison of Client Outcomes and Cost in Two Mental Health Programs

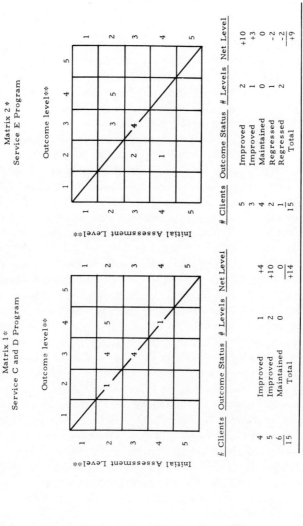

Matrix 1*
Service C and D Program

Matrix 2*
Service E Program

# Clients	Outcome Status	# Levels	Net Level
4	Improved	1	+4
5	Improved	2	+10
6	Maintained	0	0
15	Total		+14

# Clients	Outcome Status	# Levels	Net Level
5	Improved	2	+10
3	Improved	1	+3
4	Maintained	0	0
2	Regressed	1	-2
1	Regressed	2	-2
15	Total		+9

* N = 15 Adult clients ages 18-24, Time period = 90 days

** Based on 5 point scale where 1 = Extreme dysfunctioning, 5 = Normal functioning.

*N = 40 adult clients, age 18-45, time period = 60 days.

**Based on 5-point scale when 1 = extreme dysfunctioning, 5 = normal functioning.

technologies. In order to design or assess cost-effective services for resource allocation purposes, boards must have ongoing comprehensive internal management information systems. These systems should permit a marriage of accurate cost information to measures of program outcome.

Cost information in the form of unit cost of mental health care is obtained through cost finding. This procedure identifies and allocates expenses of professional time according to content and amount of activity as well as other nonpersonnel resources consumed by the organization. Unit costs of mental health care establish monetary organizational input.

Program outcome measures that are aggregated client outcomes on individuals participating in certain treatment technologies represent nonmonetary organizational output. In order to obtain the simple outcome measures discussed here, individual clients must be assessed and periodically reassessed according to a scale of social functioning throughout their treatment.

The process of relating monetary inputs to nonmonetary output measures on specific treatment programs is called cost outcome analysis. Comparing two or more sets of cost outcome data provides a measure of cost effectiveness or, put another way, demonstrates which program has the best balance of inputs versus outputs.

Additionally, boards must consider the extent to which global issues affect the quality and cost of internal program operations. A usable service information system can help to evaluate the fit between the agency's services and community needs. Such a system should include utilization data and selected performance measures illustrating how well services are being delivered by the mental health organization. This system should have the capacity to determine (1) who is being served, (2) client problems and progress in treatment, (3) appropriateness of treatment and continuity of care, (4) consumer satisfaction, and (5) gaps or duplication in services reflecting adequacy of referral networks and justification for interagency programs.

Whether boards are managing or advising a mental health system in times of financial boom or bust, cost-effective service is a desirable goal because it is simply good business practice. Cost-effectiveness data indicating efficient use of resources offer valuable support for those who negotiate with outside funders. Such data can also help the agency move toward more independent community action rather than remain in a defensive posture toward federal and state government mandates.

The guiding principles for mental health care at the local level are effectiveness, efficiency, and sensitivity to community need. Federal and state policy makers have responded to criticism of inefficiency and insensitivity by making mental health a local game. This chapter has attempted to provide information necessary to begin moving toward self-sufficiency.

REFERENCES

Beech, R. P., Fiester, A. R., & Silverman, W. H. The utilization of demographic data for mental health planning. Administration in Mental Health, 1976, 3, 166-173.

Carter, D. E., & Newman, F. L. A client oriented system of mental health service delivery and program management: A workbook and guide. Department of Health, Education and Welfare Publication # (ADM) 76-307. Washington, D.C.: U.S. Government Printing Office, 1976.

Hargreaves, W. A., & Attkisson, C. C. Evaluating program outcomes. In C. C. Attkisson, W. A. Hargreaves, M. J. Horowitz, & J. E. Sorensen (Eds.), Evaluation of Human Service Programs. New York: Academic Press, 1978, 303-337.

Karon, B. P., & Vandenbos, G. R. Cost/benefit analysis: psychologist versus psychiatrist for schizophrenics. Professional Psychology, 1976, 7, 107-111.

Luft, L. L., & Fakhouri, J. A model for a comparative cost effectiveness evaluation of two mental health partial care programs. Evaluation and Program Planning, 1979, 2, 33-40.

May, P. R. A. Cost efficiency of mental health care III: Treatment method as a parameter of cost in the treatment of schizophrenia. American Journal of Public Health, 1971, 61, 127-129.

Rocheleau, B. A. Without tears or bombast: A guide to program evaluation. De Kalb, Ill.: Northern Illinois University, 1975, 61-73.

Sorensen, J. E., & Grove, H. D. Cost outcome and cost effectiveness analysis: Emerging non profit performance evaluation techniques. The Accounting Review, 1977, 1.11 (3), 658-675.

Sorensen, J. E., & Phipps, D. W. Cost finding and rate setting for community mental health centers. Department of Health, Education and Welfare Publication # (ADM) 76-291, (Rev.). Washington, D.C.: U.S. Government Printing Office, 1975.

Wynne, Louis. Cost efficiency and staffing in mental health services. Administration in Mental Health, 1979, 7 (1), 58-68.

III

MENTAL HEALTH
SERVICES

One of the major contributions of the community approach to mental health care is the notion that solutions to psychological problems are inextricably tied to a comprehensive system of services. Probing the etiology of mental disorders means looking at ecological relationships as well as personal dynamics. Interventions are not only supplied by mental health professionals but also by natural support systems and human service agencies. No longer is it necessary to rely solely on individual psychotherapy when specific techniques and programs can be applied to particular problems.

Part III presents a cross section of the most common techniques and programs in a modern service delivery system. Since space limitations do not permit an exhaustive review, only the most important interventions are described.

Primary prevention rather than treatment or rehabilitation is the most rational approach to mental health problems. We cannot train the number of practitioners required to meet burgeoning treatment needs, nor can the public continue to pay the increasing costs associated with secondary and tertiary interventions. Zolik acquaints us with the successes of primary prevention in public health and explains how the knowledge gained in these efforts can be applied to mental health. He classifies programs and approaches to prevention under two main categories, person-oriented and social-systems-oriented, and describes many specific programs and research studies. Several major barriers to program development are cited, and Zolik offers some solutions for facilitating primary prevention efforts.

Whenever possible the natural environment is the most desirable locus for mental health intervention. It is the least disruptive place from the client's perspective, and it avoids stigmatization. Furthermore, the use of the natural setting for intervention supports the view that it is the community that should assume primary responsibility for the welfare of its citizens. Gartner and Riessman have studied one form of natural intervention, self-help mutual aid activities. They point out that for each of the special populations discussed in Part IV, one or more self-help mutual aid groups exist. These groups provide two unique features—social support and coping skills. They work on the helper-therapy concept, that is, those who help are helped most. CMHCs can be useful to the self-help movement by cultivating groups in their communities, referring clients to them, offering consultation, strengthening existing support networks and initiating new ones, and conducting research to augment self-help group effectiveness.

Many CMHC staff members would concur that the most demanding duty they perform is in the emergency unit. Because of the high level of energy expended and the physical and psychological dangers inherent in the activity, an emergency unit requires the most skillful clinicians. As Rines points out, the vast majority of clients are not in life threatening situations but are chronic, multiproblem individuals. Staff also must cope with such profound problems as substance abuse, suicidal behavior, rape, and other types of physical assault. More than any other CMHC component, effective linkages with law enforcement and other human service agencies are vital to emergency services. Workers must be given special consideration in supervision, work load, and inservice training. As a consequence of its unique demands, emergency care is relatively expensive and is usually run at a loss to the center. Administrators and board members should keep these facts in mind during their financial planning.

As we have become more knowledgeable in the field of psychopathology, we have learned that a multiplicity of factors can cause aberrant behavior. Val emphasizes the importance of a pluralistic approach toward interventions. Furthermore, the number and complexity of service and evaluation requirements needed to achieve comprehensiveness is beyond the capacity of a single practitioner. A team of mental health professionals with a variety of training and experience such as that found in CMHCs is ideal. However, even a CMHC is incapable of comprehensiveness without the aid of special-care facilities. Val presents a three-level model of care that encompasses both CMHC and specialized mental health programs. He then presents an overview of the currently available types of treatments classified by biological and psychotherapeutic interventions.

Levin stresses the key role of ideology in substance abuse programs. Because he regards these programs as the responsibility of the community rather than of professionals and government administrators, the chapter is written for boards. Levin challenges traditional approaches toward substance abuse and calls for the reexamination of widely accepted beliefs on its cause and treatment. The best approach is to maximize the number of community people who control policy formulation and planning vis-à-vis substance abuse intervention. Financial independence from bureaucratic entanglements is an important step in accomplishing this end.

The most underutilized treatment program at most CMHCs is partial hospitalization. Takei-Mejia, Ghertner, and Beigel describe why this is so and give suggestions for the use of such programs for chronic and acute clients. Partial hospitalization is useful in avoiding 24-hour hospitalization of acutely disturbed clients, reeducating and rehabilitating them, and orienting them into a new community setting.

Tertiary intervention or aftercare services to severely emotionally disabled adults have usually taken the form of drug clinics or individual sessions of supportive psychotherapy. Rubin describes alternative interventions under the rubric of a Community Support Program (CSP). This program is the responsibility of a core service agency that either directly supplies or contracts for CSP services. He presents the basic philosophy and services of a CSP and its accompanying administrative structure.

Because comprehensiveness requires CMHCs to operate interdependently with other human service agencies, coordination is essential. Agranoff and Mahler introduce new intervention approaches and attitudes toward mental health that have resulted in closer ties among agencies. They describe factors influencing linkages among agencies: resource dependency, power distribution, awareness of need, and legal mandates. They also outline board strategies for building workable interagency agreements.

12

PRIMARY PREVENTION
Edwin S. Zolik

Although interest in the prevention of mental disorders has achieved greater prominence in the last two decades, concern with prevention is not recent. Harry Stack Sullivan in 1931 wrote: "Either you believe that mental disorders are acts of God, predestined, inexorably fixed, arising from a constitutional or some other irremediable substratum . . . or you believe that mental disorder is largely preventable and somewhat remediable by control of psychosociological factors." The accelerating interest in the last half-decade has resulted in primary prevention being designated as "an idea whose time has come" (Klein & Goldston, 1977; U.S. Department of Health, Education and Welfare, 1979).

DEFINITIONS

Primary prevention in public health theory and practice is one component of a tripartite approach to control of disease, the other two components being secondary and tertiary prevention. Although the boundaries between these three areas often are not clearly delineated, there are important differences among them. Primary prevention embraces the activities concerned with the reduction of the rate at which new cases of a disorder or disease develop in a specific population. The objects of such activities are groups of persons who have not been identified as having mental problems or groups that because of various factors in their backgrounds can be considered as being at risk of developing problems. Consequently, the goal of primary prevention is to maintain and increase healthy functioning and to reduce the degree of risk of a disorder.

The focus of primary prevention is on a population of people rather than specific persons. Although some people in the population toward which a primary prevention program is directed may develop the disorder, the total number of new cases will be lowered. In public health terminology, the reduction in the number of new cases is designated as reducing the incidence of a disorder—that is, the rate at which a disorder becomes manifest in a population during a specified period of time, typically a year. The population can be a county, a community, a specified geographic area, or a high-risk group.

Secondary prevention is concerned with early detection and prompt treatment, thereby preventing disorders from becoming more serious. Successful secondary prevention lowers the prevalence of a disorder (the number of cases existing during a specified period of time) in the community.

Tertiary prevention is concerned with reducing the severity of the residual disability that results in many disorders. The residual disability is frequently permanent and is manifested in a lowered level of psychological, social, and occupational functioning. Rehabilitation is the main approach in tertiary prevention. Tertiary approaches, such as vocation or social retraining, can be initiated either during or following treatment. The goal is to minimize the effects of the disability.

Due to conceptual difficulties, primary prevention has been defined in different terminology and with different degrees of generality. These factors coupled with the lack of clarity in distinguishing between primary and secondary prevention led Wagenfeld (1972) to propose limiting the designation of prevention to primary prevention, and returning to designating secondary prevention as treatment, and tertiary prevention as rehabilitation.

On the basis of these definitions it should be readily apparent that the clinical programs in community mental health centers (CMHCs) and in other mental health facilities are concerned with secondary and tertiary prevention. In CMHCs, primary prevention typically is one of the activities carried out by the consultation and education program.

EPIDEMIOLOGY

The study of health and disease in human populations involves many scientific disciplines—among them, biochemistry, pathology, physiology, microbiology, the various clinical medical sciences, statistics, demography, sociology, psychology, and anthropology. Drawing on these fields and others, the discipline of epidemiology has evolved as a systematic approach to the study of disease in groups of persons or populations. It is the basic science on which preventative programs are based.

Epidemiology has been defined as the study of the distribution and determinants of disease prevalence in man (MacMahon, Pugh, & Ipsen, 1960). The study of the distribution of disease or health status is the concern of descriptive epidemiology, which focuses on demographic data such as age, sex, race, and various geographic characteristics. These studies help discover the rates or the extent to which a disorder is present in different population groups. Such information is useful in uncovering factors associated with a disorder. For example, Goldberger (1914) on the basis of the absence of pellagra in attendants in mental hospitals was able to strengthen the hypothesis that pellagra was due to a nutritional deficiency and to reject the commonly accepted position that pellagra was an infectious disease.

In prevention, knowledge of the distribution of a disorder must be coupled with knowledge of the determinants of a disorder. The investigation of the determinants involved in a previously established distribution pattern is referred to as analytic epidemiology. This search for possible causal factors or patterns and the subsequent evaluation of their association with a disorder, singly or in combination with other factors, can provide the knowledge base for altering linkages in the pattern of causation. As Snow (1855) demonstrated, a disorder can be prevented and even terminated before the etiology of the disorder is completely understood.

Experimental epidemiology is concerned with testing hypotheses developed from analytic studies in controlled experiments to ascertain whether modification of the hypothesized causal factors decreases the incidence of the disease. Controlled field studies on the incidence of coronary heart disease in a population that has stopped smoking, decreased its cholesterol intake, and adopted a regular program of exercise—as compared to a population that has maintained a minimal exercise program and a high level of smoking and cholesterol intake—is an example of experimental epidemiological research.

The constitution of the World Health Organization (1948) defines health as "a state of complete physical, mental and social well-being and not merely the absence of disease or infirmity." This is a comprehensive general definition. Health can be viewed as a state of equilibrium in which many diverse factors are in balance. When this equilibrium is disrupted by changes in one or more factors, the possibility of a disease occurring is increased.

In epidemiology the diverse factors involved in a disease are grouped into three main classes. Factors associated with people are called host factors; factors relating to the infecting organism, such as bacteria or a virus, are called agent factors; and the remaining factors, external to the host, are environmental factors. The dynamic interrelationship of these three components—the host, the agent, and the environment—is often illustrated by a model referred to as the epidemiological triangle. The points of this triangle represent the host, agent, or environment. This model further indicates that each class has a dynamic interrelationship with the other two, and that a change in the factors in any one of the classes will alter the state of equilibrium. The prevention of a disorder involves either maintaining the existing dynamic interrelationship in healthy individuals or modifying, eliminating, or adding factors in one or more of the components—typically factors associated with the host or the environment.

The classical example in epidemiology of terminating an epidemic without knowledge of the agent is the famous work of John Snow (1855) on the Broad Street epidemic of cholera in London. In 1854 there was some acceptance of the theory of contagion with respect to illnesses such as measles, syphilis, and smallpox, but the germ theory of disease causation had not yet been developed. An anesthesiologist with an interest in cholera, Snow inferred that tiny amounts of contaminated fecal matter were ingested by persons who subsequently became ill. Food, water, and direct contact were the possible sources of the epidemic. By determining the place where each person became ill, his attention was drawn to the common pump in Broad Street, since the area served by the pump had the greatest concentration of sick people. The small number of cases in the area of the Marlborough Street pump was accounted for when he learned that the water there was clearly polluted and residents preferred to use the more distant Broad Street pump. Within the area of the Broad Street pump, however, there were several inconsistencies in the distribution of cases. Whereas a workhouse had only 5 cases out of 535 inmates, a percussion-cap factory had 18 cases out of approximately 200 workers. The difference was accounted for when it was learned that the workhouse had a well on its grounds, and that the factory workers obtained water from the Broad Street pump. Further, there were no cases among the 70 workers of a brewery in Broad Street. Dr. Snow subsequently learned from the owner that the brewery had its own deep well, and more importantly, that as the workers were allowed to drink malt liquor, the proprietor believed the workers did not drink any water at all.

By focusing on factors in the environment and behavioral patterns and habits of the people, Dr. Snow was able to infer that the source of the epidemic was the water of the Broad Street pump. With the closing of the Broad Street pump and the subsequent drop in the incidence of cholera, Dr. Snow's analyses were vindicated. The importance of Snow's work stems from the fact that it was conducted in the pre-germ-theory period without knowledge of the causal agent, the bacillus, and dramatically illustrates that knowledge about the host and environment are often sufficient for effective prevention.

Primary prevention of malaria has focused on man the host, the plasmodium parasite which is the agent, and the mosquito vector/environment relationship. Early efforts were directed at modifying the environment in the direction of creating conditions inhospitable to the breeding of mosquitoes. Such efforts included drainage projects, often on a massive scale, filling small holes and depressions that served as breeding areas, increasing the penetration of the sun to shady breeding areas, changing the salinity of the water when possible, and after World War II undertaking a worldwide DDT spray-gun war to eradicate the mosquito. Each of these methods achieved varying and even outstanding degrees of success in reducing the incidence of malaria, as well as eradicating the disease in a small number of places in the world.

The indiscriminate DDT war was directed at wiping out the mosquito once and for all. The grand design was that if the mosquito was eradicated for a sufficient period of time, malaria then would disappear, as the parasites in infected hosts would die out in the absence of the mosquito vector necessary for transmission. Very significant successes were achieved, and some have been maintained in a few parts of the world. But due to the costs involved and what appeared to be victory, the DDT war was stopped in country after country before the mosquito truly had been eradicated. As a result, most of the victories turned out to be illusions, for when the incidence of malaria began to climb, most parts of the world also began to report the emergence of mosquito strains resistant to DDT and other pesticides.

Today, total eradication has been replaced by "integrated control" (Harrison, 1978) and many of the old methods, such as drainage programs, the use of screening, spraying with petroleum products, and other types of environmental modification, have returned. DDT and other pesticides are part of the approach, but their use is much more carefully controlled because of their danger to man and other living creatures.

At the level of the host, primary prevention is concerned first with providing specific protection against malaria through the use of various antimalarial drugs that suppress the development of malaria when the individual becomes infected, and second, education in various methods that decrease the risk of exposure to infection. Primary prevention at the level of the agent, the plasmodium, is achieved essentially through secondary prevention. Prompt, effective treatment of infected persons decreases the pool of individuals who can transmit the disease to a mosquito and subsequently to other people. Decreasing the risk of transmission by treatment serves as a primary preventative method for noninfected persons.

The successes and failures in the prevention of malaria provide a number of lessons for prevention in general, and specifically for the prevention of mental disturbances. The termination of the all-out DDT war revealed the willingness of people to settle for quickly achieved results that can turn out to be pseudovictories, and their resistance to undertaking long-term programs that are costly to sustain and need the investment of maximum participation by a population in achieving the desired goal. Of equal importance is the knowledge that for most effective prevention it is necessary to understand and intervene in the context of the host-agent-environment perspective, that is, from an ecological standpoint.

In recent years considerable epidemiological attention has been directed toward such chronic problems as coronary heart disease, diabetes, arthritis, mental disorders, and accidents. On the basis of the present state of knowledge, these conditions do not involve a single factor or agent that is a necessary precondition for their development. Paramount concern for these disorders has focused on the host and the environment and their interactions. The reader will recall that the agent is only one of the many factors in the environment that had been singled out to facilitate an understanding of primarily infectious diseases. The chronic disabling diseases that are presently receiving attention apparently result from a number of interacting factors. In recognition of this many prefer today to simply use a host-environment model.

CAUSATION IN EPIDEMIOLOGY

In the development of programs of prevention, it is most desirable to have knowledge of a causal relationship between a disorder and the factor(s) the preventative program seeks to modify or change. Such evidence, however, is very often unavailable. When experimental proof is lacking, there are three possible ways of determining a causal relationship (MacMahon, Pugh, & Ipsen, 1960). First, for a causal relationship there must be consistency in the time sequence of related events; second, the stronger the association between a suspected factor and a disorder, the greater the possibility that there is a causal relationship; and third, the suspected causal association must be consistent with the existing knowledge base. In assessing whether there is a causal relationship it is necessary to determine the possibility of a secondary noncausal statistical association being erroneously considered a causal relationship. For example, factor X both precedes and affects factors Y and Z: X is causally related to both Y and Z. Since X affects both Y and Z, factors Y and Z will be statistically associated; but the relationship between Y and Z is noncausal because changing Y does not result in a change in Z.

On the basis of the concept that "effects are never dependent on single causes," MacMahon, Pugh, and Ipsen (1960) have formulated a "web of causation" model. They state that whereas the focus is typically on a few broad classes of causal events, each of these classes of events is comprised of a number of smaller events. Each event is the result of a "complex genealogy of antecedents." The "chains" of causation consisting of a myriad of antecedent factors comprise a web whose total complexity "lies beyond our understanding." A very important implication of this model is that various degrees or levels of prevention are possible, depending on which linkages in the myriad of causal chains are eliminated. The extent to which the incidence of a disorder is reduced is dependent on the importance of the eliminated factors relative to other causal factors.

The web of causation model has considerable relevance to the prevention of mental disorders. An example of this can be found in the psychosis called general paresis. This is an organic psychosis in later life that results from an earlier untreated syphilitic infection. Although a syphilitic infection is a necessary precondition for general paresis, it is not the sole cause. Only about 5 percent of the untreated cases of syphilis develop paresis, indicating that other factors are involved. Whether they are host or environmental factors or both is unknown. Due to the successful treatment of syphilis today, general paresis is seldom seen. The fact remains, however, that syphilis must be accompanied by other important causal factors to result in general paresis.

CAUSATION IN MENTAL DISORDERS

During the past 30 years it has become possible to specify with precision underlying, predisposing, causal factors for a number of mental disorders having an organic or genetic basis. Among these disorders are general paresis, fetal rubella, Down's syndrome, phenylketonuria, galactosemia, congenital hypothyroidism, various organic brain syndromes due to poisons (lead, alcohol, environmental pollutants), and injuries and accidents. The screening of early newborns for early identification and treatment of phenylketonuria, galactosemia, and congenital hypothyroidism has prevented later severe mental retardation, behavior disorders, and seizures. The introduction of the use of hard hats in many industries has reduced the risk of brain damage from accidents and injuries. On the other hand, some of the problems in prevention are illustrated in relatively unsuccessful attempts to implement the use of seat belts and infant car restraints to prevent brain damage resulting from head injuries in car accidents.

The prevention of mental retardation, difficulties in learning, and even death from lead poisoning in children has received considerable attention in the last decade. The lead in flaking and peeling lead-based paints had been considered a major source due to the tendency of many young children to eat such material. Children who are at the highest risk of ingesting flaking paints are those who have pica. Pica is defined as a craving or tendency to eat nonedible material. Knowledge as to why and how pica develops is limited and incomplete. It is known that by eliminating lead in all paints, and renovating housing where lead paint is peeling, the risk of brain damage from this source is reduced not only for children with pica but for all children. It is estimated, however, that about half of the lead in American diets probably can be traced to food from lead-soldered cans. Unfortunately, nothing is being done about this source (Settle & Patterson, 1980).

In contrast to the successes achieved in identifying the causal factors in mental disorders with an organic or genetic basis, the predisposing and causal factors in functional psychoses, neuroses, and emotional disorders are either unknown or poorly understood. The anticipation has been that research would uncover single unitary causal factors for these disorders—that each disease has its specific cause and that each cause has its specific disease. This conception is an integral part of the medical model that has been successful in the prevention and treatment of organic mental disorders. The medical model has been extensively criticized, however, in its applicability to the field of functional mental and emotional disorders (Albee, 1968; Smith, 1968; Szasz, 1961). The adherents of the monoetiological model fail to recognize that the classification system of mental disorders does not have the precision of the classification system of infectious and other diseases. For example, when for the sake of convenience we speak of schizophrenia, we should be speaking of the schizophrenias, as we also should with cancer. Another major weakness in this model is that causation is largely restricted to biological or physical factors with the consequent failure to give significant weight to psychosocial and cultural factors.

Although the causes of some mental disorders are rooted in biological or genetic factors, the causes of the vast array of functional psychoses, neuroses, and emotional disorders are the result of a complex combination and interaction of psychological, social, biological, and environmental factors. Causality thereby is multi-factorial, that is, the result of many interacting factors.

CRISIS THEORY

The work of Lindemann (1944) and Tyhurst (1957) on the effects of disasters indicated that the adequate resolution of such a crisis has implications for the individual's future psychological well-being. Lindemann's work delineated the fundamentals of crisis theory, and its implications for mental health. Crises are brief, transitory periods of acute physical and psychological disturbance. They are a result of abrupt changes or disruptions in situations that are psychologically important to the individual and require some type of adaptation. Lindemann (1944) and Tyhurst (1957) identified specific reactions to crises, phases that a person goes through when confronted with a crisis, and psychological and social consequences of disasters. Although the initial work focused on natural disasters, the impact of all types of crises on the individual's subsequent psychological adjustment was recognized and incorporated by Caplan (1964) as a significant component of primary prevention.

Tyhurst (1957) described three overlapping crisis phases: a period of impact, a period of recoil, and a posttraumatic period. In the period of impact, physical and psychological symptomatology or disturbances are manifested almost immediately following the disaster or crisis. These typically include various disruptions or disturbances of bodily functioning, feelings of anxiety and fear, bewilderment, confusion, disturbances in thinking, feelings of powerlessness and ineffectuality, and so forth. The period of impact typically is very brief.

In the period of recoil, physical and psychological disturbances can be intensified. In addition, the person starts to express feelings and gain a clear awareness of what has been experienced. Anger, childlike dependency, and the need to ventilate feelings are characteristic. Due to the psychological disruption being experienced, the individual is open to suggestions for coping with the crisis and of ways of handling or resolving the crisis. In the posttraumatic period the person continues to experience stresses that stem from the preceding periods, as well as stresses of a social and interpersonal nature. At this point the integration of past and present experiences with the future is initiated. The individual then achieves adaptation. Tyhurst asserted that the optimal time for intervention is during the recoil period.

Caplan (1964) further developed crisis theory in a number of important dimensions, and especially in relation to the individual's future level of psychosocial adjustment. He postulated that an unsuccessful resolution of a crisis can result in a continuation of tension, varying degrees of personality disorganization, and a level of psychosocial functioning lower than the level that was characteristic prior to the crisis. An adequate resolution of the crisis and its associated problems not only has the potential to increase the level of psychosocial functioning in relation to precrisis functioning but also can increase the probability that future crises will be resolved successfully.

In addition to sudden, unanticipated, or accidental events, crises can also be precipitated at various significant, typically transitional, points in the life-span. The knowledge of the critical periods in development, and major life events can serve to develop programs for primary prevention. These efforts would be directed at population groups that had not yet experienced those crisis-producing events—for example, first day at school, marriage, parenthood, and so on. Groups can be trained to cope with potential crises through "anticipatory guidance" or "emotional inoculation" (Caplan, 1964). They can be instructed on how to handle and work through the event or transition.

A PROPOSED NEW MODEL FOR PREVENTION

Extensive research on both animals and humans has indicated that individuals are most susceptible to the emergence of a mental or emotional disturbance as a consequence of stressful experiences (Dohrenwend & Dohrenwend, 1974). The individual's reaction to the stressful experience is psychologically determined. Included among the many factors determining the individual's reaction are the personal meaning of the experience, the available repertoire of coping skills, the number and types of previous stressful experiences, the extent of social supports, and the severity of feelings of powerlessness.

The Task Force on Prevention of the President's Commission on Mental Health (PCMH, 1978) has proposed a new model for research and program development in primary prevention.

The Task Force Report (PCMH, 1978) summarizes the new model as follows:

1. Identify stressful events or experiences that have undesirable consequences in a significant proportion of the population and develop procedures for

reliably identifying persons who have undergone or who are undergoing such events or experiences.

2. Study the consequences of those events in a population by contrasting subsequent illness experiences or emotional problems with those of a suitably selected comparison population.

3. Mount and evaluate experimental prevention programs aimed at reducing the incidence of such stressful life events and/or at increasing coping skills in managing those events.

As the reader can discern, the paradigm described above focuses on stress and stressful life events as a common denominator in all mental and emotional disorders, and involves a shift of attention from predisposing factors to precipitating factors. It also deemphasizes linking specific events with specific disorders or disturbances. An example can be found in looking at the effects of a stressful event such as retirement. One person may happily adjust, another may become depressed, a third may develop psychosomatic symptoms, and a fourth may experience marital conflict.

PROGRAMS AND APPROACHES TO PREVENTION

Following the formulations and program descriptions provided by Caplan (1964), the number of program descriptions, approaches to prevention, and theoretical formulations has increased very rapidly. As space limitations preclude describing a wide variety of programs and approaches, the reader will find useful reviews and descriptions in Cowen (1973); Kessler and Albee (1975); Kelly, Snowden, and Munoz (1977); Bloom (1980); the Vermont Conference on the Primary Prevention of Psychopathology series (Albee and Joffe, 1977; Forgays, 1978; Kent & Rolf, 1979), and the report of the Task Force on Prevention of the President's Commission on Mental Health (PCMH, 1978).

Primary prevention traditionally has been viewed as consisting of two components: providing specific protection, and promoting mental health. Specific protection refers to those activities and programs that are directed at the prevention of a specific disorder. Examples would include the vaccination of women prior to pregnancy to prevent fetal rubella and the prevention of various birth defects by adequate prenatal care. Health promotion involves broad approaches of education, such as those undertaken by some of the educational programs of community mental health centers, and more specific programs such as those directed at increasing coping skills, social competence, and parent education.

Caplan (1964) classified preventative programs into two major groups: social action and interpersonal action. Social action programs work with institutions and organizations that impact on mental health. They are directed at modifying or changing policies, regulations, and so on, so as to assure an adequate level of physical, psychosocial, and sociocultural supplies or resources. Interpersonal action programs are directed at individuals or small groups—typically individuals such as clergymen, school personnel, physicians, and so on, who can have an influence on community problems. Both social action and interpersonal action programs encourage the optimal development of people, and the resolution of crises so as to maintain and promote mental health.

In contrast to the broad panorama presented by Caplan (1964), Bloom (1968), with a concern for increased specificity and clarity, proposed classifying preventative programs on a threefold basis: as community-wide programs, milestone programs, and high-risk programs. Community-wide programs include social action and community development programs. Milestone and high-risk programs are described in the following section on person-oriented approaches to prevention.

For descriptive purposes, preventative programs directed at individuals and groups will be designated as person-oriented, and programs directed toward organizations, institutions, the community, and society at large will be designated as social-systems-oriented. The following section describes several major program types in each of these two categories.

Person-Oriented Preventative Approaches

Programs for Preventing Specific Disorders

Programs for specific disorders include the prevention of lead poisoning in children; the prevention of fetal rubella by vaccinating mothers; the prevention of mental retardation and other disorders resulting from phenylketonuria, galactosemia, and Down's syndrome by providing genetic counseling, subsequent screening, and optional abortion; and the prevention of mental retardation and other disorders resulting from prematurity and inadequate prenatal nutrition and health care.

Programs for High-Risk Groups

Programs for high-risk groups are directed at individuals or groups, who as a consequence of predisposing factors in their backgrounds, are vulnerable to emotional disturbances or disorders. Examples of high-risk groups for whom programs can be developed include children of schizophrenics; children of alcoholics; individuals who have experienced a death or divorce in their family; individuals who have experienced a natural or man-made disaster; individuals who have experienced the death of a spouse or a child; parents of premature babies, babies with physical or mental handicaps, and "difficult" babies; and elderly persons who are either isolated or lack a support system.

Broussard (1976), on the basis of findings that first-born children who during the first month after birth were perceived negatively by their mothers subsequently were at risk of emotional disturbances, developed a prevention program directed at the mothers. The program was based on supplementary parenting through mother-infant group meetings and home visits. At one year of age the high-risk children in the intervention group had better scores on a series of clinical scales than the intervention-refused group and the comparison group.

Silverman (1976) developed a successful widow-to-widow program in which widow aides assisted new widows, through the bereavement process, in establishing new roles and an adequate lifestyle.

Milestone or Transitional Programs

Milestone or transitional programs focus on the major points in people's lives when they undergo an important transition. During the passage through the many transitions in life there is a potential for one's adjustment to be adversely affected or disrupted on either a short-term or a long-term basis. Important transitions include, among others, marriage, the birth of the first child, retirement, any of the transitions during the schooling process from kindergarten to college, and any of the transitional points in the life-span.

Bogat, Jones, and Jason (in press) reported significant effects in a program directed at elementary school children changing schools as a result of a forced school closing. The children who participated in the program subsequently were demonstrated to be superior to two control groups in terms of self-esteem related to peer relationships, knowledge of school rules, and teacher conduct ratings.

Bloom (1971) conducted a program directed at college freshmen, a life transition that involves an aggregate of stresses. Using techniques such as questionnaires about problems of adjustment, with subsequent feedback, and readings dealing with topics such as mental health on the college campus and human sexuality in young adults, survival rates—that is, enrollment as sophomores—were higher in the experimental group than in a comparative group.

Competency Development Programs

Competency development programs are directed at the development of psychosocial and cognitive strengths. The possession of a repertoire of competence-related skills has the potential of having a radiating effect into all areas of human functioning. A lack of competence is accompanied by low self-esteem, feelings of powerlessness, and ineffective coping strategies, which eventually can result in a lowered quality of life or emotional and mental disorders. The competency-training approach is relatively new, but on the basis of various research findings (Spivack & Shure, 1974; Jason, 1975; Gesten et al., 1978) it has the potential to become one of the most powerful approaches to primary prevention. Competency-training programs can be developed in almost unlimited settings, and for groups in all categories of the social spectrum.

A program conducted by Heber (1978) over ten years focused on developing parenting competencies in mothers with IQs below 75. Their children were at high risk of "cultural familial retardation." Starting at the birth of the child, mothers were trained in areas such as cognitive skills, nutrition, hygiene, and child development. The children received language and cognitive skill training as part of their educational program which started at three months of age. By age six, the initially high-risk children of these mothers had a mean IQ of 124 in contrast to a mean IQ of 87 for the control group.

Spivack and Shure (1974), working with four-year-old children in a ten-week Head Start program, developed skills involving the ability to identify feelings, to understand causal factors in interpersonal problems, to use means-end thinking and alternative thinking, and to evaluate consequences. The children significantly improved in social adjustment. These investigators further demonstrated that the gains were maintained, that teachers and mothers can be taught to be trainers, and that improved adjustment follows the acquisition of the skill.

Social-Systems-Oriented Preventative Approaches

In contrast to the person-oriented approaches, which focus on assisting specific populations in developing coping skills and competencies, there is a growing body of opinion that society's major problems are rooted in its systems, rather than in its people (Dörken, 1971). Societal problems such as racism, sexism, poverty, alcoholism, suicide, unemployment, illegitimate births, and alienation are viewed as indexes of society's malfunctioning. They produce emotional and mental disturbances. From this point of view primary prevention has to become involved in social system change.

Society is organized in increasingly more complex levels. The levels toward which preventative approaches can be directed are the individual level, the group level, the organizational level, the institutional level, the community level, and the societal level (Reiff, 1977). It can be readily recognized that the greatest impacts occur when system changes result at the societal level. Such changes typically involve legislation and require a long time to permeate the social fabric. The 1954 Supreme Court decision on school desegregation and Title VII of the Civil Rights Act of 1964 have had an impact. Full compliance, however, is yet to be achieved. Racism is still a prominent feature of our social system. For prevention advocates it should be readily apparent that changes at the societal level require considerable time and persistent effort. Forces resisting change are found at every level. Change in the status quo requires alterations in power relationships and in role functions.

From the above example it is apparent that the mental health professional is not uniquely equipped or trained for effecting social system changes. Depending on the specific goal, the mental health professional has to work with a coalition of other groups: legislators, political scientists, economists, sociologists, urban planners, environmentalists, and grass-roots organizations. The professional's unique contribution in such coalitions is the analysis of the effects of the current social structure on mental health, as well as the potential effects of the proposed changes.

Social system change can be implemented through programs of consultation (Caplan, 1964, 1970). Program-centered consultation can be directed toward the development of needed programs, the modification of practices in current programs that impinge on mental health, and legislative endeavors. Such consultation focuses on articulating the principles of psychological development and mental health with the goals and purposes of the organization.

A rapidly growing approach to primary prevention is the modification of social environments in organizations or institutions, an approach that at times is described as social engineering. The underlying fundamental principle is that situational and environmental factors influence human behavior—either for the good or for the bad (Sarason, 1972). Moos (1975) has demonstrated that social climate influences a person's behavior, health, overall sense of well-being, as well as social, personal, and intellectual development. But the effect of an environmental system is complex. Kelly (1976) reported that in two high schools the impact of the school environment did not appear until the junior year, and that what was adaptive behavior in one school was not adaptive in the other.

The influence between person characteristics and environment characteristics is dramatically portrayed further in a methodologically sophisticated study by Solomon and Kendall (1979) who, among other findings, reported that students with high achievement motivation and high self-confidence did best in controlled/orderly classrooms, whereas children from lower socioeconomic groups did best in relatively "warm" classrooms.

These studies suggest that it is possible to facilitate development and performance through a careful organization of settings in which the person-environment fit or ecological match is a key component. The potential for primary prevention is self-evident.

Of additional considerable importance to primary prevention is that systematic procedures can be developed to change social systems or environments. Moos (1975), using a four-step procedure, demonstrated in three psychiatric programs that treatment environments could be changed.

CONSULTATION AND EDUCATION: THE HOME OF PRIMARY PREVENTION

The Consultation and Education (C&E) Program of a CMHC is the home of its primary prevention programs. Through consultation with other community caretakers the center endeavors to maintain and improve the mental health of the people with whom they work (Caplan, 1970). By supporting and extending the mental health role of the caregivers in the community, the center is able to prevent the development of mental health problems, as well as facilitate early treatment. Other C&E activities include networking with other human service agencies to provide comprehensive services, and educating community residents about mental illness and problems.

There is an extensive range of C&E services mandated in P.L. 94-63 and P.L. 95-622. On the other hand the formula for C&E grants reveals that centers are in a double bind—that is, extensive mandated C&E services are coupled with limited financial support and manpower. Studies reveal that only 4 to 5 percent of total staff time is spent on C&E services (Snow & Newton, 1976; M. Silverman, 1978) and of this limited amount of time approximately half (44.6 percent) is spent in case consultation, an activity closely related to direct clinical services.

In a factor analytic study on the implementation of policy goals by 410 centers (M. Silverman, 1978), C&E programs were evaluated as being highly effective at 16 percent of the centers, moderately effective at 61 percent of the CMHCs, and ineffective in the remainder. Further, C&E was significantly negatively correlated with a factor called "state mental health department power." A key variable in this power factor related to increases in direct clinical services to patients in state and county mental facilities—which highlights the conflict between increasing therapeutic services or developing C&E services to meet community needs.

From the inception of CMHCs, C&E programs have been handicapped by an inadequately trained and understaffed manpower pool. These shortages are changing slowly with the permeation of the community mental health ideology through the mental health system. Training directors in the 128 CMHCs that offer internship training to doctoral students in psychology report that 53 percent of the trainees are receiving training in primary prevention and 67 percent in consultation (Zolik, Bogat, & Jason, 1980).

Since many mental health professionals have a proclivity to promote increased direct clinical services, advocating for C&E programs is a vital responsibility of board members of CMHCs. As representatives of the community, they are aware of the array of community needs. The proverb, "An ounce of prevention is worth a pound of cure," should play a major role in their policy formation and resource allocation.

The training of board members to perform their functions is a basic requirement in establishing effective CMHC programs. Silverman (in press) described a carefully designed and evaluated training program for mental health advisory/governing boards, which not only had an impact on the functioning of the board member trainee but also had an influence on the board and the center.

Primary prevention programs of the type presented in this chapter and in the cited literature are examples of approaches that can be implemented. But until resources for C&E are brought to an adequate level, through the action of boards in coalition with other groups at the local, state, and federal level, centers would be best advised to undertake limited preventative programs that are carefully designed and evaluated. This approach has the potential of demonstrating, in a safe and effective way, the results that can be achieved through primary prevention.

BARRIERS TO PREVENTION

Although it is recognized that primary prevention is responsible for having conquered most of the major diseases of mankind, the increasingly greater resources in mental health over the last three decades have been channeled almost entirely into secondary and tertiary prevention efforts. This has resulted in training more professionals for the practice of treatment and rehabilitation rather than primary prevention.

In medicine, in addition to the costs for the physician's direct service, each physician generates over $12 million of costs to the health care system over an average 40-year professional career, or $300,000 per year (Califano, 1978). The costs associated with maintaining each professional psychiatrist, psychologist, and social worker in the treatment arena are not yet known. The associated costs might be anticipated, however, to be equally appalling.

From another perspective the direct costs in 1976 for mental health care and treatment amounted to $17 billion of which 21 percent was provided by the federal government (PCMH, 1978). In contrast to the $39 billion allocated to all treatment programs (general health and mental health) supported by the federal government, less than $3 billion was allocated to prevention in general (Califano, 1978), of which only $2 to $3 million was allocated to the prevention of mental and emotional disorders by NIMH (PCMH, 1978).

These data dramatically highlight the problems involved in supporting prevention, especially in the mental health area. In addition to funding problems, there is a moral dilemma. Seeking treatment often involves an imperative—avoiding death or serious disability. Prevention often is not backed by such an imperative; it typically can be delayed without immediate dire consequences.

The constituency that prevention can mobilize is much more fractionated than the constituency for greater investments in direct treatment services. This latter constituency, furthermore, is backed by the political power of the health care industry, ranging from hospitals, the medical lobby, the pharmaceutical and nursing-home industries, the various contractors who supply health care facilities, the lobbies for specific diseases, and the health insurance lobby. Prevention does not have such a support system. In fact it is perceived at times as a threat by various components of the health care industry and its supporters, and various social or political groups.

Primary prevention has been accused of restricting freedom of choice, imposing the values of a minority on the majority, and at times possibly leading to negative health consequences. Programs for the fluoridation of water to prevent dental caries encountered each of those arguments as well as others. Consequently, when groups feel their "rights" are threatened, power groups are formed and vested interests are protected.

In addition to these barriers, there is the power of "the establishment." Well-entrenched social and political systems resist change and cannot be expected to yield passively even when confronted with dramatic evidence. As an example, the U.S. Surgeon General's Report (HEW, 1979) stated that as much as half of the U.S. mortality in 1976 was due to unhealthy behavior or life-styles,

and that improvement in health status would not be achieved predominantly through the treatment of disease but rather through its
prevention. It is clear that factors beyond cold scientific facts—
economic, political, psychological—dominate in the struggle for
social change.

Another barrier to prevention programs is the argument that
the etiologies of mental disorders are largely unknown. Consequently there is a natural resistance to reallocating limited or
scarce resources to activities that often are perceived as leading
to questionable or unknown outcomes. Underlying this is the traditional perception that prevention is directed at interrupting the action of the causative agent, and since the causative agent in emotional disturbances and mental illness is unknown, the outcome or
results of preventative activities cannot be predicted with a high degree of specificity. As Halliday (1943) has indicated, however, the
knowledge base required for primary prevention frequently is not
the same as that required for successful treatment. Complete
knowledge of the etiology of mental disorders is not necessary for
successful prevention. The reader will recall the work of Snow in
London.

A final problem, of special relevance in the modification of
social systems, is the possibility of unintended consequences. This
was illustrated in the all-out DDT war to eradicate mosquitoes. To
avoid unplanned outcomes, programs have to be developed with extreme care, be based on substantive findings, plan for potential difficulties, and be monitored at each step.

CONCLUSIONS

The primary prevention of emotional disorders is a task whose
time has come. The knowledge base is more than sufficient for undertaking a wide variety of programs on a broad scale. Although
many programs can be undertaken by mental health professionals,
other programs need allies such as educators, city planners, politicians, and so on, along with the involvement and interest of the
citizenry. Local community needs should dictate the problem areas
toward which preventative programs should be directed.

Any program that improves the quality of life and facilitates
coping at times of crisis can be considered as primary prevention.
Indeed, such efforts may sound idealistic, but primary prevention
must also be based on scientific principles. Consequently, the
greater the precision regarding what is done to what group for what
purpose, the more effective prevention will become.

There has been a reawakening among policy makers and mental health professionals to the fact that prevention rather than treatment is the basic approach to health and mental health problems. We can never train enough professionals to meet burgeoning treatment needs nor can we continue to pay the increasing costs for treatment and other health care services. Primary prevention is more efficient and more cost-effective.

Today's approach to health care economy is incompatible with prevention (Terris, 1976). Current and proposed health insurance plans are not health programs, but fiscal measures. Because they are based on a fee-for-service model, they reward the treatment of illness rather than the promotion of health. Only through a national health service coordinated through federal, state, and local efforts, can a major emphasis be placed on primary prevention. Therefore, we must divest the Social Security Administration and insurance companies of their power as the planners and financiers of service delivery.

Finally, and most importantly, primary prevention is a more humane approach. Whether the "idea whose time has come" blossoms and bears fruit in large measure is dependent on an informed citizenry. Nonprofessional members of boards of CMHCs in concert with the small group of professionals oriented to primary prevention are the key at the local level to fostering, promoting, and implementing prevention as a birthright of all Americans.

REFERENCES

Albee, G. W. Conceptual models and manpower requirements in psychology. American Psychologist, 1968, 30, 1156-1158.

Albee, G., & Joffe, J. (Eds.). Primary prevention of psychopathology: The issues (Vol. I). Hanover, N.H.: University Press of New England, 1977.

Bloom, B. L. The evaluation of primary prevention programs. In L. Roberts, N. Greenfield, & M. Miller (Eds.), Comprehensive mental health: The challenge of evaluation. Madison: University of Wisconsin Press, 1968.

Bloom, B. L. A university freshman preventive intervention program: Report of a pilot project. Journal of Consulting and Clinical Psychology, 1971, 37, 235-242.

Bloom, B. L. Social and community interventions. Annual Review of Psychology. Palo Alto: Annual Reviews, 1980.

Bogat, A., Jones, J., & Jason, L. School transitions: Preventive intervention following an elementary school closing. Journal of Community Psychology, in press.

Broussard, E. Neonatal prediction and outcome at 10/11 years. Child Psychiatry and Human Development, 1976, 2, 85-93.

Califano, J. A., Jr. Remarks of Joseph A. Califano, Jr., Secretary, U.S. Department of Health, Education and Welfare, before the Association of American Medical Colleges. Washington, D.C.: U.S. Department of Health, Education and Welfare, 1978.

Caplan, G. Principles of preventive psychiatry. New York: Basic Books, 1964.

Caplan, G. The theory and practice of mental health consultation. New York: Basic Books, 1970.

Constitution of the World Health Organization, 1948. In Basic Documents. (15th ed.). Geneva: World Health Organization, 1964.

Cowen, E. L. Social and community intervention. Annual Review of Psychology. Palo Alto: Annual Reviews, 1973.

Döhrenwend, B. S., & Dohrenwend, B. P. (Eds.). Stressful life events: Their nature and effects. New York: Wiley, 1974.

Dorken, H. A dimensional strategy for community focused mental health services. In G. Rosenblum (Ed.), Issues in community psychology and preventive mental health. New York: Behavioral Publications, 1971.

Forgays, D. (Ed.). Primary prevention of psychopathology: Environmental influences (Vol. II). Hanover, N.H.: University Press of New England, 1978.

Gesten, E. L., Flores de Apodaca, R., Raines, M., Weissberg, R., & Cowen, E. Promoting peer related social competence in young children. In M. Kent and J. Rolf (Eds.), Primary prevention of psychopathology: Promoting social competence and coping in children (Vol. 3). Hanover, N.H.: University Press of New England, 1978.

Goldberger, J. The cause and prevention of pellagra. Public Health Reports, 1914, 29, 2354. Reprinted in M. Terris (Ed.), Goldberger on pellagra. Baton Rouge: Lousiana State University Press, 1964.

Halliday, J. L. Principles of aetiology. British Journal of Medical Psychology, 1943, 19, 367-380.

Harrison, G. Mosquitoes, malaria and man: A history of hostilities since 1880. New York: Dutton, 1978.

Heber, F. R. Sociocultural mental retardation: A longitudinal study. In D. Forgays (Ed.), Primary prevention of psychopathology: Environmental influences (Vol. II). Hanover, N.H.: University Press of New England, 1978.

Jason, L. Early secondary prevention with disadvantaged children. American Journal of Community Psychology, 1975, 3, 33-46.

Kelly, J. G. The high school: An exploration of students and social contexts in two midwestern communities. New York: Behavioral Publications, 1976.

Kelly, J., Snowden, L., & Munoz, R. Social and community interventions. Annual Review of Psychology. Palo Alto: Annual Reviews, 1977.

Kent, M., & Rolf, J. (Eds.). Primary prevention of psychopathology: Social competence in children (Vol. III). Hanover, N.H.: University Press of New England, 1979.

Kessler, M., & Albee, G. Primary prevention. Annual Review of Psychology. Palo Alto: Annual Reviews, 1975.

Klein, D. C., & Goldston, S. E. (Eds.). Primary prevention: An idea whose time has come. Washington, D.C.: U.S. Government Printing Office, 1977.

Lindemann, E. Symptomatology and management of acute grief. American Journal of Psychiatry, 1944, 101, 141-148.

MacMahon, B., Pugh, T., & Ipsen, J. Epidemiological methods. Boston: Little, Brown and Company, 1960.

Moos, R. H. Evaluating correctional and community settings. New York: Wiley, 1975.

President's Commission on Mental Health (PCMH). Report to the President from the President's Commission on Mental Health (Vols. 1-4). Washington, D.C.: U.S. Government Printing Office, 1978.

Reiff, R. Ya gotta believe. In I. Iscoe, B. Bloom, & C. Spielberger (Eds.), Community psychology in transition. Washington, D.C.: Hemisphere Publishing, 1977.

Sarason, S. The creation of settings and the future societies. San Francisco: Jossey-Bass, 1972.

Settle, D., & Patterson, C. Lead in albacore: Guide to lead pollution in Americans. Science, 1980, 207, 1167-1176.

Silverman, M. Factors associated with effective implementation of policy goals of the CMHC Act of 1973. Unpublished doctoral dissertation, University of Northern Illinois, 1978.

Silverman, P. The widow as a caregiver in a program of preventive intervention with other widows. In G. Caplan & M. Killilea (Eds.), Support systems and mutual help: Multidisciplinary explorations. New York: Grune and Stratton, 1976.

Silverman, W. Self-designed training for mental health advisory/governing boards. American Journal of Community Psychology, in press.

Smith, M. B. The revolution in mental health care—A "bold new approach"? Transaction, 1968, 5, 19-23.

Snow, D., & Newton, P. Task, structure, and social process in the community mental health center movement. American Psychologist, 1976, 31, 582-594.

Snow, J. On the mode of communication of cholera (2nd ed.). London: John Churchill, 1855. Reprinted in Snow on cholera. New York: Commonwealth Fund, 1936.

Solomon, D., & Kendall, A. Children in classrooms: An investigation of person-environment interaction. New York: Praeger, 1979.

Spivack, G., & Shure, M. Social adjustment of young children. San Francisco: Jossey-Bass, 1974.

Sullivan, H. S. Socio-psychiatric research: Its implications for the schizophrenia problem and for mental hygiene. American Journal of Psychiatry, 1931, 87, 977-991.

Szasz, T. The myth of mental illness. New York: Harper and Row, 1961.

Terris, M. Prevention in today's economy and tomorrow's society. Paper presented at the meeting of the American Public Health Association, Miami Beach, October 1976.

Tyhurst, J. S. Psychological and social aspects of civilian disaster. Canadian Medical Association Journal, 1957, 76, 385-393.

U.S. Department of Health, Education and Welfare. Disease prevention and health promotion: Federal programs and prospects. Washington, D.C.: U.S. Government Printing Office, 1978.

U.S. Department of Health, Education and Welfare. Healthy people: The Surgeon General's report on health promotion and disease prevention. Washington, D.C.: U.S. Government Printing Office, 1979.

Wagenfield, M. O. The primary prevention of mental illness. Journal of Health and Social Behavior, 1972, 13, 195-203.

Zolik, E., Bogat, A., & Jason, L. Community training for interns and practicum students in CMHCs. Paper presented at the meeting of the American Psychological Association, Montreal, September 1980.

13

SELF-HELP ORGANIZATIONS
Alan Gartner
Frank Riessman

Few developments in recent years have as far-reaching potential for community mental health services as does the self-help mutual aid phenomenon. On the one hand, growing and diverse demands
for services at a time of resource constraints strain the community
mental health center (CMHC) network. At the same time there is
increased questioning of the efficacy and nature of traditional professionally provided services. These trends come at a time when
the value of large institutions is being challenged. We are seeing,
in effect, a convergence of factors in the larger society and in human
service practice.

On the other hand, partially in response to these factors, there
has been the growth of self-help mutual aid activities. The growth is
but the tip of the very large iceberg; an extensive study by the Office
of Prevention, California Department of Mental Health (Roepal,
1979), reports that while 75 percent of those queried felt getting together with persons with similar health and mental health problems
was a good idea, only 9 percent had done so. There is, it seems, a
considerable "market" for further growth of self-help mutual aid
activities.

This growth appears in both the number of groups and people
participating in them, and in the variety of problems addressed by
such groups. One recent study (Evans, 1979) estimates that there
are currently more than 500,000 self-help groups with 15 million
participants in the United States alone. The range of problems addressed by the groups continues to expand.

TYPES OF SELF-HELP MUTUAL AID GROUPS

There are groups addressed to particular mental health conditions, for example, Depressives Anonymous, Manic-Depressives Anonymous, Neurotics Anonymous, and Schizophrenics Anonymous. Evans (1979) and Gartner and Riessman (1979) offer extensive listings of self-help mutual aid groups, with the latter including an index both of type of problem addressed and geographic location of group headquarters.

There are also groups concerned with the mental health needs of various population groups. For each of the "special populations" groups discussed in Part IV of this book, one or more self-help mutual aid groups exist: older adults (see Lieberman & Gourash, 1980); children whose parents have a specific problem (Alateen); parent toward the child (Parents Anonymous); the consequences of parents' behavior toward the child (Daughters and Sons United); minority group members (Sisterhood of Black Single Mothers); mentally retarded (National Association for Retarded Citizens); women (Abused Women's Aid in Crisis and La Leche League); and chronically disabled (Center for Independent Living). Self-help groups deal with the same specialized problem areas to which CMHCs direct services such as alcoholism (the Calix Society, the National Association of Recovered Alcoholics in the Professions, and Women for Sobriety) and drug dependency (Delancey Street Foundation, Narcotics Anonymous, and Pills Anonymous).

We see that self-help mutual aid groups provide two unique features in support of prevention. They provide social support to their members through the creation of a caring community, and they increase members' coping skills through the provision of information and sharing of experiences and problem solutions. It is no surprise that the Council on Prevention of the National Council of Community Mental Health Centers has identified self-help groups as an effective, efficient model that is within the resources of CMHCs across the country (Self-Help Fostered by Community Mental Health Centers, 1979).

Another way to view the range of self-help mutual aid groups is to note those that relate to parents and children. There are groups for those who are pregnant (Self-Help Education Initiative in Childbirth). Several groups exist for parents: parents of "normal" newborns (Postpartum Education Project); those whose babies are born prematurely (Premature and High Risk Infants); and those whose children die at birth (Aiding a Mother Experiencing Neo-Natal Death) or in the first year (National Foundation for Sudden Infant Death Syndrome). Still others meet for adopted children seeking their natural parents (Adoptees' Liberty Movement Association) and for parents who have surrendered children for adoption (Concerned United Birthparents). There are groups for single parents (Parents Without Partners), mothers (Association of Professional Women Who Are Mothers), and fathers (Fathers' Rights). Still other groups give support to parents with children who are "normal" (Parent Care), handicapped, or dying (the Candlelighters). Other groups convene for those whose relatives are institutionalized (Friends and Relatives of the Institutionalized Aged) (Killilea, 1976; Gartner & Riessman, 1980).

We need not belabor the point to assure the reader that whatever the concerns of a particular CMHC, there are self-help mutual aid groups addressed to the topic. But, of course, the mere existence of such groups does not resolve the issues of the appropriateness of the CMHC in becoming involved in such activities or the ways and means of going about it. It is to these issues that we now turn our attention.

SHOULD CMHCs BE INVOLVED WITH
SELF-HELP MUTUAL AID GROUPS?

Two issues arise in terms of the appropriateness of a CMHC becoming involved with self-help mutual aid activities. First, do these groups provide useful and helpful services and second, can a CMHC play a positive role with them. As with much in the mental health arena, there are few good research data indicating effectiveness. Those groups most studied have been AA (Tiebout, 1944; Stewart, 1955; Phillips, 1973) and the weight-reducing groups. In the mental health field, those of greatest scholarly attention have been groups for ex-inpatients, Recovery, Inc. (Low, 1950; Wechsler, 1960; Lee, 1971; Grosz, 1972; Raiff, 1979; Raiff, 1980), groups for abusing parents (Lieber, 1976; Behavior Associates, 1977; Wheatt & Lieber, 1979; Lieber, 1980), and groups providing aftercare for the formerly institutionalized (Sanders, 1976; Edmunson, Bedell, Archer, & Gordon, 1980; and Edmunson, Bedell, & Gordon, 1980).

Two new books by Lieberman and Borman (1979) and Gartner and Riessman (1980) contain several essays on evaluation of self-help groups. At this writing, there have been no large-scale longitudinal studies and few with control groups. What has been found is suggestive and reinforcing of participants' reports of self-satisfaction, a clear signal for more systematic attention. With these caveats, findings worth noting here are those by Raiff (1980) concerning Recovery, Inc., and by Edmunson, Bedell, Archer, and Gordon (1980) on a program for deinstitutionalized patients in Florida.

Raiff studied the most highly "involved" participants of Recovery, Inc. —group leaders, administrators, and 'helpers." She gathered data on their medical backgrounds (more than half had been hospitalized for a nervous problem), current utilization of professionally organized health care systems, and self-attitudes regarding mental health. She reports that the "entire Recovery leadership cohort ranks high on all these health-related indicators."

In the Florida project, a Community Network Development (CND) group, a form of a self-help mutual aid group, was established among discharged patients. After ten months, one-half as many patients in the CND group had required rehospitalization as compared with a control group (17.5 percent to 35 percent), and their average total days of rehospitalization was less than a third as long (7.0 days versus 24.6 days). Twice as many CND members were able to function without any mental health system contact (52.5 percent versus 26 percent).

HOW SELF-HELP MUTUAL AID WORKS

In both Recovery, Inc. and the Florida Community Network Development Program, persons with the problem play special leadership roles. And, as we have seen in Raiff's (1980) study, they derive special benefits. This appears to be the case as well in Florida, where the effects on the groups' peer leaders were even more positive than for members as a whole—for example, no peer leader was rehospitalized.

These findings suggest that in the helping function there may be something especially therapeutic. Of course, this phenomenon is exactly what Riessman (1965) sought to capture with his "helper-therapy" concept. In its simplest form, this principle states that those who help are helped most.

Thus, an alcoholic in AA who is providing help and support to another AA member may be the one who is benefiting most by playing this helping, giving role. Furthermore, since all members of the group play this role at one time or another, they are all benefited. In a sense, this is true of all helpers, whether they be professionals, volunteers, or whatever, but it is more sharply true for helpers who have the same problem as the one who is helped. While all help-givers may be helped themselves in a nonspecific way, people who have a particular problem may be helped in much more specific ways by providing help to others who have the same problem. Dewar (1976, p. 81) points out that "It feels good to be the helper. It increases our sense of control, of being valued, of being capable."

There are numerous mechanisms postulated to explain the potential power of the helper-therapy idea. Skovholt (1974) has summarized the benefits received from helping into four factors: (1) an increased feeling of interpersonal competence due to impacting on another's life; (2) a sense of equality in giving and taking between oneself and others; (3) receiving of valuable personalized learning while working with a person in need; and (4) receiving social approval from the other. Skovholt hypothesizes that all four factors, rather than any one, make the helper-therapy principle potent.

In addition, there are at least three additional mechanisms to account for the fact that the person playing the helping role achieves special benefits: the helper is less dependent, has a chance to observe his or her own problem at a distance, and obtains a feeling of social usefulness. The entire helper-therapy concept is derived from role theory, whereby a person playing a role tends to carry out the expectations and requirements of that role. In effect, as a helper the individual displays mastery over the afflicting condition (in playing the role of a nonaddict, for example) and thereby acquires the appropriate skills, attitudes, behaviors, and mental set. Having modeled this for others, the individual may see himself or herself as behaving in a new way and may in effect take on the new role as his or her own.

While key to understanding the activities of self-help mutual aid groups, the "helper-therapy" principle does not stand alone in helping in the understanding of the processes of self-help mutual aid. The group itself is a key factor, since it provides support, reinforcement, sanctions, and norms, extends the power of the individual, provides feedback, and occupies time. While the latter might normally be regarded negatively, the addicted person's involvement in the group does help to fill time and to replace the activities involved in the addiction. It is not uncommon for alcoholics to attend AA meetings several night a week, both to give and receive help.

Katz (1970) provides a useful overview of some of the processes of self-help that are related to the group:

1. Peer or primary group reference identification.
2. Facilitation of communication because members are peers.
3. Enhanced opportunities for socialization.
4. Breaking down of individual psychological defenses through group action, open discussion, and confrontation.

5. Provision of an acceptable status system within
which the member can achieve his place.
6. Simulation of or proximity to conditions of the outside world in the groups.

These factors are particularly significant for people who have
been excluded, for whatever reason, from society's mainstream.
In the self-help setting, they can experience normal social contacts
as well as communication that is unhampered by irrelevant barriers.
Most important, they can experience the opportunity for leadership.
Although a self-help group includes professional or volunteer participation or may even be the result of a human service worker's
initial prodding, its potential for success is based on the active participation and commitment of its members. Those members must
know that there is "room at the top. "

While we have emphasized the group members' similarities,
there is a key difference between oldtimers and newcomers. In discussing the helper-therapy concept, we have noted that the oldtimers
benefit in the process of helping others. But there is benefit, too,
for the newcomers. Festinger (1954) has argued that individuals
are most influenced by persons whom they perceive as like themselves. In the statement of an oldtimer at an AA meeting that he is
an alcoholic but obviously under control, the new member sees what
he himself can become.

A further aspect of many of the self-help groups is their ideological character. Ideology goes beyond the activity of the individual
to involvement in something beyond oneself to a broader commitment and to social change. This is perhaps most obvious in consciousness-raising groups and in parent groups. But it is also op-
erative in the various deviant and stigmatized groups, such as homo-
sexuals, former offenders, stutterers, midgets, and other social
outcasts where the ideology of the group involves criticism of society
and the demand for social change. This criticism is also frequently
directed at professionals and social agencies. The ideological perspective of the self-help group gives it force and conviction in dealing with these agencies and in feeling more positive about itself and
its condition.

While part of the force powering many self-help mutual aid
groups is antipathy toward professionals and their organizations,
the great bulk of self-help mutual aid groups involves various forms
of professional participation. Recovery, Inc. was founded by a
psychiatrist, Abraham A. Low. Parents Anonymous was co-founded
by a psychiatric social worker, Leonard Lieber, and has a professional sponsor for each group (Willen, 1980). Many of the large
national health organizations, American Cancer Society (Laryngec-

tomy, Inc.; Reach to Recovery), American Heart Association (Stroke Clubs), the TB and Lung Association (Easy Breathers), the National Multiple Sclerosis Society (The Hopefuls), and the Epilepsy Foundation, sponsor self-help mutual aid groups. The National Council of Community Mental Health Centers at its 1979 annual meeting made support and development of self-help mutual aid activities a national priority.

Great impetus has been offered in this direction by the Report of the President's Commission on Mental Health (1978). The Report gives broad support to the importance of the formal mental health caregiving system in relating to community support networks. It also makes specific recommendations to CMHCs, namely, developing directories of self-help groups, encouraging referrals to such groups, training agency personnel to work with them,* and sponsoring conferences between professionals and self-help participants.

HOW A CMHC CAN BE INVOLVED
WITH SELF-HELP GROUPS

We turn now from these general areas of relationship to six specific topics by which CMHCs can relate to self-help mutual aid activities: creating self-help groups, making referrals to the groups, consulting with the groups, strengthening support networks, developing indigenous helping networks, and conducting research.

Creating a Group

There are many examples of professionals actually setting up self-help groups where none previously existed. The most usual pattern occurs when professionals spot a need among their clients and set up a situation in which a self-help group can develop. Summarizing the way professionals can help in the formation of self-help groups, Gottlieb (1979) has suggested that professionals can create new occasions for the development of mutual help groups by identifying and connecting people in similar stressful circumstances

---

*The Experimental Training Division, NIMH, funds a unique program, "Urban Training and Brokerage," at the Graduate School and University Center, City University of New York. It brings together leaders of self-help mutual aid groups and professionals interested in self-help mutual aid activities, who then train each other in appropriate techniques.

and by proposing a general scenario to be followed at group meetings. Furthermore, epidemiological tools, such as measurement
of stressful life events and usage of social indicators, can help to
identify potential group members.

Gerald Caplan has written about the process of organizing
mutual support groups. He suggests that the professional begin by
meeting with two or three people suffering with a common problem
and then introducing them to an individual who has already dealt
with that difficulty. The number of people then can be increased to
form a small group. Caplan sees the role of the professional as a
"support for the supporters" and as a provider of continuity in the
group sessions (Caplan & Killilea, 1976).

The Widow-to-Widow program typifies this pattern. It was
developed by Phyllis Silverman, a social worker, in collaboration
with Caplan and his Harvard group. Silverman's and Caplan's idea
was to prevent serious emotional problems in newly widowed women
by offering each the help of another widow. At the heart of the program were one-to-one meetings of these widow-aides and the recently widowed. Aides were trained to use their own experience as
well as what they learned in workshops. Two years were required
to prepare a widow to counsel others.

Compassionate Friends is a self-help group comprised of
parents who have suffered the death of a child. S. Neal, the social
services secretary of Compassionate Friends, describes the formation of that group:

> In 1969, our founder, the Rev. Simon Stephens, was
> acting as Chaplain to a . . . hospital where, as it hap-
> pened, two teenage boys lay dying at the same time.
> In the course of ministering to these boys and their
> parents he observed how much comfort the parents
> seemed to derive from talking to each other, and it
> was from this chance occurrence that the Compassion-
> ate Friends came to be formed. (Gartner & Riessman,
> 1979, p. 169)

The sensitivity of the professional, in this case a minister,
to the common needs of his clients was the impetus leading to the
formation of this group. Compassionate Friends has since grown
widely in England and America. At present, there are 105 chapters
throughout the United States.

Parents Anonymous (PA) was begun in 1970 as a collaboration
between Leonard Lieber, a psychiatric social worker, and two
women whom he was counseling, mothers who were abusing their
children and wanted to stop. The three established a self-help group

that has now grown to an organization comprising over 1,000 chapters, each holding weekly meetings. The format of the meetings is fairly ritualized: members admit their problem, pledge to stay free of it one day at a time, accept responsibility for their behavior, and promise to keep group matters confidential. In this sense, PA is very much in the mold of other anonymous groups.

But Parents Anonymous is somewhat different from other anonymous groups in its use of professionals. Doctors and social workers serve on PA's Board of Directors and Advisory Council. PA requires in its carefully spelled out "Chapter Development Manual" that each local chapter have as its sponsor a mental health professional "who has a profound respect for the self-help concept." PA is thus a "mixed" organization, combining some basic features of other anonymous groups with a level of professional involvement generally not tolerated by them.

Many self-help groups have involved professionals from their inception. Laryngectomy, Inc., for instance, was developed by the American Cancer Society under strong medical supervision. Daytop Lodge was begun by professionals using the basic self-help approach modeled after Synanon.

Some self-help groups, however, have been uninterested in involvement with professionals. Alcoholics Anonymous (AA), the prototype of anonymous groups, is sometimes cited as a group co-founded by a physician. This attribution is misleading: although Dr. Bob, AA's co-founder, was indeed a physician, he was also an alcoholic. His primary orientation was that of a consumer, and from its earliest origin, AA has been emphatically aprofessional.

In order to encourage patients to carry out a self-help program that would permit them to control their symptoms and to prevent relapses, a Chicago psychiatrist named Abraham Low founded Recovery, Inc. in 1937. Recovery groups were originally closely tied to the medical profession, meeting in hospitals and supervised by doctors. Often the doctors asked members to report back to them about other members' behavior at the meetings. This requirement forced the groups to move away from the hospitals and into the community.

Although Low's influence on the groups was profound in establishing the structure of meetings and setting the philosophical tone of Recovery, Inc., he himself was instrumental in keeping Recovery from being dominated by professionals. He stipulated that professionals could not become group leaders or hold office. Under Low's guidance, a training program was established that permitted members to follow the goals of Recovery without further professional supervision. The organization was expanded so that Recovery, Inc. is now the largest ex-patient group, with 15,000 members organized into nearly a thousand groups.

Making Referrals

Making referrals to self-help groups for those individuals who can benefit from them is another important function for professionals. In this regard, it is important for the professional to have specific knowledge of the correlation between a client's characteristics, the group's admission criteria, and the details of the program. An unacceptable candidate, or a person who enters a group with unrealistic expectations and then has a disappointing experience, can do more harm than good by hindering the group's progress or by "bad mouthing" the group to the referring professional. Agencies such as courts or mental health professionals are not always sensitive to the fact that there are many clients who do not respond to a group situation. However, the greatest referral problem is the ignorance of professionals as to the existence of self-help groups (Gottleib, 1979).

Consulting with Groups

Professionals can work within the self-help framework by thinking of themselves as caregivers providing services for a group of people who share the same problem rather than serving a single client. Problem-centered consultation is usually initiated by a member of a self-help group in order to get help with specific problems in programs, policies, training, administration, or any aspect of a human service. By being open and flexible and by becoming sensitive to the needs and objectives of the group, the consultant may propose a plan of action. Drawing on his or her knowledge of systems theory, organizational development, human behavior, and interpersonal dynamics, the consultant can impart information, model appropriate communication skills, facilitate problem solving, and provide support. The more consultants are able to enhance the group members' own abilities, the more effective they are as change agents.

Richard Wollert, a psychologist with self-help expertise, provided consultation services to one chapter of Make Today Count, a self-help group of cancer patients and their spouses. His suggestions were considered by group members to be instrumental in improving the effectiveness and organizational structure of their group. At the members' request, Wollert's guidelines were formalized, and have subsequently been distributed by the national organization to other chapters facing organizational difficulties.

Giving information to group members and educating people in crucial matters of concern to them can be seen as one aspect of the professional consulting function. In a group formed by parents who abuse their children, a professional can provide factual information and teach group members basic communication skills. Groups composed of people who must learn to use medically dictated contrivances like prosthetics or dialysis machines obviously must be educated in their use. Teaching groups of prospective parents how to play an active role in natural childbirth is another example of the educational function of professional consultants.

Strengthening Support Networks

Developing supportive networks is a task that has recently emerged as central to the mental health of families in crisis, as well as that of recuperating patients. Under the guidance of family therapists, the concept of family network therapy has grown out of family therapy. Most often, what happens in family network therapy is that when a family and its therapist agree that network intervention is the best approach to a problem, family members contact relatives, friends, neighbors, schoolmates, and work associates (15 to 100 people), and invite them to participate by coming to a meeting at the home of the family. Although the network has come together because of a specific problem or person, the intervener's goal is to refocus or reunite the entire network into a resource and support structure for the entire group as well as for the identified patient. The professionals are essentially trying to educate a community in ways to help itself. By creating an atmosphere of freedom so that change can take place, they build trust for the entire network. Working on this level of helping to strengthen a supportive network may be the right step in the direction of preventive services from professional helpers.

Community network therapy is an approach that combines working directly with troubled children using family systems therapy, school consultation, patient advocacy, and the nurturance of supportive networks. It begins frequently with a referral by a school for assistance with a child's behavior problem. A team of two mental health professionals meets regularly with the school's adjustment counselors, nurses, and principal. The consultant team becomes a part of the child's network, which includes extended family, neighbors, friends, school, welfare, housing, employment or court representatives, charitable or church groups, children's extracurricular activity leaders, and other professionals such as doctors or ministers. The teams see themselves neither as managerial nor as parental authorities. Rather, they are consultants whose expertise lies in the ability to describe, sort out, and coordinate relationships of a family to various service facilities in the community, and to adjust their own views and roles according to the network's influence.

The peer management approach is based on the assumption that it is therapeutic for patients to assume responsibility both for themselves and for other patients. Typically, patient groups are trained by the staff to utilize their own insights, skills, and problem-solving abilities to handle most problems of everyday life. The group then operates autonomously, with the staff primarily functioning in the role of advisors or facilitators.

The prototype for a successful peer management project of this type is the Community Lodge program for ex-mental patients developed by George Fairweather in California. This program has been in existence for more than ten years and has demonstrated its value as a very reasonable alternative to institutionalization and more traditional treatments of mental patients.

More recently, the Florida Mental Health Institute has developed an extensive peer management and support program. Under this program, patients receive training in providing mutual aid and in developing community networks. Helping chronic schizophrenics to move out of institutions and to function usefully in society is a goal for people concerned with mental health. Frequently what happens is that "cured" patients are dumped into communities. Lacking supportive networks and typically quite isolated, they very quickly wind up right back in the hospital. Using a combination of innovative methods and techniques that have proved effective in the past, Richard Gordon and his associates in Florida have succeeded in dramatically reducing the rate of rehospitalization of discharged mental patients.

The most outstanding characteristic of the Florida project is the development of a Peer Mutual Aid Network, which is begun while patients are still in the hospital and continued after they are discharged. Becoming part of this program while still in the hospital, patients are helped in peer self-management techniques. They are taught to use games that build up their technical skills, and are strongly encouraged to take on responsibilities, to run their own meetings, to develop leadership skills, and to learn lifeskills aimed at helping them when they leave the institution. The role of the staff is minimized. Staff do not problem-solve for patients, nor in any way provide traditional counseling.

Once in the community, discharged patients join in the Community Network Development (CND) program, a community-based, patient-managed leadership and support program that prepares patients for the transition from residential treatment to community life. An administrative network is set up among the patients that includes the training of area managers and an overall director.

These ex-patient personnel then carry out the functioning of other CND activities, including weekly and monthly meetings, fund raising events, and other social and supportive functions.

Developing Indigenous Helping Networks

Identifying and recruiting indigenous helpers, linking them to each other, enhancing their functioning, and stimulating local helping networks are all crucial functions. One type of professional involvement is designed to strengthen the ability of neighbors to be helpful to people who are part of their social network. The major focus is on enhancing the helpers' abilities to cope with current "clients" and with future "clients" who present similar problems. The clients in this case are friends, neighbors, and acquaintances of the natural helper.

A demonstration project recently reported by Shirley L. Patterson and her associates at the University of Kansas had, as one of its prime objectives, to "nurture and enhance indigenous helping efforts" without changing the special qualities of the natural helpers. The basic premise of the project was that the professional was to be viewed as an extension of the abilities and skills of the helper, not the reverse. "Natural helper" was defined as one to whom people turn naturally in time of trouble or difficulty. To achieve the objectives of the demonstration, the professional staff tried to support and reinforce helper contributions in helping situations. An effort was made to encourage the helper in the use of his or her own methods in dealing with difficult problems and to emphasize the attributes that the natural helper brought to the helping relationship. The role of the professional was to encourage and assist helpers to proceed in their own helping roles in their own ways (described in Gartner & Riessman, 1979).

Benjamin Gottlieb (1979) describes a program set up for the purpose of stimulating the development of natural helping networks. This project (located in Guelph, Ontario) was designed to train three groups of people—agency professionals, welfare recipients, and social service volunteers—in basic helping and human relations skills. A partial aim of this program was preventive and involved outreach into vulnerable populations in the community, for example, workshops for single parents and training in job readiness skills. Gottlieb reports excellent results toward these goals, as well as substantial cost savings.

Peer tutoring/counseling services that have developed in the last several years are another area in which professionals have become involved. One such program was developed in a large public high school. Under the supervision of the school psychologist and guidance counselor, students were trained to provide tutoring and/or counseling services to other students with academic or adjustment problems. Evaluation of this peer-counseling project indicates that it was successful in training students to serve a large number of their peers, especially on an informal, personal/social level (discussed in Gartner & Riessman, 1979).

Peer counseling in hospital settings is usually done informally with patients deriving mutual support from sharing experiences. Sometimes, however, the professional staff is instrumental in bringing together people who can benefit from exchanging experiences. Frederick Guggenheim reports case histories of patients who derived significant support from sessions planned by a psychiatrist and a nurse clinician. Each therapeutic intervention brought together two patients with a similar illness, one who had recovered from its major effects and the other who was in the initial stages of the illness. Since the task of the newly disabled individual is to contend with and develop some sense of mastery of the disability, meeting a patient who has coped successfully can be very therapeutic. It can help the recently disabled person to perceive himself or herself as handicapped rather than as an invalid. Peer counseling can cut through overwhelming anxiety and move a patient from hopelessness to motivation. It seems clear that arranging such therapeutic peer interactions is a valid and useful function for hospital personnel.

Conducting Research

There is a definite need for research of all types into the functioning of self-help programs. General articles describing the psychological properties of groups or delineating situations in which self-help groups are likely to be more effective than other types of treatment are important to undertake.

A determination of just what changes can be expected in groups is being carried out by Wollert. He speculates that self-help groups have a significant impact on their members in the reduction of feelings of helplessness, social isolation, and abnormality. Wollert also theorizes that self-help groups are a source of factual information and attitude change. Thomas Powell, a social worker at the University of Michigan, has looked at the role played by ideology in influencing people to join self-help groups.

Professionals can play an important role in assessing a group's success in achieving its goals, as well as the factors accounting for its success. Much evaluation research is currently going on in this regard. Gordon's group assessing the peer management program at the Florida Mental Health Institute has tried to specify in great detail exactly what aspects of the program can best account for the good results they have had in reducing recidivism. Gary Bond and his Chicago associates are currently conducting research into the Mended Hearts program to document the working relationship it has established with the medical community and to confirm statistically the effectiveness of the self-help group.

Since self-help groups are not usually professional creations nor controlled by any human service agency, special sensitivity and respect for their procedures and ideologies must be maintained by researchers. It seems reasonable, too, for a group to expect that research exploring its functioning will lead to important payoffs for the group itself, as well as for "science" and "education."

REFERENCES

Behavior Associates. Parents Anonymous, self-help for child abusing parents project: Evaluation report. Tucson, Ariz., 1977.

Caplan, G., & Killelea, M. (Eds.). Support systems and mutual help. New York: Grune and Stratton, 1976.

Dewar, T. Professionalized clients as self-helpers. Self-help and health: A report. New York: National Self-Help Clearinghouse, Graduate School and University Center, City University of New York, 1976.

Edmunson, E. D., Bedell, J. R., Archer, R. P., & Gordon, R. E. Integrating skill building and peer support. The Early Intervention and Community Network Development Project. In R. Slotnik and A. Jaeger (Eds.), Community Mental Health: A Behavioral-Ecological Perspective. New York: Plenum Press, 1980.

Edmunson, E. D., Bedell, J. R., & Gordon, R. E. The Community Network Development Project: Bridging the gap between professional aftercare and self-help. In A. Gartner and F. Riessman (Eds.), Mental Health and the Self-Help Revolution. New York: Human Sciences Press, 1980.

Evans, G. Family Circle guide to self-help. New York: Ballantine Books, 1979.

Festinger, L. A theory of social comparison processes. Human Relations, 1954, 7, 117-140.

Gartner, A., & Riessman, F. Help: A working guide to self-help groups. New York: Franklin Watts, 1979.

Gartner, A., & Riessman, F. (Eds.). Mental health and the self-help revolution. New York: Human Sciences Press, 1980.

Gottlieb, B. H. Opportunities for collaboration with informal support systems. In S. Cooper and W. F. Hodges (Eds.), The Field of Mental Health Consultation. New York: Human Sciences Press, 1979.

Grosz, H. J. Recovery, Inc. Chicago: Recovery, Inc., 1972.

Katz, A. H. Self-help organizations and volunteer participation in social welfare. Social Work, 1970, 15, 51-60.

Killilea, M. Mutual help organizations: Interpretation in the literature. In G. Caplan and M. Killilea (Eds.), Support Systems and Mutual Help. New York: Grune and Stratton, 1976.

Lee, D. T. Recovery, Inc.: A well-role model. Mental Hygiene, 1971, 55, 194-198.

Lieber, L. Parents Anonymous. Child Abuse and Neglect Reports, 1976, 3, 1-2.

Lieber, L. Parents Anonymous: The use of self-help in the treatment and prevention of family violence. In A. Gartner and F. Riessman (Eds.), Mental Health and the Self-Help Revolution. New York: Human Sciences Press, 1980.

Lieberman, M. A., & Borman, L. D. (Eds.). Self-help groups for coping with crisis: Origins, members, processes, and impact. San Francisco: Jossey-Bass, 1979.

Lieberman, M. A., & Gourash, N. From professional help to self-help: An evaluation of therapeutic groups for the elderly. In A. Gartner & F. Riessman (Eds.), Mental Health and the Self-Help Revolution. New York: Human Sciences Press, 1980.

Low, A. A. Mental health through will training. Boston: Christopher, 1950.

Phillips, J. Alcoholics Anonymous: An annotated bibliography, 1935-1972. Cincinnati: Central Ohio Publishing, 1973.

Raiff, N. R. Recovery, Inc.: A study of a self-help organization in mental health. Unpublished manuscript, 1979.

Raiff, N. R. Some health related outcomes of self-help participation: Recovery, Inc. as a case example of a self-help organization in mental health. In A. Gartner and F. Riessman (Eds.), Mental Health and the Self-Help Revolution. New York: Human Sciences Press, 1980.

Report of the President's Commission on Mental Health. Washington, D.C.: U.S. Government Printing Office, 1978.

Riessman, F. The "Helper-Therapy" principle. Social Work, 1965, 10, 27-32.

Roepal, C. E. A study of California public attitudes and beliefs regarding mental and physical health. San Francisco: California Department of Mental Health, Office of Prevention, 1979.

Sanders, D. H. The lodge program in community rehabilitation. In A. Katz and E. Bender (Eds.), The Strength in Us. New York: Franklin Watts, 1976.

Self-help fostered by Community Mental Health Centers. Self-Help Reporter, 1979, 3, 1-2.

Skovholt, T. M. The client as helper: A means to promote psychological growth. Counseling Psychologist, 1974, 4, 58-64.

Stewart, D. A. The dynamics of fellowship as illustrated in Alcoholics Anonymous. Quarterly Journal of Studies on Alcoholism, 1955, 16, 251-262.

Tiebout, H. M. Therapeutic mechanisms of AA. American Journal of Psychiatry, 1944, 100, 468-473.

Wechsler, H. The self-help organization in the mental health field: Recovery, Inc., a case study. Journal of Nervous and Mental Disorders, 1960, 130, 297-314.

Wheatt, P., & Lieber, L. Hope for the children: A personal history of Parents Anonymous. Minneapolis: Winston Press, 1979.

Willen, M. Parents Anonymous: The professionals' role as sponsor. In A. Gartner and F. Riessman, Mental Health and the Self-Help Revolution. New York: Human Sciences Press, 1980.

14

EMERGENCY SERVICES IN A
COMMUNITY MENTAL HEALTH CENTER
W. Brian Rines

Offering emergency services in a comprehensive community mental health center (CMHC) is a difficult but very rewarding task. The staff operates in an emotionally charged environment foreign to most mental health clinicians. Immediate decisions must be made, frequently with limited information. The police and other helping agents are often involved, while supervisors and trusted colleagues are usually absent. On many occasions, a clinical decision is reviewed by an emergency room physician with little knowledge of mental health theory or practice. And, finally, there is the pressure of time, which relentlessly pushes a decision. The emergency service is one of those arenas that draws immediate attention in the community and one that can be most easily misunderstood and misused. This chapter discusses the goals and methods of such a program, and presents some of my own views and experiences.

WHY DO WE NEED EMERGENCY SERVICES?

Emergency service is one of the five essential components initially mandated by federal community mental health centers legislation. If for no other reason, every center must have an emergency service to continue receiving federal funds. But that alone, of course, would not justify its existence. More important is the fact that an emergency unit provides a special and unique service that is usually the first and often the only one utilized by clients.

213

WHAT ARE EMERGENCY SERVICES?

A CMHC emergency unit provides a broad range of interventions. Traditionally, one of its major roles is to offer a triage or sorting mechanism in general hospital emergency rooms (ER) in order to separate those who need psychiatric hospitalization from those who do not. Under National Institute of Mental Health (NIMH) guidelines, the screening role is required. However, facilitating admissions to hospitals is a secondary function of the emergency unit. The largest amount of time and energy is spent keeping the chronically mentally ill out of hospitals through crisis intervention and by linkage to other social service agencies.

The emergency unit admits people who have never before been treated by the mental health system. Frequently, we find someone who has sat at home for months with a problem and then decides rather impulsively at three o'clock on Saturday morning that he/she has to talk to someone about it. It falls to the emergency worker to do the evaluation or at least to arrange for the client to receive an appropriate evaluation at a later time. A hospital-based emergency unit often finds itself consulting with other medical services of the hospital at all hours of the day and night.

Other social service agencies may also use an emergency unit to do their crisis work during off hours. Great care must be taken to ensure that "dumping" of their problem cases does not occur. The police, fire department, and other crisis-oriented public agencies actively call upon an emergency unit to assist them.

Specialized treatment is frequently demanded of the emergency unit for victims of assault and rape. Political issues arise in providing these services, and great sensitivity is needed if the support group that initially sought emergency assistance will continue to use it. If community groups discover that the emergency room and the mental health emergency service are staffed by males, they may choose not to use them and to implement alternative care. Emergency services should also be made available to other assault victims.

Emergencies sometimes happen to entire communities rather than to individuals, as in transportation crashes, tornadoes, earthquakes, and disastrous floods. The service provided in these situations extends through many months and involves more than immediate crisis alleviation. To deal with these catastrophies may require the involvement of the entire center. Silverman (1977) points out quite accurately that the services should be matched carefully to the cultural and social expectations of the community if they are to succeed. Davidson (1979) discusses very poignantly the provision of these services to an entire police and fire department after a catastrophic airplane crash in San Diego. In this tragedy services were needed

not only by the survivors, but also by others who were touched by
it through family or neighborhood contacts or by occupational demands such as rescue work.

Basically, an emergency unit provides short-term, immediate
relief in crises. Services that can be obtained by the potential patient or victim should be oriented to discovering the person's
strengths and weaknesses and his/her coping mechanisms. While
a portion of this discovery might occur in individual counseling
sessions, certainly assignment of a DSM II or III diagnosis is less
important than an evaluation of the person's human needs and resources.

Some centers have found it helpful to have a continuing open
group for emergency clients who essentially enter into a very short-
term treatment contract with a specially trained clinician. Patients
should be selected very carefully for such a crisis group, since
long-term treatment may be needed. Inappropriate disposition often
necessitates reuse of the emergency service. It is my impression,
however, that most of the problems presented to an emergency unit
by patients who are not chronically mentally ill are responsive to
such treatment.

The emergency unit also gives evaluation or prevention services for suicide-prone individuals. This particular activity requires a special sense of clinical judgment and is fraught with substantial peril to the crisis worker and to the CMHC. This topic will
be discussed in greater detail in a later section.

WHO PROVIDES EMERGENCY SERVICES?

The providers range from the unlettered neighborhood "natural
therapist" who practices in her/his own community to the most sophisticated mental health professional. Today one finds fewer members of either group practicing in an emergency setting. The radical bloom seems to have gone from community mental health, and
the intense involvement of indigenous "mental health field workers"
seems to have diminished markedly. Similarly, the great glory and
commitment of working in the trenches with the poor and downtrodden
seems to have lessened. Finding a well-trained clinician willing to
work actively in an emergency service is becoming harder and harder.
Monetary gain is limited, there are few immediate reinforcements,
and the work is often "dirty" as well as dangerous.

Since the emergency contact is often the first and, if not
handled appropriately, last contact with the mental health center,
an emergency staff should be chosen from among the most compe-
tently trained clinicians available. Full-time professionals work in

our unit, but we are able to rotate the duty to attract professionals
to work weekend hours. We must pay them an additional salary,
but for the quality of services received the investment is well worth
it. For afterhours (weeknight) coverage, we employ a prebacca-
laureate level individual with many years of experience in inpatient
and outpatient care. He has substantial psychological and psychiatric
backup available should he need it. In my judgment, the center's
best clinicians should be enticed in some fashion to work in this
area, since it demands the greatest sense of judgment and clinical
skill of any unit.

WHO ARE THESE CLIENTS?

The literature and our experience continue to suggest that
most clients are not emergencies in the classical sense of the word.
Most clients coming to an emergency unit are not in a life-threatening situation (only about 3 percent are), nor do they need immediate
psychiatric hospitalization. Indeed, they tend to be chronic aftercare patients who have virtually no other service available to them.
These people are neglected by society and see the emergency unit
as one of the few places mandated by law and custom to assist them.
The major problem of typical chronic aftercare clients is usually
tangentially psychological in nature. They often are without food,
shelter, and (in the Northeast) fuel. Their first response is to return to the hospital for these basic necessities, and the emergency
unit has the responsibility of deflecting that admission. These
shortages can create psychological difficulties, under which circumstances a formal intervention may be appropriate. In most of the
cases, however, screening and referral to the appropriate agencies
is indicated. This type of intervention is, perhaps, the most taxing
that an emergency worker faces. The resources are usually insufficient and require a great deal of time and energy since the direct
providers of these resources do not particularly want to give them
to the aftercare population.
    Rape and assault victims are in a special kind of crisis that
requires particular interventions. Usually these people are accompanied to the emergency site by a police officer, who may or may
not have received specialized training in coping with these victims.
Whatever his training, however, the officer has a responsibility far
different from that of the emergency clinician. He/she needs to
"close the case" by capturing the rapist or assailant, while the clinician wishes to provide the maximum psychological assistance to the
victim. There are many behavioral choices available to a victim,
and some of them are not going to make the police officer happy. In

addition to the alleviation of the immediate crisis, which may involve talking with other family members or spouses, the victim has to be prepared for a continuing series of psychological events that are quite predictable. Additionally, the victim will have to make some decisions about prosecution and the potential problems that relate to participating in that process. Burgess and Holmstrom (1974, 1979) have written the definitive books in this area, which ought to be available to all emergency workers. Specialized in-service training to deal with these crises should also be encouraged.

The "garden variety" emergency patient is someone who is seeking services for the first time, usually during off hours. It is our experience that most (approximately 80 percent) of these people do not return for further outpatient services. Nevertheless, as is the case with the medical emergency room, we have to serve those who do not seem able to schedule their lives to get the help they need in a regular and consistent fashion. Hence, the emergency worker requires special training in giving as big a dose of psychotherapeutic "medicine" as is possible. The literature indicates that when care is taken to facilitate a comprehensive personal, social, and cultural assessment, linkages to significant others can be initiated. This, in turn, increases the probability that a client will stay involved in the service system. Gersen and Bassuk (1980) in an overview of psychiatric emergencies describe succinctly the ways that these comprehensive assessments can occur.

WHEN ARE EMERGENCY SERVICES PROVIDED?

NIMH insists that emergency services be provided on a 24-hour a day, seven-day-a-week, year-round basis. As indicated above, we have one regular person on duty every night from 4:30 in the afternoon to 8:30 the following morning, and other people work a staggered rotation throughout the weekend. The weekend people are regular full-time senior clinicians who buy blocks of weekend time for extra pay. Originally one clinician covered the whole week-end from 4:30 Friday to 8:30 Monday, but we found that the demands were too much on that person if he or she was scheduled to return to work Monday morning. Now we have three shifts: one from 4:30 Friday to 8:30 Saturday morning, the second to 8:30 Sunday morning, and the third to 8:30 Monday morning. After trying a number of different time schedules, we have found this one the easiest to maintain. Our weekend people are on call with a "beeper," responding to our answering service, which receives calls either directly from clients or other emergency services.

Emergencies are unscheduled, and the myth is that most of them occur about 4:15 on a Friday afternoon. The reality is that more emergencies are likely to occur on Monday morning immediately after the center opens. The peak times are in the late night hours of Tuesday and Saturday. I suspect that Tuesday night is popular because it is located not quite in the middle of the week and people are not sure that they are going to make it through. In the case of Saturday, calls are often precipitated by romantic spats or the greater use of alcohol than at other times during the week. Also, I suspect that people have unrealistic expectations for Saturday since it is a "free" day, and when those expectations are unmet they turn to us.

There is a peak of emergency visits after the winter holidays as well as at Easter. At those times, people seem to have discovered that the magic solutions to their problems, which were to have occurred with the holidays, were just fantasies. Usage in the summertime is not particularly high, but many crises are presented by people who are returning to jobs or home lives that do not truly satisfy them. They discover that their vacations did not change the problems they had.

Winter in New England is a stressful event, and the general and emergency use of mental health services peaks between November and March. I have no experience with more constant or moderate climates, but I would suspect a flatter frequency curve. Our utilization curve has deep valleys in the summer.

WHERE ARE EMERGENCY SERVICES PROVIDED ?

During the day, emergency services can be offered in CMHC outpatient offices. After hours, however, many choices are available. Our center uses an answering service. A trained, pleasantly voiced operator informs the caller that a professional is available and that the message will be relayed for an immediate return call. The responsibility of the on-call clinician is to contact as soon as possible the potential emergency client. A large portion of those clients can be helped by a telephone conversation. They usually are chronic aftercare clients who need a friendly ear. Our on-call workers are home-based, but have offices located in the emergency rooms (ER) of three hospitals in the catchment area.

We choose to provide our afterhour services in an ER setting because of the immediate availability of medical care and around-the-clock security. The police tend to respond immediately to a call for assistance from the ER. Also, it is usually located in a fairly accessible spot in the community.

There are difficulties, however, associated with the location of emergency services in the ER. The medical and nursing staff are there to save lives or limit the damage that can be caused by traumatic injury or acute illness. They are not always sensitive to the vague, amorphous, and ambivalent complaints often presented by our clients. The ER staff do not perceive themselves as social service agents responsible for finding heating oil in the middle of the winter. They should receive at least basic training in psychological screening skills, so that they do not push away clients who might need our services.

We have also located our treatment room immediately outside of but adjacent to the medical area of the ER, so that the tension, conflict, and high drama often present there can be avoided. There is nothing more upsetting to a person with a psychological emergency than to contend with another's crises. Many problems can be exacerbated or escalated into emergencies by such an active environment. Clients should be in a quiet, comfortable area away from the hurly-burly. We have found that the presence of coffee, juice, and other nonalcoholic beverages commonly associated with relaxation is helpful.

We also provide emergency service in our county jail, as well as in the city police lockup; but we insist on adequate protection and security for our staff. In my experience, most jailers and inmates accept and are even thankful to have mental health clinicians at their call, since we take care of their noisy and disruptive emotionally disturbed inmates and offer suicide prevention services.

Our emergency unit makes few home visits. Not only is it grossly uneconomical in terms of travel time, particularly in a rural catchment area such as ours, but it also makes more problems for the overburdened emergency worker. The substantial resources and backup required for emergency evaluation are not immediately available, and the worker must be concerned with personal safety in the home of a stranger.

In summation, a telephone emergency service is a necessary but insufficient mode of emergency service delivery. A CMHC must have a location that is accessible and public, and that is also comfortably furnished, private, and secure.

We have reviewed the who, what, where, when, and why of an emergency unit. From these basic conditions arise a series of problems that we will now consider.

EMERGENCY SERVICES ARE EXPENSIVE

An emergency service unit tends to be a "loss leader." Even if staffed with the center's least expensive clinicians and put in a rent-free environment with telephone provided, it cannot make its expenses. If the emergency unit is treated as an essential CMHC component and staffed with competent, well-paid, highly trained clinicians, it is going to cost approximately $65,000 per year. Our own cost is broken down to include a full-time staff member (or equivalent) working daytime hours at approximately $20,000/year, an afterhour weeknight person at approximately $15,000/year, another $15,000/year for part-time weekend staff, and additional money, approximately $8,000 in our case, for psychiatric backup for medical coverage. The last requirement is a legal one, because our unit is ultimately seen as medical. In our state, a psychiatrist must be contacted routinely to approve an admission to our inpatient unit, and he or she must also attend to emergencies when needed. In addition to the above personnel costs are the expenses of mileage, telephone, clerical, and general support services.

Emergency services cannot be run "on the cheap." While vigorous billing practices will afford some return on the investment, emergency services, be they psychological or medical, cannot be expected to break even. An additional financial burden may be placed on the client if services are delivered at an ER. Many hospitals charge separately for the use of the ER. We have an arrangement with our hospitals whereby charges are minimal if the client clearly is there to receive only our services.

Emergency costs can also have an impact on the cost of other services in the center's delivery system. If inpatient staff is chosen to administer the emergency unit, there will be increased costs in the inpatient budget that may well be hidden. Those detailed for emergency work are in the long haul superfluous to the inpatient staff, and their cost should rightfully be charged to emergency.

If the emergency unit is located in the center's own offices, there are additional costs in lighting, heating, and security that might otherwise not be required. One center in which I worked had a duty room where the emergency worker was able to sleep when he was not active clinically. The center provided linen and white goods. On-site security was not available, so "walk-ins" were seen at the ER of the community hospital two blocks away. Occasionally, when an agitated or threatening person was at the CMHC doorstep, the police had to move him or her to the ER before the clinical intervention could occur. We undoubtedly saved expensive security costs but did not endear ourselves to the local precinct.

Thus, there are trade-offs no matter where the emergency unit is placed. A good administrative team knows the costs and benefits of each one of its components. It is perhaps easiest to be confused about emergency care because clinicians and administrators often obfuscate the cost of this unit to protect it. The fact is that emergency units are expensive and will inevitably be a cash drain on the center.

HOW TO AVOID PROBLEMS WITH THE POLICE

One of the few other agencies in the community that operates on a 24-hour basis is the police department. It is the first organization with which an emergency service ought to have a liaison. A review of the activities of any modern U.S. police department will show that approximately 75 percent of its time is spent in social service. Police have the responsibility for the handling of problems with which no other agency wishes to work, and they should be perceived as allies and not as impediments. The key problem is that policemen often view mental health clinicians as a threat to their power and role. The police have learned by experience or tradition how to work with the social problems they face. They are not interested in a scientific explanation of their own behavior or that of their clients. They are least of all interested in becoming a "shrink," whom they tend to regard as a relatively useless person who thinks about problems rather than acting on them. Policemen cannot be made into psychotherapists, or vice versa, but with care and time they can be taught to perform their duties more effectively. In turn, they have skills they can teach clinicians. Morton Bard, a psychologist and former policeman, has written extensively on this subject (Bard, 1975; Bard & Berkowitz, 1967).

One trap that policemen sometimes set for clinicians is to co-opt them into becoming plainclothes "cop-shrinks." It is very difficult for clinicians to maintain the necessary professional distance if they insist on becoming acquainted with the officers with whom they work. Clinicians have to make a very different set of decisions from policemen. Officers may wish to separate conflicting parties to terminate an argument. Clinicians, on the other hand, may wish to allow the conflict to run its course in order to expose the disputants to the experience of working it out. Policemen also prefer to isolate individuals who are causing difficulties, while clinicians may wish to bring more people into the activity in order to get all of the participants in a particular social system engaged in the solution. The community also has very different expectations of clinicians from those it has of officers. It is important to the community and to the individuals in crisis to keep those roles separate and distinct, so that the person in crisis can have more flexibility and choice. There are also times when it is a great disadvantage to clinicians to have clients perceive them as part of the police system.

INTER- AND INTRA-ORGANIZATIONAL LINKAGES

Linkages between the inpatient and outpatient programs and the emergency unit will be difficult to sustain, because daytime services and clinicians may be foreign to afterhours staff. The latter have few administrative or clinical resources to fall back on and, due the hours they work, are often absent from the routine staff, referral, and dispositional conferences that occur in the center. Their communication with regular outpatient staff to whom they are referring clients is frequently only on paper, and the relationships that are fostered over a cup of coffee during a break are usually absent. The problem is multiplied when the emergency clinician refers someone to an inpatient unit that is geographically separate from the outpatient service. This allows for another set of "cracks" through which the patient can fall. In order to facilitate transfer of patients and information, a number of steps are required. Identical referral forms should be used throughout the system. Personal contacts should be encouraged by planning special occasions when all involved can get together. Administrators should know the special demands and situations placed on the referring emergency clinician so that he or she doesn't get scapegoated for other organizational problems. In some situations, vigorous proactive steps need to be taken to ensure that interagency and intra-agency linkages are maintained. Periodic review of those procedures is also encouraged.

PROVIDING FOR SPECIAL SUPERVISORY NEEDS

Due to the afterhours work schedule of the emergency worker, supervision is usually on a catch-as-catch-can basis. Rather than classical supervision, an emergency clinician requires consensual validation. The clinician has resolved a crisis and needs someone with whom she or he can formally talk to confirm actions already taken. Regular supervisory time for emergency workers should be scheduled, and use of their supervisors on an immediate basis for affirmation should be encouraged. Obviously, this need is greater with new emergency clinicians, and supervisors should be particularly supportive to them. Validation is required far less frequently with seasoned workers, but even after years of emergency service, I sometimes find myself leaving an ER feeling uneasy about the outcome of a particular situation.

Supervisors and emergency clinicians should meet regularly to insure that new or even routine procedures are understood and are being followed. Supervision in an informal setting may be more productive than in the more formal hierarchical model. Experienced emergency clinicians do not need didactic supervisors as much as empathic, sensitive colleagues.

Inservice training for emergency staff and supervisors is often best conducted when the skills and information of the visiting instructor are paired with those of a local "expert." Numerous workshops are continuously being offered, and a week's worth of the center's fourth-class mail will provide a sample of these programs.

THE PROBLEM OF BURNOUT

There is a new concept that seems to have cropped up in the last few years called "burnout." This is a condition in which clinicians seem to become less and less effective, have increasing difficulty with their home life, and often terminate their employment. It is very important that administrators and senior clinicians responsible for an emergency unit keep a close eye on the scheduling of emergency clinicians. Expectations should be realistic and be reviewed constantly with the staff to insure that they do not set them too high or become involved in rescue fantasies. The emergency clinician works alone; the controls that a group of colleagues can place are frequently absent. Burnout prevention workshops are available around the country, and the condition is analyzed in the scientific literature. Administrators and supervisors should become aware of the phenomenon and develop ways to combat it.

WHAT DO YOU DO WITH THE INTOXICATED AND STONED CLIENT?

It is virtually impossible to get anywhere therapeutically with someone who is intoxicated. Encourage the ER staff to allow the client to sober up or come down. In the late 1960s and early 1970s, a great deal of excitement was generated around the issue of acute drug intoxication. This problem has lessened somewhat over the years as emergency staff have learned to deal better with it. When this situation presents itself, a clinician may spend hours with someone simply reassuring that person that the process is chemical and will go away. The National Institute of Drug Abuse (NIDA), the National Institute of Alcohol Abuse and Addiction (NIAAA), and other organizations have prepared exhaustive protocols for working with these crises. It should be possible to procure portions of this specialized literature from the regional office representing these agencies. Such literature should be made available to the emergency staff.

These clients present many unique problems beyond mere behavioral control. The clients test our personal value systems regarding taking responsibility for oneself and subjecting one's body to damage. They are frequently repeaters and certainly tax our patience since they consume significant portions of the treatment resources in the community. Clinicians sometimes have to decide to deny anything but emergency medical services to these chronic abusers who repeatedly use our emergency services. It is often self-defeating for clinicians to become involved in trying to change the behavior of someone who continues to use services inappropriately or act routinely in a self-destructive manner.

THE SPECIAL PROBLEMS RELATING TO SUICIDE AND SUICIDE PREVENTION

While only 3 to 5 percent of emergencies involve a threat of suicide, such threats are among the most difficult problems with which lay and clinical people deal. Philosophical concern about whether people have the right to end their lives under certain circumstances is sometimes balanced against the general cultural belief that anyone who wants to die has to be mentally disturbed. In our statutes the state is usually allowed to assume control of a person who threatens suicide. The assumption is that reason will prevail after a period of time. This time is often spent in an involuntary commitment in a psychiatric treatment facility.

Most of the suicide attempts that an emergency unit faces are not lethal in their intent, although they may have approached lethal proportions. The client may have ingested a deadly amount of drugs with the intent of "crying out for help." The emergency worker must evaluate each situation on its merits. One of the most taxing is deciding whether a person's condition merits hospitalization, or whether that person should be allowed to follow through with voluntary outpatient treatment.

There are some clinical rules that emergency workers may wish to follow as they make their evaluations. These include assessing the potential lethality of the event, as well as reviewing the history for other suicide attempts. The motives of the client should be carefully examined, and the worker should question whether the material or instrument is still available in the event that suicide is attempted again in the immediate future.

Physicians and emergency room personnel typically take the conservative treatment approach and advocate involuntary hospitalization when the precipitant crisis and clinical situation do not merit it. Sometimes their motive (of which they may not be aware) is to hospitalize the patient as punishment for the fear and anger that the patient's act has created in themselves—the healers and lifesavers.

Case law exists, however, that states that emergency workers must use the most prudent approach available. Should a client commit suicide while under the care of emergency personnel, those workers may, in some jurisdictions, be subject to suit.

Auerbach and Kilman (1977) have reviewed extensively the outcome literature on crisis intervention and suicide prevention services. They have found that, although the services are usually well motivated and well meaning, documentation of their effectiveness is severely lacking. This article is written in scientific jargon but merits review by those who are responsible for emergency services. Regardless of the potential problems in a suicide protocol, the emergency staff should reflect on their own feelings about suicide and develop a consistent protocol for evaluation of their clinical activities. In this area, the supervisory model of consensual validation is often most helpful to the responsible clinician.

A word of caution, however, is appropriate, since there are some people who are determined to kill themselves and, no matter what services are placed at their disposal, will succeed. It is important that clinicians be prepared for this eventuality.

There are some community ramifications to a suicide, and emergency personnel should be prepared for them. A realistic community understands that people will kill themselves, and emergency workers should not be overwrought with guilt when they do. When suicides occur, realistic and consistent review by the center helps reassure the community. It also provides emergency staff with a sense of closure and a greater awareness and understanding of the suicide phenomenon.

PROBLEMS FACED BY EMERGENCY
SUPPORT STAFF

Secretaries and other support staff are usually the first contact for emergency service clients. They will frequently have to provide crisis intervention before the clinician can arrive. Their attitudes are very important in setting the tone for the intervention that will follow. Thus, support staff should receive specialized training of their own. Often, the best approach that a secretary can take is to offer coffee and a listening ear while awaiting the arrival of the clinician. At our center, we make conference money available to our support staff so that they too can receive training that allows them to perform their nonclerical roles more effectively.

LEGAL ISSUES FOR THE EMERGENCY UNIT

Emergency workers occasionally face legal questions. They may have to report criminal offenses such as child abuse, rape, and assaults. Certainly, the emergency crew should have a clear grounding in their legal responsibilities and be familiar with the statutes. Involvement with these cases sometimes necessitates a substantial time commitment after the immediate crisis is controlled. Rape victims frequently require extensive services to prepare them for prosecution, should they choose that route. The clinician will often be required to prepare and appear for court testimony. In many states, these activities are not reimbursable, and thus represent a further drain on the center's cash flow.

Problems with patient confidentiality should be carefully noted. The referral of a client to another agency in the middle of the night may be precluded if some interagency arrangement has not been previously prepared regarding the transfer of clinical information. The clinician will still be required to obtain appropriate releases even under those circumstances. Most state laws have a "good samaritan" clause that allows emergency workers under certain circumstances in life-threatening situations to review and transmit clinical information without the patient's consent. Administrators should be aware of those situations and have the emergency staff well briefed.

There are some situations in which an emergency clinician may be threatened with legal action by a reluctant client. Thus it may be helpful if the center has on call an attorney versed in mental health law.

Emergency personnel should be aware of policies regarding the circumstances under which a clinician may sue or cause the arrest of a client. Occasionally, emergency clinicians will be assaulted, and they deserve the same protection of the law as do other citizens. There are mitigating circumstances where the client should not be held responsible for his actions, but clinicians should know about those possibilities in advance.

The American Bar Association Commission on the Mentally Disabled publishes an excellent journal, Mental Disability Law Reporter, which should be a useful resource to administrative and clinical staff. Numerous patient self-help groups and professional groups have become interested in the interface of the law and mental health. Other publications available from the NIMH, the American Psychological Association, and the American Psychiatric Association are available. This area of the law is becoming better defined, and new case law is being made daily.

PROBLEMS ASSOCIATED WITH
INVOLUNTARY ADMISSION

Occasionally, emergency services screen for involuntary state hospital admission. There are legal issues that require emergency workers to know the statutes and case law particular to their state. These are also program issues in that one of the primary functions of a CMHC is to offer community services and deflect clients from state hospitals. In spite of CMHCs' success, there are people who will become psychotic, will not be able to care for themselves, and will require hospitalization regardless of how well emergency services are maintained and delivered. One should keep an eye on the admission rate, but it alone should not determine the scope of emergency programs.

State institutions are reluctant to admit people because they are facing declining budgets. An active linkage at all clinical, supervisory, and administrative levels is encouraged to insure that patients are not harmed in the political struggle for resources.

Emergency clinicians may hesitate to admit people to state hospitals, because they believe that these hospitals are ill-managed or that they deliver services in "cracker jack" small inpatient units. They may well be right, but there are patient needs that occasionally require facilities that are not available anyplace else. The center's moral and ethical responsibility is to call for improvement in the quality of those services, while carefully monitoring client's progress in the state facility.

Board members should be aware of situations in which other pressure groups in the political arena attempt to place mental health centers and state institutions in adversary roles, thereby creating a "let's you and him fight" situation. As long as we are fighting with our natural allies, it is more difficult for us to receive our fair share of legislative or Congressional appropriations. Board members can do a great service to their organizations if they assist in a process that develops a comprehensive, coordinated, and continuous range of services and creates a unified philosophy of treatment for all the consumers of mental health services.

I have attempted to summarize the structure and function of an emergency unit and to delineate some of its special problems. I have found, for personal, organizational, and systemic reasons, that such a service is invigorating, in addition to being helpful to clients. In terms of administering our unit, meeting with other directors, and reading the literature, I found that having a staff who see people as members of families and social systems invites the most success. But staff members who set reasonable expectations for themselves and hold reasonable views of their own limita-

tions will do best, for no matter how hard or how well an emergency
unit works, it will still not resolve every crisis it encounters.

ABOUT THE ROLE OF THE BOARD

The most important role that a board member can fulfill in
the administration of a mental health center—and especially its
emergency service—is to ensure the development of a treatment
philosophy for all of the center's services. If that philosophy en-
hances coordination, continuity, and comprehensiveness of services,
then the emergency service will prosper. Administrative practice
and routine should follow implicitly from that philosophical statement, as should the goals of the organization. A method for resolving administrative financial and clinical issues about specific objectives should also be included. There will be substantial resistance
to creating such a "constitution," since social service organizations
prefer to deal with more mundane operational problems, rather
than tackling this large and difficult one. All board members should
push strenuously for such a set of overall principles for the administration of their center.

Again, board members need to understand that emergency
services are going to lose money for the overall delivery system.
The rewards are not financial, and financial viability is not the only
criterion by which our services are evaluated. The emergency unit
offers a significant special service to the community that probably
is not available through any other resource. It also provides an
active, informal liaison and consultative assistance to other agencies. These are hard to cost out, but they certainly have substantial intrinsic value to the entire service network, as well as to the
center.

An emergency unit is the one service most visible to the other
providers in the community. The people in this unit should have a
sense of professional confidence that reflects well on the center.
This may create a dilemma for the board, since members of such a
unit may be internally validating "loners" who are listening to the
beat of a somewhat different drummer. It is important, nevertheless, that they be integrated members of the entire treatment team;
substantial individual differences and foibles can be tolerated if that
basic condition is met.

In setting policies, the board should insure that administrative
clinical support is available to the emergency unit. This may include the assistance of an attorney and other professionals for back-
up. Personnel rules may be flexible in that special leave arrangements can allow for "recharging batteries" that are rapidly depleted

in crises. Some centers have an informal classification known as
"mental health days" that allow an emergency clinician to use such
time on a limited basis.

Perhaps the most important role that a board can take vis-à-
vis the emergency unit is to work actively for continued funding for
comprehensive mental health services. It follows that no such package can exist without the inclusion of an adequate emergency unit.
Legislators at all levels must be made aware of the consequences
if such a service is not present and of the distinct social and economic advantages that accrue when a good emergency service is
available to the community.

You will also face situations where other political action
groups attempt to create the "let's you and him fight" situation described above. In these very difficult financial times, those fights
can look very appealing to an agency wishing to preserve its power
and responsibility. But entering into a struggle with your natural
allies is very dangerous and usually results in all being losers.
Every effort should be made to build a comprehensive system that
includes all participants in the mental health delivery system.

In summary, this chapter has discussed the emergency services unit as an integral and necessary part of a CMHC. Patterns
of staff and client usage have been described, with recommendations
about location, special training, supervisory needs, support staff,
and expenses. Special client issues such as intoxication and suicide
have been reviewed, as well as related legal issues and problems
with involuntary admission. For the reader who wishes to learn
more, the regional NIMH office should be able to offer a substantial
bibliography from which to choose further reading. For professionals with more technical interests, the use of The Psychological Ab-
stracts is encouraged.

REFERENCES

American Bar Association. Commission on the Mentally Disabled.
    Mental Disability Law Reporter. Washington, D.C., 1976 to
    present.

Auerbach, S., & Kilman, P. Crisis intervention: A review of the
    outcome research. Psychology Bulletin, 1977, 84(6), 1189-1218.

Bard, M. The function of the police in crisis intervention and con-
    flict management. Washington, D.C.: U.S. Department of Jus-
    tice, 1975.

Bard, M. , & Berkowitz, B. Training police as specialists in family crisis intervention: A community psychology action program. Community Mental Health Journal, 1967, 3, 315-317.

Burgess, A. , & Holstrom, L. Rape: Victims of crisis. Bowie, Md.: Robert Brody Company, 1974.

Burgess, A. , & Holstrom, L. Rape: Crisis and recovery. Bowie, Md.: Robert Brody Company, 1979.

Davidson, A. Air disaster: Coping with stress. A program that worked. Police Stress, 1979, 1(2), 20-23.

Gerson, S. , & Bassuk, E. Psychiatric emergencies: An overview. American Journal of Psychiatry, 1980, 137, 1-11.

Silverman, W. H. Planning for crisis intervention with community mental health concepts. Psychotherapy: Theory, Research & Practice, 1977, 14(3), 293-297.

15

ADULT SERVICE DELIVERY
Eduardo R. Val

In the planning, development, and evaluation of mental health services, an understanding of systems theory is of the utmost importance. The goals, structures, and priorities of each service program are interdependent. Likewise, the advisory/governing functions of each mental health board are influenced by the totality of forces interacting in the system. One of the central tasks of mental health boards is to mediate among the different parts of the system to bring cohesion and balance to competing needs and priorities.

Until the 1960s, needs and priorities in mental health services were determined by professionals or those officials representing citizens through county, state, or federal health agencies. The enactment of the Community Mental Health Centers Act of 1963 and its subsequent amendments has drastically changed both planning and implementation. Some observers have referred to this change as a revolution. Others see it merely as a reshuffling of priorities and power, a fad with no fundamental alterations in policy. Perhaps it depends on how one defines revolution.

The Community Mental Health Centers Act, in introducing the concepts of continuity of services, bound to a geographically defined area on a nondecline basis, and with direct community input, brought about an alteration in perspectives and a reordering of service priorities. This, indeed, has been a revolutionary change when one compares it to the public mental health system of just 15 years ago. Patients were then sent to isolated and distant state hospitals and often given erratic aftercare. Most of the services provided were administered by city, county, or state agencies, with little coordination and a total absence of direct neighborhood accountability or

231

participation. It is the radical departure from this situation that has made the community mental health movement a novel event. It is not the treatment aspects that have been revolutionary but the system in which they are embedded. The major task and challenge for mental health programs is to institute modern therapeutic practice within the context of a community-oriented organizational philosophy.

The 1965 Community Mental Health Centers Amendments required the delivery of five essential services: inpatient, outpatient, partial hospitalization, emergency, and consultation and educational services. Further amendments in 1975 mandated the addition of such services as care for children and the elderly, aftercare for post-hospitalization, and halfway houses. These newly required services corrected the neglect of long overlooked sectors of the population. However, it also created an added burden for community mental health centers (CMHCs). Can a CMHC with a defined population of 75,000 to 200,000 provide all these services to its catchment area efficiently and effectively? Since this seems highly improbable, a fundamental task is to develop harmonious and optional delivery systems with service components of appropriate size and functions (see Spiro, 1969). At times there will be service demands and objectives that fall outside the scope of a given CMHC. There may be limitations of staff skills or size, a low frequency of occurrence of a particular problem, or financial constraints. The provision of a full array of services would then be a poor use of resources resulting in negative impact on quality of care.

It is, therefore, advisable to delineate services in terms of district size, locale in which the functions are to be carried out, and affiliate or alternative service arrangements. Taking these variables into account, a conceptual distinction can be made between a comprehensive community mental health program and a CMHC. The former is more inclusive and encompasses the CMHC and other specialized mental health services. This concept as originally proposed by Spiro is outlined in Table 15.1.

This model allows for the utilization of resources, placing emphasis on continuity of care. Depending upon community needs, special programs can be placed under the leadership of a small agency, a large affiliate, or the CMHC. This decreases overlap and prevents "service overkill" for a specific community and its problems. The model also has implications for the constitution, scope, and type of board representation to the complex of service delivery agencies. For instance, representation may be viewed as layers in the sense that each neighborhood center sends delegates to the CMHC board, and the CMHC board designates citizens to represent its interests to a tertiary care program. According to this

TABLE 15.1

A Comprehensive Community Mental Health Model for a CMHC
and Specialized Mental Health Services

Factors Influencing Level of Care	Primary	Secondary	Tertiary
Locus of functions	Comprehensive health center, or neighborhood satellite clinic of CMHC	CMHC	Specialized wing of CMHC, or state hospital, or nursing home system
District size	15,000–30,000	70,000–200,000	140,000–1,000,000
Service functions	1. Early case finding 2. General intake 3. Outpatient care 4. Day care 5. Home visiting and care	1. Emergency services 2. Inpatient services 3. Partial hospitalization 4. Intensive rehabilitation	1. Categorical care (drug abusers, alcoholics) 2. Specialized inpatient care (residential child care)
Consultation functions	1. Primary physicians 2. Neighborhood programs and local agencies	1. Superordinate agencies (school system, social welfare agencies) 2. General hospitals 3. Other consultation through primary care facilities	1. Agencies relevant to categorical programs 2. Other consultation through primary and secondary care facilities

Source: Adapted and modified from H. Spiro, Beyond mental health centers, Archives of General Psychiatry, December 1969, 21, 550–559.

model, each unit of the care delivery system must be designed to impact upon other subsystems in a clearly differentiated, yet integrated, fashion. This assures that each community mental health program is unique by virtue of its goals and functions.

ADULT SERVICES

In the previous section we emphasized the importance of a systemic view in establishing the structure and function of mental health programs. Planning services around such age parameters as children, adolescents, adults, and the elderly can also be accomplished within the same system view. This means that various stages in the life cycle require different resources, because each group expresses its needs in different ways. For instance, children and adolescents are part of an educational system that is usually accessible in terms of catchment area boundaries. The adult group is more mobile and, therefore, less accessible. Adults work in private and public enterprises frequently located outside the district. Early detection, active follow-up, and access to their daily social network interaction become far more difficult and complex.

Nevertheless, the adult sector between the ages of 18 and 65 receives the bulk of mental health services. Several reasons may account for this. First, it is a reflection of the relative political and economic power of adults vis-à-vis children and the elderly. Second, the incidence and number of episodes per disorder is most frequent between ages 20 to 60. Third, although the rate of increase of illness episodes accelerates after age 65, especially for men, the concurrent decrease in life expectancy decreases demands for service to this group. Perhaps the main factor for the disproportionate amount of service to adults is that major mental disorders have their onset in young adulthood and that these disorders contribute to subsequent episodes. This age group is also at relatively high risk for many types of stress, such as suicide, divorce, and widowhood, as well as for medical conditions affecting brain behavior, such as diabetes, cardiovascular accidents, metabolic disorders, and brain tumors.

PSYCHOPATHOLOGY

Human behavior is the result of the multiple interactions of biological, psychological, and social factors. Likewise, mental disorders as expressed by abnormal behavior are a consequence of these multiple etiological factors.

Perhaps the greatest consensus existing among mental health professionals is that mental disorder is a collective term for a variety of different conditions. In terms of causation, those disorders that seem to have more of a biochemical involvement are behavioral disorders resulting from brain tumors, metabolic disorders, and some schizophrenic and affective disorders. In schizophrenia and some of the affective disorders, genetic vulnerability is a necessary, but not a sufficient, condition: an environmental contribution is required for its expression. Disorders that are the result of psychosocial factors with minimal or no biological predisposition are the psychoneuroses, personality disorders, and marital and family disturbances. Included in this group of disorders is vulnerability in personality organization, usually produced by stress during crucial periods of development. Even in those disorders where biological factors are implicated, life experience and environmental factors affect the presentation of symptoms and influence relapses and the course of the disorder. For example, the incidence of schizophrenia is unrelated to social class status. However, the lack of social and treatment systems available to the poor accounts for the greater prevalence of schizophrenia in lower socioeconomic classes.

In view of the multiplicity of factors involved in producing psychopathology, one must have a pluralistic approach toward interventions. While the use of psychopharmacological agents is required for biologically based disorders, they are not sufficient. Psychological management must also be included in the form of rehabilitation for the individual, family, group, or a combination of them. For those disorders based on psychosocial factors, psychotherapy is the primary form of intervention.

The most essential phase of service intervention is the diagnostic evaluation. The clinician must know the source of the problem(s) before therapeutic tools are used. Unfortunately, in some programs, adherence to a particular modality of treatment takes precedence over clinical needs. A single specific form of treatment that alleviates all forms of mental disorder is a myth. Multiple causation of emotional disorders necessitates a comprehensive evaluation of each individual and his or her environment, a process generally referred to as the diagnostic evaluation. A great deal of controversy has plagued the mental health field over the necessity for diagnosis. Some have criticized the negative effects of labeling a person with a diagnostic category, while others have claimed that sorting out clinical entities is useless since treatment interventions are nonspecific. For instance, it has been argued that using treatments A, B, or C for disorder X did not yield any different results. With the recent advances in the use of medications and more sophisticated evaluation of psychotherapy, this has ceased to be a valid criticism. Although the field is still more an art than a science, a greater number of our decisions can be based on scientific data rather than on clinical intuition.

Because a pluralistic approach to intervention and evaluation requires a team effort, CMHCs are better equipped than the private practitioner. A team effort entails a division of labor requiring two fundamental aspects: specialization among the members so that each offers a unique service, and the integration of all of these members into a system (see Cumming, 1968). This division of labor is most needed at the diagnostic phase. Members of a clinical team contribute in specific ways related to the unique functions of their respective disciplines or expertise. Historically, the psychiatrist has assessed status, medical conditions, and longitudinal history, while the psychologist has investigated individual psychological aspects of the clients, and the social worker has examined family constellations and social networks. These areas of specialization do not necessarily have to be assigned by disciplinary boundaries, but the responsibility for them must be clearly defined and skillfully applied. Once the diagnostic phase is accomplished, interventions can be assigned in a more universal manner, depending more on areas of interest and skills than on traditional disciplinary lines.

We want to emphasize the importance of linkage and integration of services for diagnosis and intervention with the community primary physician and with neighborhood medical clinics. Of the 15 percent of Americans affected by emotional disorder, 60 percent are under the outpatient care of primary physicians or primary care facilities. Only 15 percent are seen by mental health professionals (Eaton, unpublished manuscript). Recent studies also have demonstrated that about half the patients with emotional disorders have some type of major physical illness, either concurrently associated with the mental disorder or, in the minority of the instances, causing the disorder (Koranyi, 1979). Thus, primary practitioners are the logical target for early detection efforts.

TREATMENT APPROACHES

In this section some of the more commonly encountered therapeutic approaches will be briefly discussed. The treatment of mental disorders can be divided in two major categories: biological interventions, sometimes referred to as organic therapies, and psychological interventions, commonly known as the psychotherapies.

Biological Interventions

Electroshock

This procedure was widely used before antipsychotic and anti-depressive drugs were available. Electroshock attempts to provoke tonic (spastic-like) and clonic (jerking-like) convulsions by passing a current of electricity for a few seconds between two electrodes applied laterally on the forehead. Under short-acting anesthesia, this is a painless procedure, and the patient experiences amnesia of the treatment episode. A series of 12 to 15 treatments is usually required to achieve results; treatments are usually administered three times a week. Currently, this mode of treatment is almost exclusively used for severe depression unresponsive to antidepressive medication, and for lifesaving situations involving highly suicidal patients. Its effectiveness is far superior to that of drugs. While electroshock has been criticized because of the possibility of producing brain damage, the evidence is contradictory. Nevertheless, it should be used only in extreme circumstances under secure hospital conditions. A sound policy is to have its prescription supported by the agreement of two independent specialists (see Salzman, 1977).

Drug Treatment

Before the 1950s only a handful of drugs, such as barbiturates and chlorohydrate, were available and they were used primarily for sedation. These types of compounds did not provide relief of the specific target symptoms of any of the major conditions. The new drugs have a specific action on target symptoms without altering the patient's consciousness. While the use of drug treatment preceded the establishment of CMHCs, drugs have greatly altered clinical practice. An initial polarization between the sociotherapeutic model sponsored by community mental health advocates, and a biological orientation proposed by the drug treatment advocates, has over the years been modified into a more integrated eclectic view. This approach views behavior as a complex biopsychosocial phenomenon, and favors selecting optimal treatment modes without focusing on one specific behavioral aspect to the exclusion of others.

The psychopharmacological agents can be usefully classified in terms of the primary clinical disorders they treat: (1) anxiety disorders, (2) psychotic disorders, and (3) mood disorders.

1. Anxiety disorders:

Anxiety is the experience of fear without the presence of real threat or danger. A state of anxiety is common in a variety of conditions, including psychosis, depressive disorders, psychoneurosis, and medical conditions. Only when the most predominant disturbance is anxiety does one consider it an anxiety disorder. About 2 to 4 percent of the general population has experienced an anxiety reaction. This large number, approximately 4 to 8 million people, may explain the extensive use and abuse of antianxiety agents. Drugs in this group are the benzodiazepines, which include such brand names as Valium, Librium, and Ativan. In general, these drugs should be prescribed only when there has been no response to psychological treatment or when anxiety interferes with the patient's level of functioning. They should be used only on a short-term or "as needed" basis, as they have powerful addictive properties.

2. Psychotic disorders:

The term psychosis denotes a group of behavior disturbances characterized by impairment in reality testing. They include the presence of delusions, hallucinations, ideas of reference, incoherence, or derailed types of thinking.

In some instances psychotic disorders are due to organic brain pathology caused by vascular accidents, tumors, drug abuse, metabolic disorders, or senility. In the majority of instances, however, psychosis is not clearly related to a definable organic condition; consequently, these types of psychotic disorders are referred to as functional disorders. For the younger adult group, schizophrenia accounts for the majority of psychotic occurrences. Other types of psychosis are the so-called brief psychosis and atypical psychosis, which share some features with schizophrenia. However, they have a short duration and are more likely to be related to stress conditions.

Some of the essential features of schizophrenia are delusions, hallucinations, and a particular type of thought disturbance. The current tendency is to restrict use of the diagnostic category of schizophrenia to avoid inclusion of psychosis with better prognosis. Schizophrenia is a chronic illness with varying degrees of severity and a tendency to remissions and relapses. The first episodes of schizophrenia tend to occur between the ages of 15 and 35; it affects women and men in equal proportions. The importance of this disorder in planning adult services is evident. Even when using narrow diagnostic criteria, its prevalence has been estimated from about 0.5 to 1 percent of the general population. In other words, for a typical CMHC with a catchment area of about 200,000, approximately 1,000 to 2,000 cases will need treatment annually.

A large group of drugs is effective in the treatment of psychosis. Some of the brand names are Thorazine, Haldol, Stelazine, and Prolixin. These compounds tend to have the same degree of effectiveness; however, individual patient response varies widely, so that laboratory tests and examinations for side effects are essential. Under standard clinical conditions, these drugs require two to three weeks of treatment with increasing dosages before symptoms begin to abate. In general, delusions, hallucinations, and thought disturbances require longer interventions of six to eight weeks for improvement, while acute cases of schizophrenia, particularly during the first episode, may require medication for a period of six to 12 months. Findings indicate that up to 70 percent of these patients relapse within a year after discharge with no medication, while only 30 percent with medication do so. The majority of the relapses take place within the three months following an episode, pointing to the value of active treatment follow-up after hospitalization. More than one relapse may call for the use of medication for several years, with periodic "drug holidays."

Certainly, medication does not cure schizophrenia, but it is effective in preventing relapses, minimizing the need for frequent hospitalization, and facilitating psychotherapy and rehabilitation. Research studies have shown conclusively that medication and psychotherapy, used in conjunction, augment each other and facilitate better social rehabilitation.

3. Mood disorders:

Research data suggest two large groupings of mood disorders: primary affective disorders and secondary affective disorders. Primary affective disorders are so named because they are not associated with any other psychiatric illness or medical condition. Primary affective disorders are further subclassified into those with a tendency to oscillate between depression and mania (bipolar affective disorders), and those with a tendency to have only a depressive episode in a recurrent fashion (unipolar affective disorders). The secondary affective disorders are found in association with other types of mental disorder or medical conditions. The following diagram summarizes the classification.

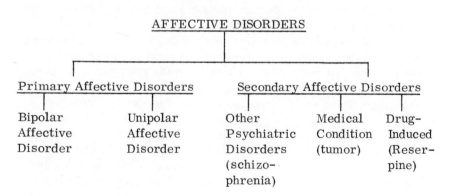

AFFECTIVE DISORDERS

Primary Affective Disorders / Secondary Affective Disorders

| Bipolar Affective Disorder | Unipolar Affective Disorder | Other Psychiatric Disorders (schizophrenia) | Medical Condition (tumor) | Drug-Induced (Reserpine) |

Both groups of primary affective disorders, unipolar and bipolar, exhibit a high degree of family incidence, especially the bipolar type. This relationship has implications for the prevention and treatment of these disorders, since they respond therapeutically and preventively to specific drug management.

Affective disorders are one of the most overlooked and undiagnosed of all conditions. Their prevalence is the highest among mental disorders. It has been estimated that about 20 percent of the adult population has experienced at least one major depressive episode. About 0.4 to 1.2 percent of the adult population has exhibited a bipolar condition. For a typical catchment area, this suggests the presence of 20,000 major depressive cases and 1,200 bipolar cases. Since affective disorders correlate highly with the incidence of suicide, their early detection and proper management carry dramatic preventive implications.

Drugs with antidepressants, Elavil, Tofranil, and Norpramine, are included in this group. These drugs are given ten days to two weeks before clinical improvement is observed. It is advisable to keep many of these patients on maintenance doses for at least six to eight months. This group of drugs has also been demonstrated to have preventive capabilities for depressive episodes.

A second group of drugs for the treatment of depression are the Mono-Amino Oxidase Inhibitors (MAO-I), so named because of their inhibiting action against enzymes that break down norepinephrine, a cathecol-amine implicated in the biochemistry of depression. The use of these agents is restricted to depressions that have not responded to the tricyclic drugs, or to cases in which a quick response is warranted. Some of the brand names are Marplan, Nardil, and Parnate. Since these compounds are far more dangerous, they need to be handled by psychiatrists familiar with their therapeutic effects and complications.

Lithium carbonate, a natural salt, is the drug of choice in the treatment as well as prevention of manic episodes. There is a narrow margin between the therapeutic and toxic levels of lithium that requires close monitoring of blood levels.

Mood drugs have proven to be effective both in the treatment and prevention of episodes. However, several research studies also indicate that their effect is mainly on the prevention of the cardinal symptoms of mania or depression, having little effect on the psychological and social aspects of these disorders. Therefore, psychotherapy is indicated in conjunction with medication when there are psychosocial disturbances. Refractory cases or those that have concomitant medical problems should be referred to a clinic specializing in the treatment of affective disorders. A candidate for any of these medications should have a thorough history taken and a

physical examination and pertinent laboratory evaluation performed
before they are prescribed.

Psychotherapy

Over the last several years psychotherapy has been under
close scrutiny by third-party payers and concerned consumers because of its cost and efficacy. The effectiveness of psychotherapy
has been considered in the recent report by the President's Commission on Mental Health (see Parloff, 1979). The bulk of the evidence demonstrates that psychotherapy works. What remains to be
answered is what kind of psychotherapy works most effectively for
what kind of condition.

There are some basic factors common to all psychotherapies
for producing a successful intervention. They include (1) a good
patient-therapist relationship, (2) allowance for ventilation, (3) reinforcement through implicit/explicit approval or disapproval,
(4) facilitation of a corrective emotional experience, (5) identification with the therapist, (6) support, (7) persuasion, (8) rehearsal
of new coping techniques, and (9) acquisition of cognitive insight
(Marmor, 1966).

Psychotherapies may be classified in a variety of ways. The
schema can be based on numerous factors: ideological or theoretical
formulations, for example, behavioral, psychoanalytic, transac-
tional; length, for example, brief, short-term, long-term; goals,
for example, crisis, focal, conflict, insight-oriented; or targets of
intervention, for example, individual, group, family psychotherapy.
In the following section, we will use the target classification to describe some of the most common psychotherapies.

1. Supportive psychotherapy:
This type of psychotherapy is aimed at helping the individual
gain and sustain equilibrium by using encouragement and direct advice. It avoids the encouragement of regression or free association
as well as lengthy and frequent sessions. The object is to establish
a therapeutic alliance. The therapist offers his/her reactions and
views. A problem-solving approach is used to enhance self-esteem
and test reality. This type of treatment is generally adjunctive to
medication. Its use should be restricted to cases with clear evidence of low coping abilities, since one of the risks of employing it
indiscriminately is that it fosters dependence.

In order to provide high quality supportive care, the therapist
must have a great deal of experience and sophistication. Unfortunately, supportive psychotherapy is usually assigned to the least

trained member of the team, and many chronic patients are produced in this manner. Cases should be referred to a more active, growth experiencing psychotherapy as soon as possible.

2. Intensive psychotherapy:

Intensive psychotherapy is an umbrella term covering many types of theoretical orientations to individual psychotherapy. Their common denominator is the attempt to produce growth and change beyond the initial resolution of the presenting symptoms or complaints. The term denotes either a short-term or long-term therapeutic involvement with at least once-a-week sessions and a central focus on the patient-therapist relationship. Some of the schools of thought belonging to this modality can be divided, albeit quite arbitrarily, into the two large groupings of dynamic and existential psychotherapies. The mode of change in dynamic psychotherapy is mainly through the revival of past conflicts by way of regression, confrontation, and exploration of feelings in the context of the patient-therapist relationship. The ultimate goal is the achievement of insight, that is, intellectual and emotional knowledge. The main therapeutic tool is the clarification and interpretation of transference phenomena. This group encompasses approaches such as psychoanalysis, insight-oriented psychotherapy, and focal psychotherapy.

The primary means to change in existential psychotherapies is a similar encounter between patient and therapist, but with emphasis on shared dialogue, dramatization, and playing out of feelings. Their major goal is the actualization of self-growth, authenticity, and spontaneity. Although the existential approach is centered on the therapeutic relationship, it leans more toward a mutually permissive or gratifying process in contrast to the more indirect and frustrating ambience of the dynamic psychotherapies. Existential analysis, Logotherapy, client-oriented therapy, and Gestalt therapy are some of the schools within the existential group. The fundamental assumption of all these intensive psychotherapies is that growth and change occur through learning via identification in the context of the relationship (see Karasu, 1977).

Intensive psychotherapy is indicated for chronic or persistent disturbances of self-esteem, such as neurotic conditions and a variety of personality disorders in which a major reorganization of life patterns, attitudes, self-perceptions, and interpersonal relations is required. In order to become a skilled therapist in this mode of treatment, a great deal of supervision and clinical experience are needed; the therapist is even required to undergo his or her own individual treatment experience. By and large, too many patients in community mental health programs never receive intensive psychotherapy, in part due to lack of qualified staff and to unavoidable limitations in caseload size for each psychotherapist.

3. Behavioral therapy:

This mode of intervention represents a recent development in the field. It is based on the idea that abnormal behavior is a function of conditioning or learning, so that altering behavior consists of extinguishing certain behaviors and replacing them with others through the strategic use of reinforcement. As was previously pointed out, reinforcement factors are present in each psychotherapy: in behavioral therapy they are the primary means of treatment through the use of manipulation, education, reward, or desensitization. Behavioral therapy has proved to be the most effective mode for treating avoidant disorders, especially phobias, as well as sexual disturbances.

4. Group psychotherapy:

Group psychotherapy is increasingly chosen not only because it uses staff and resources economically, but also because it is an effective treatment with a wide range of applicability. It is particularly effective in aftercare programs. Group psychotherapy can be short- or long-term, supportive, exploratory, or task-oriented. Indications for group psychotherapy are impulsive behavior, self-observing deficits, social withdrawals, and immaturity. For people with impaired reality testing, group pressure and support are powerful assets (see Grunebaum & Kates, 1977).

5. Family therapy:

Originally conceived for the treatment of families with a schizophrenic member, family therapy has become one of the most rapidly growing and accepted psychotherapy treatments. The central assumption in family therapy is that the family is an organized system. Normal behavior is viewed as the result of complementary roles that serve to keep the family system in balance. The more closed and rigid the system, the greater the chances for disequilibrium in adapting to internal and external stresses. The family provides the opportunity for each offspring to become a separated and autonomously functioning individual. When this does not occur, it is usually because parents and offspring need each other to perform some psychological function without which they would feel incomplete and handicapped. This results in self-differentiation problems and psychological symptoms.

Disordered behavior within a family system is not always caused by pathological role functions. In some cases pathological interactions are triggered by changes in a particular member. Take the example of a young girl who develops an incapacitating neurological disease. This stress may launch a healthy and well-balanced family into adaptations that promote growth, or it may result in a catastrophic disruption of the entire family system. Thus, the therapist views the family as a dynamic system that both produces behavior and adapts to random life events originating independently of the family system (as, for instance, mental retardation, parental loss, or medical illness). Therapeutic goals may be directed toward solving basic tensions and conflicts or toward facilitating better coping styles.

Hospitalization

Modern hospital services provide the treatments previously outlined, but integrated into the hospital milieu. Hospital programs can be grouped into full-time and part-time treatments. Full-time programs can be further divided into short-term (from one to 30 days), intermediate (from one to four months), and long-term (beyond four months). Short-term and intermediate programs are located at the secondary care level and should be sited in the community. Long-term hospitalization is tertiary care, most likely available at a state hospital facility.

There is no correlation between diagnostic categories and type of hospitalization. The evaluation of need for hospitalization depends upon a multiplicity of psychological, sociological, and biological factors such as self-care ability, the presence of homicidal or suicidal risk, need for close medical monitoring, or lack of support systems and residential facilities. Recipients of long-term treatment are individuals who are refractory to short-term interventions and tend to be significantly disturbed. This group consists of patients who display psychotic symptoms and intermittent disturbances in their reality testing. Drug therapy and accessibility to CMHCs have greatly diminished the need for long-term hospitalization.

Partial hospitalization can consist of day and night hospital programs, but the latter are rare. Day hospitals provide alternatives to 24-hour inpatient care, act as transitional care centers, provide rehabilitation for chronic patients, and develop a specific service as defined by the community (Astrachan, 1970). In practice, all these functions cannot be served by a single facility. Currently, the first two functions—alternatives to inpatient care and transitional care services—are most frequently associated with day hospitals. The term "day care center" is reserved for the treatment of chronic patients in a more structured ambulatory center with daily activities. Day care centers fall either within the primary care functions in the neighborhood or, if they are designed for a particular clientele (as in the cases of mental retardation and residential care for adolescents), are part of the tertiary service level.

Day hospital programs are used to prevent full-time hospitalization or to reduce length of stay. As an alternative to full-time inpatient care, day hospitals avoid the stigma and economic burdens of full-time hospitalization and prevent patient isolation from the family and the social network (see Silverman & Val, 1975). There is some evidence that those patients using partial hospitalization tend to use inpatient facilities less frequently.

CONCLUSIONS

In this chapter we have discussed the importance of planning and implementing community mental health programs and services from a systems view and the need to delineate these programs into components of appropriate size with defined tasks. The role of the center is to integrate and monitor the subsystems of a comprehensive mental health system through their advising and governing functions. The community mental health approach has introduced a radical departure from previous service delivery systems. Its unique contribution is not so much its forms of interventions, but the ways these interventions are delineated and prioritized. A review of the most commonly utilized modes of treatment has been presented.

Community mental health centers are now fully entrenched into the health care system of this country. The future challenge for public mental health programs is to offer modern treatment methods to its clients with sufficient numbers of competent and skillful personnel. A basic difficulty is economics, since mental health services are one of the most costly of all human services. Informed consumers as well as third-party payers will demand quality care provided by well-trained personnel, one consequence being that manpower costs will continue to escalate. The improvement of mental health care and the greater accessibility of services to the poor and minorities were the main issues of the 1960s and early 1970s. For the 1980s, the task is to continue those laudable goals and strive toward offering diversified, appropriate, up-to-date and high quality services.

REFERENCES

Astrachan, B. M. , Flynn, H. R. , Geller, J. D. , and Harvey, H. H. Systems approach to day hospitalization. Archives of General Psychiatry, 1970, 22, 550-559.

Cumming, E. Community psychiatry in a divided labor. In J. Zubin and F. Freyhan (Eds.), Social Psychiatry. New York and London: Grune and Stratton, 1968, 100-113.

Eaton, J. The role of the primary care physician in the management of affective disorders. Unpublished manuscript.

Grunebaum, H., and Kates, W. Whom to refer for group psychotherapy. American Journal of Psychiatry, 1977, 134, 130-134.

Karasu, T. Psychotherapies: An overview. American Journal of Psychiatry, 1977, 134, 851-863.

Koranyi, E. Morbidity and rate of undiagnosed physical illnesses in a psychiatric clinic population. Archives of General Psychiatry, 1979, 36, 414-419.

Marmor, J. The nature of the psychotherapeutic process. In G. Usdin (Ed.), Psychoneurosis and Schizophrenia. Philadelphia: Lippincott, 1966, 66-75.

Panzetta, A. F. Community mental health: Myth and reality. Philadelphia: Lea and Febiger, 1971.

Parloff, M. Can psychotherapy research guide the policymaker? American Psychologist, 1979, 34, 297-306.

Salzman, C. ECT and ethical psychiatry. American Journal of Psychiatry, 1977, 134, 1006-1009.

Silverman, W., and Val, E. Day hospital in the context of a community mental health program. Community Mental Health Journal, 1975, 11, 82-90.

Spiro, H. Beyond mental health centers. Archives of General Psychiatry, 1969, 21, 646-654.

16

THE ROLE OF THE COMMUNITY MENTAL HEALTH BOARD IN A SUBSTANCE ABUSE PROGRAM
Joseph Levin

INTRODUCTION

The most important task of community boards is to develop and implement an ideology of the community. While professional staff of community mental health centers (CMHC) and substance abuse programs are becoming more sophisticated and technically competent, and administrators are likely to be well trained in business management and rehabilitative aspects of program direction, neither group is trained to deal with the ideology of the community. Ideology is the scaffolding of values, beliefs, philosophy, ethnic styles, and cultures that give a community its unique characteristics. Even though mental health and substance abuse professionals may be concerned with ethics in their professional or personal lives and may be deeply committed to individual patients, they are not likely to be committed to the community. Their concerns are usually in terms of business ethics, issues of confidentiality, responsibilities of patients, colleagues, and profession, not with the survival and enhancement of the community.

The responsibility of a CMHC board in substance abuse is to ensure that community interests are being served by government bureaucrats who influence policy, and hospital and center staff who determine day-to-day operation. Each of these groups has its own allegiances. Hospitals have to keep their beds filled and their doctors happy. Staff identify only with their professions and their own jobs. Government bureaucrats are committed to maintaining and expanding their own power. All of these groups strive to make the community dependent upon them as elite providers.

The role of the CMHC board member is to see to it that the needs of the community are being met in the most humane, cost-effective way. Board members attempt to minimize the community's dependence upon elite professional groups, and also have the responsibility, where appropriate, of looking outside the organized health industry toward the self-help movement for solutions to problems.

They must be aware that all the solutions presented to the board may involve an outside group of specialists coming in to solve community problems. These specialists have no appreciation of the community's history, nor any commitment or investment in its future. To the extent that professional staff do not identify with the community, they are not likely to be sensitive to community needs. They tend to see substance abuse problems, not health, social, economic, or political problems. Consequently, the application of their solutions is likely to have little positive effect even on problems of substance abuse. Because board members have knowledge of and commitment to their communities, they should take a primary role in planning substance abuse services.

Many people in our society approach mental health problems in general, and substance abuse services in particular, with the following misconceptions:

There is a universally accepted definition of what substance abuse is.
All unpleasant social events such as substance abuse can be labeled as "sick" behavior or a "health/disease" problem. This justifies building an economic and/or political agency around it and labeling it a treatment program.
The solution of all substance abuse problems is contingent upon a bureaucratic system, publicly financed and staffed by specialists.
All substance abuse problems can be solved in a fraction of the time that they took to develop.
The quality of substance abuse programs is determined to a great extent by the way it is delivered and not by success rates.
Better social living through chemistry is acceptable if the chemical is legally available.
Solutions to problems are of value in direct proportion to their size, cost, and visibility. The more expensive, large, and fancy they are, the better they are.
People who earn a living in the alcohol or drug abuse field are technically knowledgeable about substance abuse and also know what's best for the community.

So long as we hold these beliefs, we are chained to approaches that are generally archaic and unworkable. The object of this chapter is to examine these issues in the light of current research and to provide guidance for board members whose responsibility it is to establish and monitor policy as it affects substance abuse programs. The remainder of this chapter will answer the following questions: (1) What is the nature and extent of national substance abuse problems? (2) How have substance abuse services been affected by traditional approaches to health care delivery? (3) What treatment alternatives to the traditional model of health care delivery exist for chemically dependent persons? (4) How can the board be trained in substance abuse? (5) What are reasonable substance abuse treatment goals? (6) What are the real targets of substance abuse programs? (7) What can be done to prevent substance abuse? (8) What role should the board play in selecting a director of substance abuse services? (9) How does finance affect ideology?

WHAT IS THE NATURE AND EXTENT OF SUBSTANCE ABUSE PROBLEMS?

Substance abuse is most often defined by the number and distribution of cases in the community at any given moment and over a period of time. Since we have not as yet learned to differentiate use from abuse, statistics are often confusing. Some substance abuse problems are self-limiting, while others are best limited by more efficient law enforcement. Epidemiological studies (those investigating the prevalence of a "disease or event in a particular time and place") of substance abuse can provide useful information that, when interpreted in light of a community's values and priorities, may result in more realistic planning and evaluation.

The estimated national rate for narcotic addiction is 21 per 100,000 population, while the estimated national rate for alcoholism is 9,000 per 100,000 population. Approximately 10 percent of the physicians and other professionals and managerial personnel are alcoholic. In addition, the rate of narcotic addiction among physicians is approximately 1,500 per 100,000. It is estimated that each alcoholic disrupts the lives of four other people in his or her social network. Therefore, we assume that 45 percent of the population is adversely affected by alcoholism, although about 47 percent of the population imbibes only one drink or less per month. The rate for alcoholism increases with income and education; conversely, rates are lower in rural areas than in urban and suburban communities. It should be noted that approximately 90 percent of those who drink alcoholic beverages are not problem drinkers.

The other focus of substance abuse involves legally prescribed minor tranquilizers and sedatives, and accounts for an additional 15 percent of the population. It is estimated that approximately half of such persons are physiologically dependent upon these drugs.

The recreational use of licit and illicit drugs is not usually associated with other health or social problems. This is important because CMHCs often come under pressure to create programs to "do something" about substance abuse in response to a concerned, articulate citizenry.

What can be done? First, become aware of the problem. More important than the rates for the total age span of men and women is the problem of substance abuse among children and senior citizens. The most serious health hazard to children is increased use of alcohol and tobacco. Since the aged in our society are usually the victims of neglect by all health, welfare, and educational agencies, as well as private citizenry, their problems of substance abuse are only minimally recorded. Medical errors in prescription and a lack of patient education in the use of prescribed and over-the-counter drugs are serious problems of substance abuse. While such problems could easily be remedied with minimal allocation of resources, the task of treating and preventing the abuse of these substances may be difficult because of the lack of concern about these populations by a large part of our society.

The ranking of substance abuse priorities is well within the province of a CMHC board. For example, there is evidence that at least a quarter of the population under 25 years of age has tried marijuana. At the same time there is still little evidence that the moderate use of this drug by itself constitutes a health or social problem. Yet substance abuse programs often come under pressure to deal with "the marijuana problem." It is perhaps due to our national hysteria that we equate use with abuse. If board members are committed to serving their total community and their most serious health problems, they will have to take some unpopular stands. It is not likely that people will thank them for ringing the alarm on alcohol and tobacco abuse or on community dependence on addiction specialists. But in the 1980s these are likely to be the most pressing problems, and they ought to be the main targets of community-based programs. In order to understand the direction of substance abuse problems, it might be useful to look at the recent history of substance abuse in its relation to the health care delivery system in general.

HOW HAVE SUBSTANCE ABUSE SERVICES BEEN AFFECTED BY TRADITIONAL APPROACHES TO HEALTH CARE DELIVERY?

The superstructures of government, the professions, and social agencies take their form and function from both history and

the economic nature of our changing society. The health care delivery systems approach to substance abuse is the result of these
and many other forces. The ideology of the superstructure appears
to include an absolute faith in the wisdom and knowledge of specialists, centralization of national power, and the commercialization of
most human services. Several specific factors affected the response to substance abuse by the health professions. The first of
these arose out of legal constraints imposed upon the medical profession by the Harrison Act of 1914, which, among other things,
stopped private physicians from treating opiate addicts and discouraged their future involvement in the substance abuse field. Second,
the health professions did not know how to treat effectively in a traditional medical system either substance abuse patients suffering
from a chronic illness or those manifesting behavior problems.
Third, and perhaps most important, was the fact that treatment of
addicts and alcoholics was not financially profitable. The health
profession did not consider alcoholics and addicts suitable patients
until the late 1950s and early 1960s. Until then, church-based agencies typically offered programs for the chemically dependent. Professionals still often see alcoholics as evil, weak-willed, hopeless,
and uncooperative people who fail to pay their bills.

In spite of these conditions, other factors contributed to the
development of health care delivery for substance abusers. An increasing number of alcoholic patients gave witness to their unmet
alcohol treatment needs and concurrent hostile and demeaning responses they received in hospitals and doctors' offices. A growing
number of politically aggressive and sophisticated ex-drug addicts
were successful in having legislation passed and funds allocated.
Finally, substance abuse became "good press," and the public
secret—that substance abuse is a serious problem—brought it out
into the open.

Mental health professionals generally started treating substance abusers in the late 1960s. When money for treatment services became available, an interesting structure, the corporate
medical model, evolved, in which professional health staff were
paid on a salary basis. At the same time, service was delivered
to a great extent by paraprofessional ex-patients. Physicians often
served as "fronts" for services, signing charts and insurance forms.
In many drug programs, paraprofessionals with less than a college
education managed the agencies with the power to determine medication, admissions, discharges, and treatment programs.

From the late 1960s until the present, alcoholics and addicts
have been treated in specialized programs apart from the mainstream medical or mental health programs. Because of this segre-
gation, fragmented care often resulted. In addition, strong antag-
onism between alcohol and drug abuse "kingdoms" developed at

federal, state, and local levels. These empires, in turn, developed their own separate bureaucratic divisions. Some agencies worked with alcohol and others with drugs. There was sharp competition for funds, separate training of staff, and different rules and regulations governing treatment. Thus, research, planning, treatment, and evaluation have all suffered.

Hospital care for alcoholics, in contrast to treatment for addicts, was organized in one of three ways. Some people were hospitalized as undesignated admissions, by which the sequelae of alcoholism were treated but not the presenting alcoholism. Since patients were handled as physicians' private property, it was virtually impossible to shed light on the neglect of alcoholic patients in such units. In a study of physicians' practices, Froom (1975) found that only 10 percent of alcoholic patients under the care of their private physicians were identified as alcoholic. Physicians in teaching hospitals do no better in differentiating alcoholic patients than the general medical patient population (Block, 1975). A second mode of hospital care was to assign alcoholic patients to "designated" beds reserved for them and to offer them various alcohol treatment programs. Finally, some alcoholic patients were treated in specialized programs that focused primarily on the patients' alcoholism.

Although treatment for addicts through the 1970s has usually been isolated from mainstream medical care, there is no rational basis for segregating alcohol from drug patients, or for segregating substance patients needing medical care in either of these categories from other medical patients. This isolation has encouraged the development of alternative approaches to substance abuse services.

WHAT TREATMENT ALTERNATIVES TO TRADITIONAL
MODELS OF HEALTH CARE DELIVERY EXIST FOR
CHEMICALLY DEPENDENT PERSONS?

When professionals abdicated their role in treating the chemically dependent population, self-help models emerged. Alcoholics Anonymous developed a spiritual, life-restructuring, self-help movement. Drug programs evolved from the Synanon-Daytop Village model of communal living, coined a "junkie monastery." Social (nonmedical) detoxification programs aimed at the most physically debilitated alcoholics were developed at a fraction of the cost of medical programs. They used no professional staff. Such efforts have demonstrated that with even the most medically needy and, consequently, highest (medical) risk group, 95 percent did not require hospitalization for their alcoholism.

While it might be tempting to posit an either/or approach to substance abuse services, that is, the self-help model versus the professional bureaucratic model, this writer advocates combining both. The combination offers a high potential for community control, providing that both self-help and professional bureaucratic organizations are completely autonomous and have an egalitarian relationship. Organizational and treatment diversity can create multiple intervention models and prevent self-serving concentrations of power.

Whether or not the CMHC board is advisory or governing, it should be morally and politically accountable to the entire community. While the professional staff identifies needs and carries out the day-to-day operations of the program, the board in consort with the director and staff should determine the goals and direction of the substance abuse program. To do this, the board should develop expertise in the area of chemical dependency, as well as in community organization. The state of the art is such that, aside from the purely medical aspects of treatment, any knowledgeable layperson with a reasonable amount of time and energy can master the rudiments of planning and evaluation of a substance abuse program.

HOW CAN THE BOARD BE TRAINED IN SUBSTANCE ABUSE?

The education of board members in stewardship of a substance abuse program may proceed along two parallel paths. The first leads to the development of an appropriate ideology, the second to familiarity with the technology of substance abuse treatment.

Two social critics whose writings may provide a launching point for ideological development are Illich (1976) and Lasch (1978). Illich, a philosopher, examines in a partisan and critical way the hazards and consequences of investing what he calls an unbridled power in the hands of the medical elite. Lasch, a historian, describes modern American society and details the consequences of our particular ahistorical and self-centered ideology. Two short pieces describing a religiously based health delivery system are by Tubesing and the Kellogg Foundation. Community people who are philosophically oriented might be enlisted to form a task force to examine the ideological imperatives of the community vis-à-vis substance abuse. There are many excellent technical publications on substance abuse that are either inexpensive or free. (Sources are listed at the end of this chapter.)

WHAT ARE REASONABLE SUBSTANCE
ABUSE TREATMENT GOALS?

It is clear that if eradication of substance abuse were a goal of the CMHC, it would not be achieved. Our society is chemically dependent on caffeine, nicotine, alcohol, and minor tranquilizers, and there will always be a vast array and quantity of mind-altering drugs available. A reasonable first stage substance abuse program for a CMHC would consist of acute medical care and emergency services, long-term treatment, training, and evaluation. Obviously, these are parallel to the other comprehensive health services every community needs. All of these services do not have to be delivered by the CMHC, since contractual arrangements and affiliate agreements can be made. Negotiation then must consider the continuity of services.

WHAT ARE THE TARGETS OF
SUBSTANCE ABUSE PROGRAMS?

The public inebriate is the most visible chemically dependent citizen and represents 0.3 percent of the population. Six percent of the adult male population is alcoholic, living at home, and holding down a job. Women, teenagers, the elderly, and health and service professionals (M.D.s, R.N.s, police, clergy, teachers) are subgroups that appear to have a significant number of unidentified, untreated, chemically dependent people. It should be noted that the two chemicals that cause the most serious health problems—including killer diseases that affect large numbers of adolescents and adults—are alcohol and tobacco.

If the above populations are not appearing in the utilization reports of the CMHC substance abuse programs, it is reasonable to assume that the CMHC is not treating them, that adequate outreach programs have not been instituted, and that there is a lack of concern among staff. A major reason for this is that substance abuse staff often define themselves as specialists such as methadone counselors, alcoholism counselors with or without A.A., counselors with or without chemotherapy, polydrug workers, and therapeutic community counselors. This makes as much sense as classifying physicians as penicillin doctors, hospital specialists, or head-cold-with-or-without-complications specialists. Usually, alcohol and drug abuse workers are so narrowly trained that they lack the perspective to see how they might function in a broader-based treatment program.

Because of the division of substance abuse into alcohol and drug abuse "kingdoms," federal and state funds are usually allocated to treat one category of patients or the other—rarely, if ever, both. Board members should be aware of the narrow ahistorical perspective of the staff and the bizarre nature of federal and state funding, and must serve as a watchdog and advocate for community and patient needs. When they do, they are bound to find gaps in service. But if the board asserts its leadership role and the staff accepts its responsibility to carry out the board's policies, the staff can adapt basic intervention skills to new problems and populations. The failure to apply creativity and dedication in substance abuse programs is clearly seen in the area of prevention.

WHAT CAN BE DONE TO PREVENT SUBSTANCE ABUSE?

Prevention efforts in substance abuse have been akin to "bringing goodness to the world." Rarely have these programs defined goals, objectives, or criteria for success or failure. It is entirely reasonable for a CMHC board to expect a staff to define in a concrete, objective way any project for which it asks money.

The effectiveness of prevention might be measured by the change in the number of new patients entering the pool of substance abusers before and after a new program is instituted. This is usually not possible for many reasons—among them, not having sufficient rapport with this pool to obtain reliable measures, not knowing how people leave the pool aside from treatment through death, migration, or self-cure, and case counts often biased by socioeconomic variables. So program evaluators often count the number of people requesting treatment service and the incidence of certain medical indicator or law enforcement data, and assume that they reflect a constant fraction of the number of new patients. It is important to recognize that this approach would have us focus exclusively on the use of chemicals and substance abuse services that are rendered for a fee. This would result in focusing on symptoms, without understanding root causes or fundamental forces that contribute to the existence and spread of substance abuse problems.

Another approach is to look at substance abuse as a predictable characteristic of a culture in which the media portray an ultra-individualistic society, a philosophy of consumerism, and better living through drugs. Additionally, our society makes a wide variety of cheap mood-altering drugs available. A keystone of such a culture is that people feel incompetent to solve their own drug and alcohol problems, so that they must rely on an elite of professionals. Naturally, the utilization of professional services reinforces the culture's dependence on professionals.

An alternative approach to prevention is to set a goal that maximizes the number of people from all strata of the community who exercise control over substance abuse planning and policy. Boards must become trained in substance abuse, exercise their stewardship, and reproduce themselves geometrically. That is, they must multiply by many fold the number of citizens who are capable of assuming policy making and planning roles in substance abuse organizations. This is necessary because our technology continues to produce an ever-increasing number of mood-altering drugs whose abuse will generate individual and community problems.

An additional role that local citizens can take in the prevention of substance abuse is that of political activism. For instance, they can support employment opportunities for recovering substance abusers and oppose availability of mood-altering drugs in the community. Treatment programs are wholly dependent upon job opportunities for the successful rehabilitation of their clients. In the absence of decent jobs, all treatment efforts are a waste of time and money. Rehabilitation and living "on the dole" are mutually exclusive.

Funding in alcoholism and drug abuse is usually for a welfare program rather than a substance abuse program. Such narcotic maintenance programs, using Methadone and LAAM (1-alpha-acetyl methadol), provide a system for keeping addicts pacified under supervision, but without the opportunity to be employed. To the extent that unemployment is a general community or specific substance abuse problem, it requires political action. The staff of the CMHC cannot generate the political pressure necessary to bring about change. Most important is that participating in that struggle is the ultimate self-enhancing experience for substance abusers.

It is an unfortunate fact that community boards rarely exercise their power to alert citizenry to the availability of alcohol, tobacco, and minor tranquilizers to high-risk groups. Substance abuse programs often become aware of such problems, and citizens can observe elementary and junior high school students smoking and drinking. There is evidence that the most widely abused chemical by high school students is alcohol. Often by merely asking students which merchants sell alcohol to minors, one can elicit the information. Law enforcement could be much more effective and supplies curtailed if there were more citizen cooperation.

In addition, or as alternatives to the broad approaches described above, there are less controversial activities that can enhance the substance abuse prevention activities of a CMHC, including educational activities and service to special groups. Although knowledge of what mood-altering drugs are and how they affect the body is a legitimate part of science education, it is not likely to be sufficient to prevent the recreational use of drugs. While valid biological information is necessary, accurate sociopsychological information is also needed. The portrayals of the life of addicts and alcoholics often glamorizes substance abuse to young people. Science teachers, librarians, and mass media specialists are best equipped to deal with public information about drugs. Professional staff and the board can act as advocates to see that these agencies are carrying out their responsibilities in education and public information.

Two special groups with problems of substance abuse prevention and treatment that are generally neglected are women and the elderly. In both populations, the abused substances are legally prescribed drugs and alcohol. Neither group currently has enough power or status to command the concern for study in a systematic way. Prevention of these substance abuse problems is likely to come about if physicians can be educated not to mask or deny the problems in living of their female and elderly patients with the prescription of minor tranquilizers. Local pharmacists and medical societies can take a leadership role in reeducating physicians in responsible prescribing practices.

All of the issues related in this chapter can be more easily dealt with if the substance abuse director is sympathetic with the ideology herein described.

WHAT ROLE SHOULD THE BOARD PLAY IN SELECTING A DIRECTOR OF SUBSTANCE ABUSE SERVICES?

When choosing a director of substance abuse services, a board will naturally examine resumés and recommendations. However, these rarely reflect the personal or professional philosophy of the candidate. A personal interview, supplemented by the candidate's publication record, can elucidate his/her creative and managerial skills.

During the selection of a director, the board should be able to rely on the CMHC director's competence to assess the candidate's technical skills and to determine how well his or her personal work and leadership styles will fit into the existing staff. As the substance abuse field develops, advancement in technology is likely to concern itself with the development of management information systems (paperwork) and biochemical monitoring equipment (surveillance). These areas serve bureaucratic and technocratic rather than community needs. In the field of substance abuse, we have a curious blend of medical management and law enforcement in which neither is done well. Competent administrators of substance abuse programs may be better at generating data to justify expenditures and documenting the need for more money than designing treatment and prevention programs. Therefore, the board must insure that the director of this program has a philosophy that is congruent with that of the CMHC. Naturally, this assumes the existence of a CMHC philosophy that is explicit and coherent, and reflects community beliefs and values.

HOW DOES FINANCE AFFECT IDEOLOGY?

To rehabilitate a chemically dependent person, one must break the dependency upon the chemical and have the person actively engage in his or her own self-determination. The same is true for communities dependent upon drug abuse monies.

As Americans we share a set of myths and experiences that addict us to government money the way junkies depend upon dope and alcoholics upon the bottle. The source and nature of funding are usually major determinants of intake, treatment, and discharge policies. As the federal government pressures programs into the numbers game, they pay less attention to the quality of care and more attention to admission, utilization, and discharge rates.

In a survey of drug treatment agencies in Chicago, the author found that a major and growing portion of treatment agency budgets went for administrative expenses rather than for treatment. Many program administrators reported that accepting federal funds reduced their creativity and risk taking in developing new approaches to treatment and prevention. A major inhibiting consideration was how changes would affect funding.

In truth, there is no "free" government money. The direct cost of $100 in government funds is, on the average, $116.40 to voluntary agencies (Hartogs & Weber, 1978). The total price that has to be paid is often greater than the benefits that accrue from accepting it. One alternative to current trends is to limit government funds for substance abuse services to purely medical treatment and to have self-help community groups provide the rehabilitation.

CONCLUSION

If CMHC boards prove successful in addressing major ideological issues, they could be part of a renaissance in participatory democracy. They may, for instance, promote decentralization of government by refusing federal funds. Giving up federal alcohol and drug abuse money can be as painful for communities as giving up chemicals can be for addicts and alcoholics. But the elimination of this dependence is a prerequisite for local autonomy. Why? Because it reduces the number of rules and regulations that serve bureaucracies rather than patients and communities. A board and its citizen committees may become knowledgeable about the technology of substance abuse treatment, planning, and evaluation. The board may develop a concern for ideology and insist that substance abuse programming be consistent with its system of beliefs, attitudes, and values. Success in this area is more likely to follow from an ongoing process of "best fit" than from fixed and immutable ideological assumptions. An appropriate ideology will not be situational, expedient, or technologically based, but will reflect a codified definition of "the good life" as envisioned by the community. The board may be instrumental in unifying medical services for alcoholics and addicts within general medical services. In short, the board may see its role as part of a larger movement to return power to the smallest unit of government, and using professionals and their organizations to serve rather than direct communities. If people want to have a say in how their communities and agencies are run, they may make small organizations an element in their ideologies (Schumacher, 1975). The CMHC board can serve as an advocate and enabler in this process.

REFERENCES

Block, P. Evaluation of the management of the alcoholic patient in a general hospital. Community Medicine Rotation Project, University of Pittsburgh School of Medicine, 1975.

Froom, J. Medical Bulletin. National Council on Alcoholism, March 15, 1975.

Hartogs, N., & Weber, J. Impact of government funding on the management of voluntary agencies. Greater New York Fund, United Way, 1978.

Illich, I. Medical nemesis. New York: Bantam, 1976.

Lasch, C. The culture of narcissism. New York: Norton, 1978.

Schumacher, E. Small is beautiful. Harper Colophon, 1975.

Tubesing, D. A. An idea in evolution. Hinsdale, Ill.: Society for
   Wholistic Medicine, 1978.

The wholistic health centers: A new direction in health care.
   Battle Creek, Mich.: W. K. Kellogg Foundation.

APPENDIX

Sources for Substance Abuse Literature

Drug Abuse Council
1828 L Street, N.W.
Washington, D.C. 20036

National Clearinghouse on Alcoholism
N.I.A.A.A.
5600 Fishers Lane
Rockville, Maryland 20852

National Clearinghouse for Drug Information
5600 Fishers Lane
Rockville, Maryland 20852

National Drug Abuse Center for Training and Resource Development
1900 North Moore Street
Rosslyn, Virginia 22209

Periodicals

The U.S. Journal of Drug and Alcohol Dependence
2119 A- Hollywood Blvd. , Hollywood, Florida 33020

Drug Abuse and Alcoholism Newsletter
Vista Hill Foundation
7798 Starling Drive
San Diego, California 92123

The Journal
Addictions Research Foundation
33 Russell Street
Toronto, Canada

Medical Letter
56 Harrison Street
New Rochelle, New York 10801

17

PARTIAL HOSPITAL PROGRAMS
Bea Jean Takei-Mejia
Stuart J. Ghertner
Allan Beigel

The movement to provide care to the seriously mentally ill in a partial day program, rather than through 24-hour hospitalization, began in the Soviet Union in the early 1930s. Initially developed because of constraints imposed by limited hospital space, it soon became clear that these partial hospital programs could be the treatment modality of choice for many psychiatric patients. The Russians emphasized a work therapy model. When the movement spread to England, this emphasis changed, and a social-milieu support focus emerged.

In 1946, the first North American day hospital, established by D. E. Cameron in Montreal, Canada, developed an approach that was more psychotherapeutic in nature. Even a decade later, Cameron remained nearly alone as an advocate for this psychotherapeutic modality of treatment and rehabilitation, until those in the United States, slower to follow, incorporated all three modalities (work therapy, social-milieu, and psychotherapy) into their concept of day treatment program or partial hospitalization.

In 1958, the American Psychiatric Association legitimized the partial hospitalization concept in this country by recommending day treatment centers as an alternative to expanding inpatient treatment beds in state and county mental health facilities. Since that time, day treatment centers and other types of partial hospitalization programs have had the continued support of the American Psychiatric Association and the National Institute of Mental Health.

In 1963, the Community Mental Health Centers Act (P.L. 88-164) established partial hospitalization as one of the five essential services to be required in any federally funded community mental health center. Succeeding amendments to the Community Mental

Health Centers Act in 1965, 1968, 1970, 1975, and 1978 retained
this mandate. Additionally, the movement toward deinstitutionalization of patients from state mental health hospitals during the past
15 years has also contributed to the increased attention that partial
hospitalization programs have received as potential resources for
care and treatment of this population.

Ongoing surveys by the Joint Information Services (sponsored
by the American Psychiatric Association and the Mental Health Association) and other public and private studies have documented the
continued importance and value of rehabilitating chronic patients
through the use of partial hospitalization strategies (Glasscote,
1968; Beigel & Feder, 1970; Ettlinger, Beigel, & Feder, 1972).
Although few large-scale research projects have been designed to
evaluate partial hospitalization programs, many smaller investigations have reported significant improvement among patient groups
as exhibited by increased integration in family, community, and
social subgroups following discharge from day treatment programs.

Working at the Manhattan After-Care Clinic in New York City,
Kris (1961) compared 17 patients with severe psychotic relapse who
were treated in a day hospital with ten patients who had been rehospitalized in a state mental health institution. All 17 of the day
hospital patients were discharged after two to six weeks of treatment and three years later remained in the community, while eight
of the ten rehospitalized patients continued as inpatients for the entire three-year period.

In a VA treatment center in Brooklyn, New York during the
1960s, 33 day treatment center patients were compared to 36 similar
patients assigned to conventional outpatient or aftercare services
(Meltzoff & Blumenthal, 1966). They were followed for a period of
18 months with ratings of interpersonal relations, family interactions, self-concept, affect control, mood, and motivation. Day
treatment patients maintained or improved their adjustment, while
outpatients showed a general decline in all areas.

Most recently, in 1978, the VA completed a large-scale study
that further indicated that day treatment programs significantly delayed relapses, reduced symptoms, and changed attitudes leading
to improved social functioning in this chronic population (Linn,
Caffey, & Klett, 1979). However, in spite of these and other studies, there continues to be four times the number of inpatient psychiatric treatment facilities (beds) as there are partial hospitalization or day treatment programs (spaces) in this country.

A major problem plaguing the development of sophisticated
day treatment programs is the perception by the public, and sometimes by the helping professions, that a day treatment program is
not a viable approach. It is believed that discontinuity of care

occurs as a result of allowing patients to maintain themselves in
their own family or community setting for extended periods of time
while concurrently being actively engaged for several hours a day
within a treatment program.

In addition, the public, including legislative representatives,
often require that programs and services that seek funding demonstrate their ability to "cure" individuals if the program is to receive financial assistance. In fact, though, this "cure" orientation
is not valid because most day treatment programs focus on the more
realistic goal of rehabilitation. Rehabilitation is defined as helping
a client acquire skills and behaviors necessary to control his/her
disability and to function outside an institution while maintaining a
maximum level of personal satisfaction, happiness, independence,
and community productivity. Since the concept of rehabilitation is
less well understood than the concept of cure, public funding bodies
are often reluctant to support such programs out of fear that the cost
will continue to escalate as the treatment remains open-ended.

Similar concerns are also present within the insurance industry. Many companies have been reluctant to include partial hospitalization as a benefit because of fear that this coverage will lead to
longer treatment at an ever-increasing cost. Moreover, federal reimbursement programs, such as Medicare, do not currently provide
for reimbursement of partial hospitalization, although this is presently under reexamination at the highest levels of government.

Further complicating the issue and also inhibiting the development of partial hospitalization programs is the attitude of the clients
themselves, who frequently prefer the less demanding environment
of "inpatient" status to assuming the responsibility for personal
needs, transportation, and the other duties of independent living required by many partial hospitalization programs. When these considerations are added to the harsh reality of identifying problem
areas within their lives, beginning the transition to independent living, and learning new problem-solving mechanisms, it is understandable that many patients shy away from the more intense contact involved in the partial hospitalization programs and prefer the
more dependent environment of the inpatient service.

For other patients, who often deny the severity of their illness
even after a period of intensive hospital treatment, referral to a day
treatment or partial hospitalization program is a less acceptable alternative to continuing aftercare through infrequent outpatient visits.
These patients often believe that their hospital discharge indicates
that they are no longer ill and, therefore, no longer require treatment. Understandably, they are anxious to put the experience of
hospitalization behind them. These patients are often less willing
to accept the more structured environment of a day program than
the less frequent contact in an outpatient clinic.

DEFINITIONS: PARTIAL HOSPITALIZATION, DAY HOSPITAL, DAY TREATMENT, DAY CARE, AND TRANSITIONAL SERVICES

Within the mental health professions and the public at large, considerable confusion often exists regarding the concept of partial hospitalization, primarily because of the multiple terms that are used, sometimes erroneously or interchangeably, to describe different aspects of partial hospitalization services. In this section, some of the more frequently used terms will be defined.

Partial hospitalization is the term most often used as an umbrella concept for the entire range of services incorporated within the definitions of day hospital, day treatment, day care, and transitional services. Public laws and regulations consider partial hospitalization services to include any service that is offered on a more frequent basis than services currently available in an outpatient environment, but which is also less intense than a 24-hour environment such as a hospital. Furthermore, there is the understanding that, within a partial hospitalization program, the principal focus of the therapeutic orientation is on the structured milieu. Rather than individual psychotherapy, milieu therapy or other forms of group therapy are the primary modes of treatment.

Day hospital is the term most frequently and appropriately used to describe a partial hospital setting found in a general hospital or a private psychiatric hospital. In the day hospital setting, which may be in the same part of the facility as the inpatient unit or in a separate part of the hospital, patients, many of whom have recently been 24-hour residents of the hospital, participate in ongoing treatment of the type described above. Most commonly, the day hospital—in contrast to other partial hospitalization modalities—is psychiatrically and medically oriented.

Day treatment is the type of partial hospitalization service that is most often encountered within community mental health programs outside a hospital setting. Within the day treatment setting, which is often less medically oriented than the day hospital, an array of milieu and support services is offered to clients within a structured daytime program. However, within this broad framework, day treatment programs include a variety of therapeutic philosophies and approaches, as well as a diverse psychiatric population. Some programs focus on patients with more acute histories of illness, while others emphasize the care and treatment of the more severely ill, who are long-term patients. The lack of uniform guidelines within this category may be a major contributor to the confusion that exists among many professionals regarding the concept of partial hospitalization.

Day care programs most often emphasize socialization activities with a focus on occupational and recreational endeavors. They are less structured than day treatment programs, and clients often come more infrequently and according to a less structured schedule than patients in a day treatment program. Within this environment, which is more oriented toward sustaining care rather than active treatment, protection is offered to the patient who often possesses very dysfunctional daily living and social skills. Many day care programs are not a part of or related to formal mental health settings, but instead are adjunctive to the mental health service delivery system. That system uses these programs as referral resources for patients who require additional support beyond that available within the formal mental health setting. Within most day care programs, emphasis is clearly on chronically mentally ill persons rather than the acutely disabled. As a result, staffing patterns often have less medical input, as well as a decreased emphasis on active treatment by skilled mental health professionals. Often, many of the staff in day care programs are volunteers who work under the supervision of a mental health professional.

Transitional services, while they may incorporate day treatment, partial hospital, or day care services, more commonly refer to programs that offer residential alternatives to inpatient hospitalization. Predominant in this category are halfway houses and night hospitals, where patients receive living accommodations during nonworking hours, along with a structured therapeutic program. These services are often used by patients who are making the transition from inpatient care to independent living during a time when they do not have a viable residential environment. These individuals are usually able to work, go to school, or engage in volunteer activities during the day, and then return to the transitional service environment in the evening.

INDICATION FOR AND USES OF PARTIAL HOSPITALIZATION SERVICES

There are numerous programmatic descriptions and evaluation studies of the following groups of mental health clients, for whom partial hospitalization services can be beneficial.

The Seriously Impaired Client Who Would Otherwise Require Inpatient Hospitalization

For this population, the advantage of partial hospitalization is that care takes place in the community, and the client is not ostracised. At the same time, it provides an ongoing treatment process that leads to daily confrontation with those stresses of independent living that may have contributed to the illness in its earlier stages. Furthermore, partial hospitalization services enable the patient to maintain family ties and encourage family interaction as a way of providing an additional support system to the client while he or she strives to change or improve living skills.

Acute or Chronically Impaired Clients Who Require Assistance When Moving from the Hospital to Independent Living in the Community

For this population, a partial hospitalization service affords opportunities for limited and gradually implemented reorientation to the community. When partial hospitalization services are used in this manner, the patient may remain for a period of time on the inpatient service during the evening and at night, while participating in the day treatment program that is often located in another setting. In this manner, the patient may gradually relearn or reassume responsibilities for daily activities (such as public transportation) and begin a gradual reintegration into the community before being discharged from the hospital.

Clients Who Have Ongoing Social and Vocational Deficits as a Result of Chronic Mental Illness

For this target population, the partial hospitalization setting offers a reeducation and rehabilitation program in which chronically mentally ill persons may begin to regain social and vocational skills that have been seriously impaired as a result of a psychosis. Within most partial hospitalization programs individualized treatment plans and schedules may be developed which address the specific needs of each chronically mentally ill person. Included within these programmatic strategies may be rehabilitation training and educational programs delivered either within the partial hospitalization setting or through a local community college.

Acutely Depressed and Neurotic Clients

A partial hospitalization service can provide a structured activity program in which controlled social interactions may assist the acutely depressed or the neurotic client who, prior to coming to the partial hospitalization service, was becoming more withdrawn and on the verge of an acute crisis in an independent living situation. Within the partial hospitalization service, pressures of daily living can be ameliorated, and the client can be assisted to work through the conflicts that precipitated the acute depression or crisis. The presence of a peer group process can often stimulate patients to address their problems more quickly and readily than they would in an outpatient setting.

In addition to these specific target populations for which partial hospitalization services are most applicable, some programs have recently developed additional uses for this type of service setting, which could be adopted by any mental health delivery system. For example, many community mental health programs have a great deal of difficulty in properly assessing some clients. In this regard, the partial hospitalization service can provide an important mechanism for more adequately diagnosing those clients who present continued problems. In this environment, patients can be evaluated over a lengthy period of time, as opposed to the more typical one-hour intake that generally occurs. Persons can be observed in numerous types of social interactions to determine stress levels and personal competency. In this way, the partial hospitalization program can provide a diagnostic service without the necessity of involving an inpatient service.

Another innovative use of partial hospitalization services by some mental health programs has been to experiment with utilizing a partial hospitalization setting on a limited basis as an adjunct to outpatient therapy for chronic mentally ill persons. In this regard, partial hospitalization, while serving the patient only two or three days a week (day care), can provide additional support to individuals who would otherwise decompensate and require rehospitalization.

For these populations, the successful partial hospitalization program must have access to an inpatient service in the event that any of the clients become so highly agitated that they are dangerous to themselves or others, and thereby require supervised medical intervention and temporary 24-hour care. Additionally, partial hospitalization services must also have the ability through their access to a 24-hour setting to remove those clients who cannot adjust to the program, so that the entire program, which emphasizes a milieu approach to treatment, is not impaired as a result of the actions of a few.

ADVANTAGES AND DISADVANTAGES

Regardless of the target population being served or the specific purpose for which the partial hospitalization program is being used, there are multiple advantages to partial hospitalization programs in contrast to outpatient settings and inpatient services. At the most fundamental level, the partial hospitalization service allows an individual to maintain those independent activities of which he or she is capable in spite of ongoing mental disability. This discourages excessive dependency, which may result from full-time hospitalization, and further allows the client to maintain individual dignity without encountering the social stigma of inpatient treatment.

Within partial hospitalization settings, patients are also encouraged to remain within the family setting or another independent living environment. In this way, the structure of the partial hospitalization service most closely resembles the five-day work week, thereby assisting the client in making a later transition to employment or volunteer work.

The partial hospitalization setting creates less social frustration for the patient since there is not a prolonged period of forced absence from social interaction or sexual activity, and support systems can continue to operate within the individual's life structure without significant interruption. This also encourages the patient to continue to work through any daily problem or stress areas since he or she has to return to a "normal" environment at the end of each program day. As a result, the patient finds it more difficult to deny daily problems of living when participating in a partial hospitalization service.

In offering a more active therapeutic experience, the partial hospitalization service also creates an awareness in patients of their own strengths and abilities. An inpatient service often does not encourage this because patients are frequently confined to bed and are more often confronted with their weaknesses than their strengths.

By making part-time jobs available to clients on evenings and weekends, partial hospitalization services also lend themselves more readily to nonmedical and social-vocational rehabilitation strategies. Because partial hospitalization services work hand-in-hand with existing community support systems such as those found within parks and recreation departments, local churches, and other social agencies, they can provide a smoother transition for the client from the characteristic medical model orientation found in an inpatient setting to the independent role of a functioning community member.

Clearly, partial hospitalization services are also easier and less expensive to staff than inpatient services, since there is a regular five-day work week, with most staff working a traditional eight-hour work day from 8:00 A.M. to 5:00 P.M. Finally, the partial hospitalization service provides a continued opportunity to observe medication reactions and other psychotropic effects, which would not be as available in an outpatient setting.

At the same time that this list of advantages for partial hospitalization services is provided to the reader, certain disadvantages also must be acknowledged. For example, the partial hospitalization setting does not completely remove the patient from the community or family environment, which may be precipitating the disturbance; thus, increases in symptomatology may continue for a longer period of time than if the patient were hospitalized. With the increased independence that patients experience while participating in partial hospitalization services, a higher risk for assaultive or suicidal behavior may be seen. Additionally, the open systems approach of partial hospitalization services provides less structure than an inpatient setting and, therefore, the dropout rate of patients from partial hospitalization is likely to be higher than it would in inpatient settings. Similarly, because more intensive therapeutic involvement is required of patients in day treatment programs, these partial hospitalization services will also experience a higher dropout rate than those that serve on an outpatient basis.

Finally, for staff who choose to work in partial hospitalization services, there is considerable personal stress as a result of the intensive interaction with often seriously disturbed clients. Staff turnover may be high unless support systems are also provided to staff.

UTILIZATION OF PARTIAL HOSPITALIZATION SERVICES

In 1968, a Joint Information Service survey indicated that most partial hospitalization programs were underutilized (Glasscote, 1968). At that time, one out of every five programs had fewer than ten clients. Although the census of partial hospitalization programs has increased during the past 12 years, the percentage of clients currently being treated in day treatment programs, when compared to inpatient settings, remains low, as documented in a 1976 survey conducted by the Biometrics Branch of the National Institute of Mental Health. In this survey, 3,495 psychiatric facilities of all types were queried regarding the types of services they provided. In only 1,458 (42 percent) of these facilities were partial hospitalization services present. Of 183 private psychiatric hospitals surveyed, only 70 (42 percent) had partial hospitalization services. A similar trend of underutilization was noted in other types of psychiatric facilities. Specifically, partial hospitalization programs were present in only 38 percent of VA psychiatric facilities, 58 percent of VA general hospitals, 22 percent of public general hospitals with psychiatric units, 20 percent of nonprofit, private mental health programs, and only 30 percent of residential programs.

In considering alternate explanations for this low utilization of partial hospitalization programs despite the continued research reports of their positive impact, it is important to determine whether financial considerations have played a role. Available data, however, appear to indicate that partial hospitalization programs are fiscally feasible and cost efficient and that financing considerations should not necessarily be a contributing factor in partial hospitalization underutilization.

For example, a recent evaluation of federally supported treatment programs in a Veterans Administration hospital revealed not only the efficacy of the day treatment program in preventing further hospitalization and in improving the quality of life for its participants, but indicated that this was possible through a decreased average length of stay. In conclusion, this study pointed out that the use of partial hospitalization is significantly more economical than inpatient treatment. For the 65 patients involved in this study, there was a reduction of 12,772 days of inpatient care and an estimated savings of $1.4 million (Guidry, 1979).

Another study that supports the cost effectiveness of partial hospitalization programs was conducted by a private insurance company in Washington, D.C. that provides group health coverage to its clientele. This company was interested in discovering whether partial hospitalization services could be cost effective from an insurance perspective and would serve as a means of controlling the costs of psychiatric inpatient care. Findings revealed that approximately $1.7 billion could be saved if the hospital stay of each mentally ill patient covered could be reduced by one day. As a result, they recommend that day hospital programs be more equitably reimbursed by health care insurance programs (Tischler, 1978). Unfortunately, this recommendation has been ignored by many insurance carriers who continue to contribute to the increase in cost of inpatient care by excluding partial hospitalization coverage from their policies and to the underutilization of partial hospitalization programs.

In spite of the proven clinical effectiveness of partial hospitalization programs and the fiscal advantages noted above, the low rate of utilization of these programs continues. Consequently, one must look elsewhere for factors that may be contributing to this pattern of underutilization.

Resistance on the part of clients and their families toward using partial hospitalization services occurs during times of crisis. In many instances, both clients and their family members prefer inpatient hospitalization because it offers a more "effective" way of reducing anxiety within the patient and the family. Family involvement in the treatment process is limited since the patient is in the hospital on a 24-hour basis. At the time of acute crisis, many family members are concerned about self-destructive behaviors or actions that can be dangerous to others. In this context, inpatient hospitalization is preferred even though there is no evidence to suggest an increased incidence of self-destructive behavior among patients treated in partial hospitalization programs.

As noted earlier, clients often prefer inpatient hospitalization to partial hospitalization because of the relative comfort which the dependent environment of the inpatient service offers and the removal from daily community pressures which this environment insures. Also, many hospital administrators exert pressure to maintain a high level of occupancy for psychiatric inpatient beds.

Most private psychiatrists are unfamiliar with day treatment settings because they have never worked within them. Consequently, it is difficult for them to identify clearly what types of patients could be served effectively by this type of program.

A concerned, but often misinformed, public exerts social pressure in favor of institutionalization. This is particularly true with regard to persons with chronic mental illness, who are often better served in partial hospitalization programs but are placed in outpatient environments because the community has little understanding and considerable fear regarding their presence in the community.

There is continued resistance on the part of third-party payers to reimburse for partial hospitalization services as a lower cost alternative to full-time inpatient status. In this regard, efforts are being undertaken to allow for a replacement, on a two-for-one basis, of partial hospitalization services for inpatient services in insurance coverage.

CONCLUSION

Advisory and policy-making boards of community mental health programs should recognize that an effective system of mental health services cannot be available without the implementation of an adequate range of partial hospitalization programs. At the same time, the attainment of this objective is not easy. Concerned citizens can play a vital role through community education and liaison with governmental and nongovernmental policy makers to insure that a more adequate understanding and recognition of the benefits of these types of services are achieved. Community board members can also be helpful in developing specific strategies that address some of the negative factors playing a role in the underutilization of partial hospitalization services. While these services have achieved increased recognition during the past 15 years, it is clear that universal acceptance of the benefits of this type of service delivery mechanism has not been achieved and that further efforts are required.

REFERENCES

Beigel, A., & Feder, S. L. Patterns of utilization in partial hospitalization. American Journal of Psychiatry, 1970, 126, 1267-1274.

Ettlinger, R. A., Beigel, A., & Feder, S. L. The partial hospital as a transition from inpatient treatment. A controlled follow-up study. The Mount Sinai Journal of Medicine, 1972, 34, 251-257.

Glasscote, R. Partial hospitalization programs for the mentally ill. Washington, D.C.: Joint Information Service, 1968.

Glasscote, R., & Cumming, R. E. Rehabilitating the mentally ill in the community: A study of psychosocial rehabilitation centers. Washington, D.C.: Joint Information Service, 1971.

Guidry, H. S. Evaluation of day treatment center effectiveness. Journal of Clinical Psychiatry, 1979, 40, 221-226.

Kris, E. Prevention of rehospitalization through relapse control in a day hospital. In M. Greenblatt & C. C. Thomas (Eds.), Mental Patients in Transition. Springfield, Ill.: Charles C. Thomas, 1961.

Linn, M. W., Caffey, E. M., & Klett, C. J. Day treatment and psychotropic drugs in the aftercare of schizophrenic patients. Archives of General Psychiatry, 1979, 36, 1055-1066.

Meltzoff, J., & Blumenthal, R. The day treatment center. Springfield, Ill.: Charles C. Thomas, 1966.

Tischler, G. L. Another reason for underutilization of partial hospitalization. American Journal of Psychiatry, 1978, 135, 1428-1429.

18

TRANSITIONAL AND LONG-TERM SERVICES FOR THE SEVERELY EMOTIONALLY DISABLED ADULT POPULATION
Marshall Rubin

The objective of this chapter is to present a framework of program principles for the development of community-based transitional and long-term services and facilities for the severely emotionally disabled adult population. It should be understood that specific agency and service system structures will vary from community to community and must be taken into consideration when planning for service delivery.

This chapter will attempt to develop a set of program principles for serving the severely emotionally disabled that can be helpful to laypersons, mental health administrators, planners, and educators as they meet the transitional and long-term needs of this traditionally underserved population.

DESCRIPTION OF TARGET POPULATION AND THEIR NEEDS

The phrase "severely emotionally disabled adult" does not mean the same to all readers. The recent Community Support Program (CSP) definition of service functions is the best current description of the population and their needs. A CSP is defined as "A net-work of caring and responsible people committed to assisting a vulnerable population to meet their needs and develop their potential without being necessarily isolated or excluded from the community" (National Institute of Mental Health, 1977, p. 329).

There are currently 20 states funded for CSP demonstration and strategy planning projects under NIMH. The NIMH guidelines describe a "core service agency" as necessary to a CSP. They define the "core service agency" as follows:

There must be a "core service agency" within the community that is committed to helping severely mentally disabled people improve their lives. Frequently, this agency will itself provide a number of the basic CSP components, such as psychosocial rehabilitation services and indefinite duration supportive services. Regardless of how many direct services the core agency provides, it must take responsibility for the following integrative functions without which the clients who are most severely disabled will easily become isolated from the community:
—providing a staff who enjoy working with severely disabled people, and who are skilled in helping them develop their potential;
—offering a therapeutic community milieu in which rehabilitation and supportive services can be provided;
—helping those clients who lack meaningful community ties to make friends, and encouraging clients to help one another;
—providing or stimulating others in the community to provide opportunities for clients to assume and adjust to normal social roles, such as resident, worker, club members, etc. [p. 329]

Many types of organizations could assume the "core service agency" role. Part of the CSP project nationally is to study the effectiveness of different types of agencies in assuming this role. Whatever the type of agency, its role is to assume leadership for improving services for the target population. The CSP guidelines list ten essential services, some of which are provided directly by the "core service agency," while others are contracted. The ten components are listed by Turner and Tenhoor (1978):

1. Identification of the target population at risk, whether in hospitals or in the community, and outreach to offer appropriate services to those willing to participate

2. Assistance in applying for entitlements

3. Crisis stabilization services in the least restrictive setting possible with hospitalization available when other options are insufficient

4. Psychosocial rehabilitation services

5. Supportive services of indefinite duration, including supportive living and working arrangements, and other such services for as long as they are needed

6. Medical and mental health care

7. Backup support to families, friends, and community members

8. Involvement of concerned community members in planning and offering housing or working opportunities

9. Protection of client rights, both in hospitals and in the community

10. Case management, to ensure continuous availability of appropriate forms of assistance

EVOLUTION OF PUBLIC POLICY VIS-À-VIS THE SEVERELY EMOTIONALLY DISABLED

It would be helpful to examine public funding and service delivery policy as they have evolved during the past decade with special attention to NIMH and the Rehabilitative Services Administration (RSA). During the past decade, there has been a convergence of NIMH and RSA goals relative to the severely emotionally disabled. There are three important realizations that seem to characterize shifts in both NIMH and RSA policy. First, the chronic psychiatric population needs long-term availability of supportive services. This has not been a priority by Community Mental Health Centers (CMHCs) over the last decade. Second, funding to support necessary services for the chronic psychiatric population cannot be the responsibility of any one agency alone. Third, rehabilitative services for the chronic psychiatric population must go beyond those who have clear vocational goals.

Psychosocial rehabilitation services and supportive services of indefinite duration have special relevance to the issue of long-term services. Since writing the guidelines, CSP staff have tended to view these two components as continuous. The thrust of the CSP development is thus consistent with what Olshansky (1968) describes as "the myth of transitionalism":

> One of the misperceptions is that many ex-patients require a network of transitional facilities within the community to restore them to normal participation in the labor market. Some of the transitional facilities considered necessary are sheltered workshops, social clubs, and halfway houses. By far the largest part of this visible group requires these facilities not as transitional, but as long-term, facilities that would permit many of them to stay out of the hospital, or to improve their performance while in the community. [p. 372]

These conclusions were more recently supported by Test and Stein (1978) in their review of research on community treatment of the chronic patient. They state:

Modest gains in psychosocial functioning in the community can be achieved, then, through direct and intensive intervention in specific activities of daily living in the community with gains being sustained as long as treatment lasts. That is, chronic mental illness may be a life-long disability that requires life-long supports and direct and ongoing interventions if maintenance or improvement is to occur. [p. 360]

Only recently has there been a shift toward coordinating efforts and funding for the psychiatrically disabled. Until recently, a philosophy of "let the other agency pay" has led to a lack of coordination of funding. The categorical nature of public funding to meet the multitude of needs of this highly vulnerable population causes professionals great difficulty in negotiating the separate eligibility rules for each entitlement. A 1977 GAO report states that almost every service needed by mentally disabled persons in communities can be financed wholly or partly with federal funds. Often the funds are not used because agencies are not aware of the deinstitutionalization goals or how to foster them.

Deinstitutionalization of the mentally disabled has been a national goal since 1963, with the advent of federal legislation creating CMHCs. Although these centers were given the task to work with the severely psychiatrically disabled, funding for rehabilitation was one of the five nonmandatory services. Therefore, those services that did develop for the chronic patient, with few exceptions, included only aftercare and partial hospitalization day treatment on a time-limited basis.

The Community Mental Health Centers Amendments of 1975 (Public Law 94-63) still did not place an emphasis on long-term rehabilitation services. In fact, rehabilitation was deleted as one of the possible services, and transitional services, mainly residential in nature, were added to the new mandated services. However, there now seems to be hope as a result of the 1978 President's Commission on Mental Health, which cites the CSP effort and places a priority on long-term services to the chronic mentally ill. This recommendation has been incorporated into the Carter Administration proposal for a new Mental Health Systems Act. Hopefully, we should soon begin to see a change in planning, with more funds going to CMHCs and other agencies that are ready to give priority to the chronic patient for both long-term as well as transitional needs.

All human beings strive to establish support systems: this is essential for both individual and community stability. Since the severely emotionally disabled have not been successful in establishing adequate support systems for themselves, it is precisely this type of help they need. However, if time limits are given, then regression is sure to occur.

There has been a growing recognition by rehabilitation authorities that the chronically disabled's rehabilitative needs are broader than just vocational. Mary E. Switzer, Commissioner of RSA for 17 years, explains the growth of the philosophy of rehabilitation quite well (Glasscote, 1971, p. 28):

> Vocational rehabilitation, like many other aspects of human affairs, has evolved through three stages of public attitudes—compassion without action, followed by willingness to act for economic reasons, followed by willingness to act for social reasons. It seems to me that we are at a transitional stage between the last two, with almost universal acceptance of the economic soundness of returning disabled people to employment and a slowly growing philosophy that an advanced civilization like ours should so order its systems that all disabled people will be restored as fully as possible, regardless of any economic benefits to anyone.

This enlightened statement was made 15 years ago. Since then, RSA policy has gradually shifted in the direction Switzer inferred. In 1967, the word "vocational" was dropped when the name of the federal agency was changed to Social and Rehabilitation Service (later to Rehabilitative Services Administration). In 1973, the Vocational Rehabilitation Act placed a priority on service to the severely disabled. As one of these groups, the severely emotionally disabled population was eligible but at the discretion of each state. The Comprehensive Rehabilitation Services Amendments of 1978 strengthened potential funding for the severely mentally disabled by stating clearly that RSA had a responsibility to this population. This responsibility was extended even to those without a clear potential for independent competitive employment. States have the option to establish centers for independent living. Funding for this is pending, but the mandate for RSA funding of nonvocational rehabilitation services has now been established.

Under the leadership of the CSP staff, an NIMH/RSA Cooperative Agreement was signed in May 1978. That agreement paved the way for establishment of formalized working relations on the state and local levels. The first project of this agreement was the funding of a Research and Training Center for the rehabilitation of mentally handicapped individuals. This center does not limit its research to vocational aspects of rehabilitation.

The importance of the CSP effort cannot be overemphasized. At the federal level, CSP staff have worked closely with HUD, RSA, and ACTION to coordinate efforts on behalf of the severely emotionally disabled. On the state level, similar coordinating efforts to maximize planning and entitlements for this population are undertaken. At the local level, demonstration sites attempt to actualize the efforts of the federal and state planners into coordinated and comprehensive service.

A PHILOSOPHICAL FRAMEWORK FOR DEVELOPING A CORE SERVICE AGENCY

The CSP guidelines stress that whatever type of agency is designated a core service agency, its role is to improve services for the target population. In so doing, a core service agency must take on some of the ten functions that compose a CSP. It is my contention that for the core service agency to be most effective, psychosocial rehabilitation and supportive services of an indefinite duration, including living and working arrangements, must be offered directly by the core service agency. The agencies that were first developed to deliver these services were known as psychosocial rehabilitation centers. In general, they can be characterized as free standing, nonprofit private social agencies, nonmedical in orientation (although most have psychiatric consultants); they serve the severely emotionally disabled (primarily a chronic schizophrenic population), who use the centers voluntarily; they derive income from a mix of funding sources; and their major service offerings are vocational, social, and in some cases residential. The first of these centers, Fountain House, was established in New York City in 1948.

I have increasingly become more comfortable with the term "settlement house" when describing this type of community support program because I feel the term broadens the psychosocial rehabilitation center concept and strengthens community identification. One of the guiding principles is to strive toward normalization. That is, services should be delivered in a manner that is consistent with culturally normative methods and settings, reduce stigma, and create roles for clients that are consistent with adult functioning in the community. Because the title "psychosocial rehabilitation center" carries a stigma with it, it is much easier to identify as a member of a settlement house or community center and, thus, achieve a little more distance from one's patient status.

I wish to discuss the settlement house movement, as I feel that it sheds light on the development of the community support program. Settlement houses and workers predated social work as a profession. The movement coincided with a shift by charity organizations in the late 1890s and early 1900s from an emphasis on almsgiving to the worthy to helping people help themselves. The settlement houses assisted large numbers of new immigrants in making the adjustment to and becoming functioning members of their new communities. Often they were organized on a nationality or other ethnic basis and so became communities of special interest within the larger society. Persons leaving mental institutions can be thought of in much the same manner as the new immigrants of an earlier era. Both have had to face an initial community response of "they are different, who needs them, send them back." Fortunately, the settlement house response was "we need and want you, come join us."

The settlement house gave direct help with housing, food, job development, and language skills; it offered assistance in getting medical and legal services; and it organized their members (both the advantaged older settlers and the newer more disadvantaged) to coalesce around social issues faced by their constituency. How different is this, really, from the roles that a core service agency should take on in dealing with the variety of service, organizational, and social issue tasks that must be faced if deinstitutionalization is dealt with in a manner that fosters rehabilitation and maximizes community adjustment? Landy (1960) speaks of the rehabilitation process as one of acculturation. This is surely what the settlement house movement dealt with, while at the same time strengthening the identity of its constituency as a legitimate and vital part of the larger community.

A core service agency philosophy can be developed and compared to a settlement house in five major ways: (1) members are viewed as needed citizens; (2) prime attention is given to creating opportunities for members; (3) community organization and advocacy to gain rights and access to opportunities is a major function; (4) members are active participants in the service delivery and development; (5) a core service agency is not primarily a treatment facility, but rather helps its members gain access to resources to meet their needs. A major focus is to help members view themselves predominantly in the healthy roles of friend, worker, and roommate, rather than as patient.

Having discussed the target population and their needs, the evolution of public policy, and a philosophical framework for developing a core service agency, I shall now discuss basic program principles of transitional and long-term service for the severely emotionally disabled. These program principles form the basis of the community support program implemented by Fellowship House, the agency directed by the author, which serves the severely emotionally disabled in Dade and Broward Counties, Florida.

PROGRAM PRINCIPLES FOR TRANSITIONAL AND LONG-TERM SERVICE DELIVERY

There are four major roles that a core service agency, committed to the philosophical framework described in the preceding section, must undertake: intake and outreach by staff and members; direct provision of transitional and long-term supportive services; ongoing case management intervention and advocacy; and community organization. I will discuss each of these four major areas, highlighting principles that are crucial to the maintenance of a philosophy consistent with the preceding sections.

Intake/Outreach by Staff and Members: Encouraging Involvement

The initial contact a potential member has with an agency may well determine whether the individual will get involved or drop out. We must overcome the negative attitude potential members have developed as a result of past experiences with social agencies and hospitals that put them through repetitive diagnostic and eligibility interviews. The thrust of intake should be to establish relationships, one of the main difficulties of the severely emotionally disabled population. Some suggestions follow:

1. Approach the intake situation with an attitude of screening in, rather than screening out.
2. Convey a message that potential recipients are "needed members," rather than patients or clients.
3. Have current members host, tour, and explain the program to prospective members. This can resemble a "Welcome Wagon" approach. Membership cards can be given out and the benefits available to members fully explained.
4. Hold orientation groups on days that a social program is happening so that prospective members can stay for it and for lunch.
5. Develop pre-discharge relationships with patients at local and state hospitals. Promote regular visits to the core service agency for program involvement prior to discharge.

6. Develop regular outreach, undertaken jointly by staff and members, to board-and-care homes to attempt to form relationships with prospective members.
7. Determine what segments of the target population are underserved by the core service agency (and mental health system) and develop a plan to increase service to them.
8. Encourage staff and members to work together to reach out to drop-outs or no-shows.
9. Pay special attention to assisting prospective members in obtaining decent housing, food, and other necessities. Do not leave this up to another agency! Veteran members can take an active role in helping new members apply for entitlements when routine procedures have been established, for example, escorting new members to the Food Stamp Office.

In summary, intake staff and veteran members play an important role in setting the attitude of the settlement house—"You are now a citizen, and you are entitled."

Direct Provision of Transitional
and Long-Term Services

A concerted effort must be made to render direct service offerings attractive. There should be no time limits, not only because it is impossible to predict who will and who will not be successful, but also because communities are made up of individuals with varying skills and abilities to contribute. To try to segregate individuals into "fast" and "slow" impedes the ability of members to help and to learn from each other, while creating a self-fulfilling prophecy of failure for those designated as less likely to succeed.

The program should be designed to create opportunities for members socially, vocationally, and residentially, so that they can take advantage of any combination of services based on their changing needs. Involvement should not be sequential, since rehabilitation does not happen in a sequential manner, and programs should seek to respond to members' needs as they occur. To set up rigid steps for involvement would be a disincentive to developing relationships.

Maximizing Social Opportunities

Social skills are part of all human tasks; therefore, helping members use vocational and residential opportunities entails attention to interpersonal skills. An important part of the support system

for all human beings is to have healthy leisure experiences, which
can best be accomplished by providing social opportunities (or rehabilitation) through a community center. The community center
concept developed from the settlement house movement. To belong
to a community center is an adult and normal role. The principle
to follow is to offer programs that appeal to adults rather than just
to patients. The social program offered by a core service agency
should have a duality of function: to create and maintain a community in which the severely emotionally disabled can have friends and
a sense of belonging; and to help members to function socially in the
outside community. I will briefly discuss seven purposes that I feel
social programming for an adult severely emotionally disabled population should address.

1. To break the cycle of social isolation and rehospitalization:
    Staff and members should welcome new members and reach
out to old members who do not attend. Agencies should hold "regular" community center hours. As an example, holding a dance on a
Saturday evening is normal, while holding one on a Tuesday afternoon is stigmatizing. Many types of activity groups should be created,
so that members can take on different roles and responsibilities. We
all need alternatives to choose from, and get tired of doing the same
thing. Make the community center comfortable and attractive, so
that a sense of dignity is conveyed.

2. To improve social skills of members and learn new ones:
    Staff, volunteers, and other members should serve as role
models. Recruit staff and volunteers to represent different ethnic
groups, ages, and sexes, so that there is a variety of role models
from which to learn and with which to identify. Intervene openly
when inappropriate behavior occurs, so that members get direct
feedback and others can learn by example. The message should be
given neither hostilely nor solicitously, but with normal human concern. Encourage members to give feedback to each other openly,
as their concerns are valid ones.

3. To help members learn how to relax and enjoy themselves:
    Set an atmosphere that is busy but not boring. This sets up
the expectation of not dwelling on problems. There should always
be a variety of things to do, and there should be both structure and
flexibility. Some persons participate by watching. Many severely
emotionally disabled individuals are like tourists, needing encouragement and instructions to enjoy new leisure pastimes.

4. To maximize the potential of each member:
    Offer opportunities for individual private efforts through hobby
activity and opportunities for efforts before an audience through
group participation and leadership.

5. To help members become more self-directed in their interactions with others:

Encourage individual decision making—how to use one's free time, when to come, what to do, and with whom to do it. The program should be organized so that there are decisions to make regarding what roles to undertake. An individual may choose to be part of planning on one night and to be a cook for a group meal another night. This gives the individual an opportunity to find satisfaction from different roles and to learn how others relate to him or her in those roles.

6. To create a long-term support system:

A core service agency social program is a major part of the long-term support system that maintains a sense of belonging. For example, holidays should be celebrated on the right day; family, friends, members, and staff should all be welcome. Planning should attempt to maintain tradition without staleness. Members look forward to traditional activities, but the program must always grow. As the core service agency community matures, more traditions should be added.

7. To introduce members to community resources:

This can be done through guest speakers, performers, and field trips to community activities. Since members' resources are limited, events planned should be affordable on a limited budget, so that members can return on their own or with friends.

Vocational Programming

The prime principle in developing vocationally oriented services is to involve recipients in activities that create a realistic feeling of being needed and productive. This can best be accomplished by involving members during regular working hours in prevocational work activities that are needed for the functioning of the agency, and employment in the business community.

Prevocational Work Activity

A core service agency involves members in activities consistent with the objectives of psychosocial rehabilitation. Feeling needed is healthy. A daytime vocationally oriented program helps members develop skills needed in every job situation. The focus should be on helping members feel useful by taking on responsibility at the agency. Members can prepare food, publish a daily newspaper, collect data for statistical reports, clean and repair the facility, and maintain the landscaping. For those members who do not have employment goals, being productive in their settlement house is important to maintaining a needed citizen image.

Creating Opportunities for Employment
in the Normal Business Community

A major goal of vocational rehabilitation is to enable individuals to maximize their productive capability and achieve paid employment in the business community. Fountain House in New York City is the first successful program of this type and conducts a national training program to help staff develop community-based services for the chronic psychiatric patient. A major emphasis has been on training to develop transitional employment.

This is an employer-paid program designed to meet both employers' needs for productivity and members' needs for successful work experience. Wages are paid only for real work, and the agency guarantees job performance. When a member is placed on the job, a back-up member is also trained. If both members are absent, a staff person reports to work.

Members hold the same transitional position for three to six months, after which they participate in the training of a replacement. Members receive considerable benefits from working a transitional employment job, the major bonus being real pay to supplement their incomes. They also receive a reference from the employer after successful completion of the position. In 1979, 955 members of 67 different psychiatric rehabilitation facilities participated in transitional employment, involving 361 employers. Their annual earnings are reported at $3.5 million.

It is my feeling that a core service agency should not offer specific job training programs. There are agencies in most communities whose function is to offer these services. If a member is ready for training, the core service agency should refer her/him to a good training program. The job of the core service agency would then be to provide a back-up support relationship to enable that member to complete the job training program.

Residential Services

The basic principle in the development of residential services is to provide members with the best housing for their housing dollar in the least restrictive setting. It is necessary to have a continuum of residential choices ranging from the highly supportive and transitional to the less supportive and long-term, possibly permanent. Members possess different levels of living and coping skills, and these are expressed differently at particular points in their lives. Three residential options that seem to meet the range of supportive needs of most severely emotionally disabled individuals are group homes, supervised apartments, and satellite apartments.

The three residential options are presented here in order of decreasing supervision:

1. Group home. Members can utilize this residential program when they are in need of a high degree of supervision and support. Twenty-four-hour on-premise staff supervision helps members learn living and interpersonal skills needed to live in the community and then to move into a supervised or satellite apartment.

2. Supervised apartments. For those in need of less structure and no in-house staff supervision, supervised apartments can be most helpful. Groups of two to four members share a number of apartments. A staff member lives in an apartment located in the same complex and works with the members in their apartments, helping them in cooking, cleaning, bus travel, and getting along with others.

3. Satellite apartments. The satellite apartment concept, first developed by Fountain House, is for members who have the basic skills necessary for more independent living. Satellite apartments are leased by the core service agency in clusters, so that a social network is formed among members residing there. Since costs are shared by roommates, even people on public aid and social security can afford this type of housing. Members may live in a satellite apartment as long as they maintain it, get along with their roommates, and pay their bills. The core service agency holds the lease and guarantees payment of rent to the landlord. This is an incentive both to the landlord and to the members, who would otherwise not have the references or funds necessary for a deposit. The apartments can be attractively furnished from donations of furniture and household items through community contacts. By living in a decentralized apartment, the member resides in a manner that is consistent with the surrounding community, minimizing stigma and community unrest.

Members living in any of the three options spend normal workday hours either in the core service agency vocationally oriented program or in their own productive work. They are encouraged to take advantage of the weekend and evening social programs. Members' time spent in a residential facility should be focused on home management and family living activities. Social and vocational rehabilitation activities should not be conducted in their homes. This is consistent with the principle of normalization. It also avoids what I refer to as the "bedroom slipper syndrome," in which members leave their rooms only to eat and participate in the vocational and social programs, without venturing out of the building.

Ongoing Case Management Intervention
and Advocacy

The severely emotionally disabled have needs that must be
met at different locations and by different agencies. The purpose
of case management is to provide the personalized help that allows
members to organize their lives to meet their ever-changing needs.
A system of case management should effectively reduce the disruptive effects that fragmented service delivery has on the lives of members. A case management system should be based on the following
assumptions: It is best done by the individual who has the strongest
relationship with the member; it is most effective when there is back-
up responsibility by a team of staff; and, it is most effective when
performed by an individual or team from which the individual is receiving other services.

Too often, agencies have set up separate case management
systems exclusively for tracking. Case management should foster
the core service agency's primary task of maximizing the potential
of all members.

Community Organization

Comprehensiveness and continuity of service are major goals
for a core service agency. They require an active role in organizing the community, including resource development, planning/advo-
cacy, and public education and promotion. These tasks can be performed by the core service agency administrators, by specialized
community organizers, or by CMHC consultation and education staff.
Board members and community groups can also expand the scope of
influence of the core service agency.

Resource Development

It is important to develop as broad a range of financial support
as possible, which includes both private and public sources. Agencies that depend on a limited scope of support risk financial distress.
Much can and has been written about resource development. To
cover this subject adequately would require more space than the
scope of this chapter allows. What I will do is offer some suggestions. (1) Resource development is as much a matter of attitude as
it is knowing lists of specific government and private funding sources.
Each contact should be viewed from the standpoint of "what can this
person or agency do for the severely emotionally disabled of our community?" (2) Resource development is a two-way street. A resource

relationship must be maintained and ways found to reciprocate and give recognition. (3) Board members must be helped to see their roles as fostering resource development. To do so, they must be educated about the agency service program so that they can believe in and interpret its goals. (4) Continual resource development means accountability, both in terms of taking care to use resources appropriately and to report results accurately. (5) One resource should not be expected to cover all areas. Government agencies and private resources have different areas of interest and dispense their monies accordingly.

Resource development also includes the development of sources of income maintenance for the members served. Many of the severely emotionally disabled require maintenance benefits over a long period of time. At best, they are intermittently employed, employed in less than full-time positions, or working at jobs that pay minimum wage. The deinstitutionalization effort is hindered by lack of adequate and consistent financial assistance to enable the chronically disabled to buy decent housing, food, and other basic necessities. It is unfortunate that basic health and income maintenance benefits are removed when severely emotionally disabled individuals become low-wage earners. In doing so, we only invite further deterioration and rehospitalization.

We can maximize the number of potential maintenance resources, and insure that the resources are used at the appropriate time. For instance, emergency county welfare funds may shorten a person's stay in the hospital but should be supplanted with S.S.I., Office of Vocational Rehabilitation maintenance funds, earned income, or family assistance, as the individual becomes eligible for these benefits.

Income maintenance entitlements are often difficult to assess. Community organization staff should spend considerable time developing formalized agreements with agencies that control such benefits. These agreements then become the tools that case managers utilize in helping members receive entitlements.

Planning and Advocacy

A major community organization role for a core service agency is leadership in planning and advocacy. Those involved in community organization functions at a core service agency must take major responsibility on a local and statewide level to effect changes that will promote opportunities for the severely emotionally disabled population.

Once again, space only allows for a few examples of the types of planning and advocacy tasks that a core service agency can undertake through community organization efforts:

1. Formalize linkages between the core service agency and other local agencies so that the target population can benefit from the services of each agency and avoid duplication.

2. Encourage and take leadership roles with local and state mental health, vocational rehabilitation, and other health service authorities in planning to meet the target population needs.

3. Offer technical assistance to other agencies in the community who relate to the service or entitlement needs of the severely emotionally disabled.

4. Develop state-wide and local organizations representing service providers, families, and ex-patients who can together act as an advocacy coalition to affect state and local planning priorities for the severely emotionally disabled.

Public Education and Promotion

A final community organization role is public education and promotion. It has been well documented that the lay community has many fears and misconceptions about the severely emotionally disabled. There are many opportunities to present the facts about mental illness to civic and community groups. Whenever possible, involve the severely emotionally disabled themselves in presentations. Members enjoy these opportunities to take on another needed role. Often, speaking engagements lead to volunteer help, funding, and referrals of members who otherwise would go unserved because the core service agency was unknown to the referring agent or because the symptoms were not recognized as mental illness.

District mental health boards, health planning councils, health and rehabilitative advisory boards, and mental health associations are all bodies that plan for mental health and rehabilitative services. They are not necessarily knowledgeable of, or place a priority on, the needs of the severely emotionally disabled population. Core service agency staff must be present at the meetings of these boards to educate them and increase their sense of priority for the target population. Education of our community is a never-ending task.

CONCLUSION

The emotionally disabled adult population has the same needs as other adults. Each of us needs friends, meaningful work, and a secure place to live. In addition, we need to have access to quality economic, health, and life-sustaining resources. We all strive to organize our lives so that we meet these needs and create support systems for ourselves and people we care about. Severely emotionally disabled adults are more vulnerable to stress and, therefore, need assistance in developing the interdependent relationships that establish and maintain support systems. However, the process and problems associated with developing support systems for this population are the same as those associated with developing our own supporting communities. We grow and mature if there is a community commitment to acceptance and cooperation in seeing human needs.

It is hoped that this discussion has added to the understanding of the program principles involved in establishing a community support system for the severely emotionally disabled adult population. It is a challenging, comprehensive, and rewarding process.

REFERENCES

Comptroller General of the United States, General Accounting Office (GAO). Returning the mentally disabled to the community: Government needs to do more. Washington, D.C.: U.S. Government Printing Office, 1977.

Glasscote, R. M. Rehabilitating the mentally ill in the community. Washington, D.C.: Joint Information Service of the American Psychiatric Association and the National Association for Mental Health, 1971.

Landy, D. Rehabilitation as a sociocultural process. Journal of Social Issues, 1960, 16, 3-7.

National Institute of Mental Health. Community support guidelines. Washington, D.C.: U.S. Government Printing Office, 1977.

Olshansky, S. The vocational rehabilitation of ex-psychiatric patients. Mental Hygiene, 1968, 52, 556-561.

Test, M. A., & Stein, L. I. Community treatment of the chronic patient: Research overview. Schizophrenia Bulletin, 1978, 4, 360.

Turner, J. C., & Tenhoor, W. J. The NIMH community support program: Pilot approach to a needed social reform. Schizophrenia Bulletin, 1978, 4, 329-330.

19

MENTAL HEALTH SYSTEMS AND
THE COORDINATION OF SERVICES
Robert Agranoff
Julianne Mahler

System development and coordination of mental health services are among the most significant activities that board members and administrators of community mental health agencies undertake. If the leadership of the mental health center were able to operate independently, insuring that the right services were brought to those clients in need through its organization, the job would be relatively simple. It is now recognized, however, that the community mental health center must operate interdependently, because the right services mean ensuring that clients receive the services of other mental health and human services agencies. In fact, a study measuring citizen board accomplishment (Meyers, 1972) suggested that one of the dimensions of its success is coordination. Similarly, the report of the President's Commission on Mental Health identified coordination efforts as significant. Two of its major recommendations were to "develop networks of high quality, comprehensive mental health services, throughout the country, and to coordinate these services more closely with each other, with general health and other human services, and social support systems."

The aim of this chapter is to review the current trends in systems development and coordination, and to explore the responsibilities of community mental health boards in developing interagency linkages. The potential for interagency coordination and its pitfalls are discussed next, followed by an examination of strategies for

The authors wish to acknowledge Alex Pattakos for his helpful suggestions and revisions.

coordination among mental health agencies and between mental health and other human services. The chapter concludes with a list of tactical suggestions for boards to encourage greater coordination among local agencies.

System development and coordination are distinct but related concepts. System refers to regular or patterned sets of interactive activities by diverse agencies within identifiable boundaries. In the case of mental health systems, we are referring to the attempt to develop such regular or patterned activities between mental health service organizations as well as with other human services agencies. Coordination is the means by which such systems are developed. It involves individual or mutual accommodation of the policies and/or procedures of two or more agencies. Thus, mental health agencies may modify their programs or management operations in order to improve working relations with other agencies and programs. The means or mechanisms for coordinating programs and operations are termed linkages, and can include such diverse mechanisms as informal staff contacts, written agreements, and ongoing formal policy councils. These and other linkages are discussed in detail later in this chapter.

THE EMERGENCE OF COORDINATED
MENTAL HEALTH SERVICES

Several trends in mental health have led to an increased emphasis on coordination of services. Board members should acquire a basic familiarity with these trends. New intervention approaches and attitudes toward mental disability are factors that have prompted closer ties between agencies. Most prominent of these has been greater preference for nonmedical treatment approaches, a growing awareness of the connection between societal values and mental illness, and the realization that little evidence exists to demonstrate the effectiveness of traditional treatment methods. These new approaches and attitudes have been reflected in public policy through formal requirements for greater coordination. For example, the 1975 Amendments to the CMHC Act mandate increased comprehensiveness of services, while the Special Health Revenue Sharing Act of 1975 requires states to offer a variety of services from different agencies to those in danger of hospitalization. These examples are only suggestive of the greater attention program coordination is receiving in the rules and regulations community programs must follow.

Two related trends of importance to coordination are deinstitutionalization and community support. While community-based treatment is essential in maintaining residents in the community after discharge from state facilities (Burgess, Nelson, & Wallhaus, 1974), CMHC services alone have not had a significant impact on helping people return from mental hospitals to communities (GAO, 1977), particularly without a community support system.

Developing the means to maintain people in the community, then, requires that the necessary supports be available to help people in need function in the community. These support systems are based on "a network of caring and responsible people committed to assisting a vulnerable population to meet their needs and develop their potentials without being unnecessarily isolated or excluded from the community" (Turner & Dean, 1978). According to the NIMH Community Support Program, an adequate community-level support system must perform the following ten functions: identification of the population, whether in the hospital or in the community, and outreach to offer appropriate services; assistance in applying for entitlements; crisis stabilization services in the least restrictive setting possible, with hospitalization available when other options are insufficient; psychosocial rehabilitation services, including transitional living arrangements, socialization, and vocational rehabilitation; supportive services of indefinite duration, including sheltered living arrangements; supportive work opportunities, and age-appropriate, culturally appropriate daytime and evening activities; medical and mental health care; back-up support to families, friends, and community members; involvement of concerned community members in planning, volunteering, and offering housing or work opportunities; protection of client rights, both in hospital and in the community; and case management, to insure continuous availability of appropriate forms of assistance (Turner & Dean, 1978, p. 17).

An equally significant trend can be seen in the growth of newer forms of community treatment, such as nursing homes and psychiatric units of general hospitals. These forms have been fostered by public policies that confine income maintenance and social services to residents of community inpatient facilities while excluding those in state hospitals.

Despite the sweeping changes in outlooks and techniques for treating mental disability, the range of treatment modes and settings in many mental health agencies remains quite limited (Kaplan & Bohr, 1976). Mental health personnel, being clinically trained, are naturally oriented to those therapeutic approaches with which they are most familiar. Moreover, the everyday pressures of dealing with clients remain predominantly oriented toward providing direct treatment. To achieve the broader objectives of community-based care, however, it is generally agreed that it is necessary for these organizations to break out of a strict, classical treatment mode, offer new types of treatment, and build community support structures. One important means of smoothing the way toward innovation (Ilfeld & Lindemann, 1971; Warren, 1971) is for the board to develop or use its broad-based community and political support to encourage linkages with other organizations. In other words, the community leadership represented on mental health boards are encouraged to take the lead, using their wide contacts to help the staff to move to a more comprehensive focus in programming, and broader goals. In many mental health organizations, board members possess a broader perspective than the staff do, and this can be used to encourage staff toward the emergent concepts of treatment. This leadership function in system development will be discussed in greater detail later in this chapter.

BOARD RESPONSIBILITIES IN COORDINATION

Coordination and system development requirements are increasingly being woven into laws, rules, and guidelines governing community-based mental health programs. Boards have distinct responsibilities in these areas, including policy formation, monitoring access to treatment, identifying needs for clients, and developing service agency coalitions.

Policy Making

The establishment and oversight of mental health agency policy, that is, goal-directed courses of action, are important board functions. It is essential that boards understand as many courses of action as possible, so that they can select those policies that best serve the needs of their communities.

Following Courses of Treatment

Boards must be aware of the various courses of treatment and the services offered by other agencies and programs that might meet the needs of the mental health center's clients. This may involve some familiarity with other mental health services, such as day treatment programs, respite care, peer-groups, sheltered workshops, group homes, and other such programs. Likewise, it may require familiarity with nonmental treatment programs, such as income support, vocational training, physical health, public housing, and others. Of course, boards should also have some familiarity with the service operations of their own centers.

Understanding the Regulations

Since most centers have multiple-source funding with concomitant spending and program constraints (Agranoff, 1975), board
members should be familiar with rules and regulations, especially
those regarding system development/coordination. For example,
the Illinois Department of Mental Health requires its funded agencies
to link with the education, health, welfare, and general social services in each planning area. The standards for services for developmentally disabled individuals of the Joint Commission on Accreditation of Hospitals require that some person be responsible for coordinating an individual client's program (1978). This involves a
wide range of concerns, including the total spectrum of individual
needs (housing, family relationships, social activities, education,
mobility, protective services, and so on).

Using Community Contacts

Board members usually represent the community in other
areas. They tend to be activists in local politics, as well as in
neighborhood development, education, housing, and health planning.
These activities not only tend to give community mental health board
members broader perspectives, but they provide useful contacts
with other agencies. Their contacts can open doors for the staff to
create the types of linkages needed to coordinate services. The
ability of the board to increase the visibility and political power of
the mental health program is often neglected by agencies (Warren,
1971).

Issues of Service and Strategy

In considering coordination for system development, the staff
and the board must consider basic issues of service and strategy.
Issues of service refer to questions of what should be done for
clients. First, what should the program do for an individual's needs?
Should the client receive intensive psychotherapy, counseling, medical treatment, occupational training, help in personal grooming, and
so on? Second, who should serve the client? Are highly trained
specialists necessary, or can some human services generalists provide the necessary services? Third, what resources can be made
available to serve the client's needs? Will clients be totally economically dependent during the course of service, or will some form
of employment relieve the burden? Can volunteers serve the client

as effectively as paid staff? Fourth, how far should the mental health center go with clients before they become the concern of other agencies? Does the client receive substance abuse services, or is the problem really a correctional issue? Finally, how much can an agency do for an individual in crisis? Should the agency focus on his/her emotional needs and frustrations, or more immediate formal problems?

Issues of strategy refer to how particular client problems should be approached. Another way of posing the issue is to ask, at what level does the program organize to meet client needs? If it is at the individual level, then education, therapy, or a job may be necessary. It may be at the interpersonal level, requiring family counseling, peer groups, or self-help groups. The problem could be a group problem, requiring special training programs, youth employment programs, or skill development programs for the disadvantaged. The problem may dictate an advocacy strategy, requiring speaking out for clients' housing or legal rights. The problem may be a societal problem, requiring a social or political strategy, as in the case of long-term solutions to such problems as poverty, delinquency, domestic violence, and substance abuse (Agranoff, 1974).

Before considering the particular strategies that boards and agencies can pursue, the general interorganizational context is examined. The conditions that have been found to encourage interagency ties provide a basis for examining the likelihood of success.

FACTORS INFLUENCING LINKAGE
BETWEEN AGENCIES

The evolution of interorganizational coordination and appropriate linkage mechanisms has been studied in a variety of state and local agency settings. The value of this research is that it alerts us to the conditions that facilitate or impede efforts to forge cooperative and accommodative ties among interacting agencies. The research also illustrates some of the pitfalls of coordination. Though it may smooth the development of interagency programs and augment the effectiveness of the cooperating agencies, coordination can also be costly, threaten an agency's autonomy or identity, and be of marginal value. In this context, at least five conditions have been found to affect the likelihood of successful interagency coordination. These include: (1) resource dependency, (2) agency power, (3) awareness of dependency, (4) uniform procedures, and (5) legal mandates for coordination.

Resource Dependency

When one agency relies on another for services, personnel, clients, or information, a state of resource dependency exists. Dependency has been identified as the principal basis for coordination. Without it, there is little reason for agency interaction and insufficient incentive to expend the effort to coordinate (Lytwak & Hylton, 1962; Lytwak & Rothman, 1970; Schmidt & Kochan, 1977; Hall et al., 1977). Resource dependency results from several circumstances. The universal scarcity of resources and the limits of the individual agency's service capacity makes every agency to some extent dependent on others.

Among mental health agencies, specialized children's programs and substance abuse treatment agencies often depend on mental health centers, local hospitals, or crisis centers for referrals. In these cases, however, the possibility of mutual or reciprocal dependency exists, and an exchange of services can provide a basis for coordination. Mental health centers and hospitals depend on the special treatment agencies in order to fulfill their obligation to provide a full range of treatment under funding regulations.

Some agencies are much more independent than others because they have a separate funding base or their own interest group to help them secure resources. For example, Lytwak and Hylton (1962) show how the American Cancer Society, because of the strength of its appeal to most people, was able to enforce its priorities on other Community Chest agencies. Thus, we would expect that independently funded or backed mental health agencies would be better able to forestall unwanted but mandated coordination or integration.

New laws, regulations, and funding requirements established at any level of government can change the balance of dependency rapidly. The Health Planning Act of 1974, for example, gave local health planning agencies the authority to sign off CMHC and other mental health program applications. Federal community support programs give added weight to the priorities of formerly weak service agencies whose cooperation is now needed by more independent agencies. By stipulating greater real authority for existing agencies, by establishing new agencies with powers to enforce coordination, or by devising tangible and enforceable penalties for noncooperation, changes in laws and regulations can be used strategically to encourage coordination. Global pronouncements about the value of coordination, if not backed by changes in the balance of interdependencies, is unlikely to have the desired effect.

Another source of interagency dependency is the degree to which other local agencies can provide similar or related services. As the number of organizations increases and programs change, the service environment becomes too complex and unstable for the successful functioning of any one agency. Agencies then must establish joint objectives and definitive relations to avoid unexpected policy shifts or agency alignments (Emory & Trist, 1965; O'Brien, 1971; Metcalfe, 1978).

In summary, the existence of interdependence among agencies in the service network is a prerequisite for coordination. Interdependencies may stem from a variety of conditions including resource scarcity, statutes and funding requirements, and environmental characteristics. However, the network of agencies may be unbalanced, so that some agencies are much more dependent than others (Schmidt & Kochan, 1977). This does not necessarily rule out the possibility of coordination. In some extreme cases, the dependency of one agency on another may become so great that merger rather than coordination results. Exclusive service contracts may lead to merger, for example. The most probable set of circumstances for coordination are cases in which agencies are partially dependent upon each other (Lytwak & Hylton, 1962; Lytwak & Rothman, 1970).

Agency Power

Related to the issue of interdependency is the level of resources an agency has on hand as a basis for independent functioning and/or cooperative exchange. A resource base external to and independent of the local agency network is the clearest example of such power. Local offices of state departments or federal programs are often immune to local pressures to cooperate (Lytwak & Hylton, 1962; Benson, 1975). A constituency that supports an agency's position is another power source, especially when it is faced with cutbacks. Developmental disabilities agencies, for instance, often mobilize families to oppose state budget reductions.

As stated above, asymmetric power relations among agencies do not necessarily rule out coordination. Schmidt and Kochan (1977) found that interaction and resource exchange can still occur if the weaker agency is perceived as having goals consistent with the stronger one, or is seen as being prestigious or effective. Under these conditions, the weaker agency can pursue coordination through aggressive bargaining, often mobilizing professional support to make linkage attractive to stronger agencies.

Awareness

Agencies must be aware of the state of scarce resources and the need for interagency cooperation for coordination to take place.

The possibility of interagency referrals, for example, must be acknowledged before agencies can see linkages as mutually beneficial (Lytwak & Hylton, 1962). While referral linkages may be fairly obvious in most cases, it may be much more difficult for agencies to see how their respective resource allocation and treatment decisions affect the overall effectiveness of the service network. Unilateral agency policy decisions about client eligibility or payment for care may create unacknowledged service gaps and overlaps that reduce the effectiveness of the whole care system. Evaluation research and local planning studies have been an important source of information about these effects of agency interdependency, as have the policy councils established under federal, state, and local cooperative planning programs. There may also be a kind of cyclic effect between coordination and awareness, such that initial coordination efforts to smooth one kind of interdependency puts agencies in closer contact and raises their conscious awareness of other areas of interdependency.

The other side of the awareness problem is that agencies may, in reality, be _less_ interdependent than they believe themselves to be. This may result when agencies want to board the services integration bandwagon even though the local network is not so complex that it requires elaborate coordination mechanisms. In these cases, agencies are expending previous resources on an organization function, coordination, which is needed at a lower level than is practiced. The implication, of course, is that there should be a balance between the level and type of interdependency and the elaborateness of the linkages.

Related to the issue of awareness is the extent to which there is consensus among the agencies in the network about the proper role, goals, and jurisdiction of each agency (Benson, 1975; Wamsley & Zald, 1976). If there is disagreement about which agency should perform a particular service, where, or for whom, agencies may find themselves competing for clients and jurisdictions. This establishes an additional roadblock for coordination since domain issues and the terms of cooperation must both be managed under the linkage. However, despite these difficulties, coordination may still be seen as useful if competition is draining agency resources and reducing effectiveness.

Uniformity of Procedures

The fourth factor commonly identified as facilitating linkage is consistency among agencies in work approach (Lytwak & Hylton, 1962; Lytwak & Rothman, 1970; Benson, 1975). In mental health service agencies, this means the consistency of problem definitions, diagnosis, categories of client care, and other agency management operations. The more agencies share a common language and treatment technology, the better the prospects are for devising successful ways to link services, personnel, evaluation and information systems, and planning.

Legal Mandates for Coordination

The effect of laws, regulations, and special programs to establish and enforce coordination among agencies is conditioned by the factors discussed so far. If no clear benefit accrues to an agency from coordination, that is, no dependency or basis for communication exists, and if agencies have the power base to resist encroachments on their jurisdiction or resources, then legal mandates for coordination can become costly and futile exercises.

O'Brien (1971) points to one particular aspect of this problem. He examines mandated linkages on the basis of whether they establish formal mechanisms for decision making and conflict resolution, thereby providing a structure and specific resources for managing the agency linkages. He argues that mandated linkages with managed structures are the most stable, while voluntary unmanaged links are usually transient and limited in effect. Serious problems arise when linkages are mandated with no resources or decision structures. These linkages often result in "paper policies" that create more interagency conflict than they resolve.

The consideration of all five of the conditions for interorganizational coordination suggests some useful principles for linkage. In brief, agencies can be viewed as balancing the likelihood of benefit from coordination for its level of resources, its prestige, or its clients, against the costs of coordination, including reduced autonomy and the direct costs of the personnel needed to maintain the linkage (Pondy, 1974). Within this perspective, the key characteristics of the linkage are its costs and its efficiency. Linkages that are too elaborate and time-consuming relative to the benefit derived from them will be difficult to form and maintain. Agencies may resist them.

What this analysis suggests is that coordinating agencies might be most successful if the elaborateness of the linkage mechanism closely matches the elaborateness of the interdependency among them. Weekly meetings among agency heads will not be seen as a good investment if the only problems they consider are specific client referral difficulties.

There are a variety of possible forms of linkage that can be developed, however, that will be appropriate to the level of coordination needed. The most common and successful approaches build on the informal, problem-specific contacts among agencies, gradually making them more formal and elaborate as agencies become more willing to share resources. The variety of linkage mechanisms being developed by coordinating agencies and service organizations is considered next.

BOARD STRATEGIES FOR COORDINATION: BUILDING MENTAL HEALTH LINKAGES

There are at least three strategies, broadly conceived, that boards or other agency actors concerned with building coordination can consider. First, at the agency level, the concept of service may be expanded and client-centered links to other services built into the treatment regime. Second, boards may encourage the development of linkages among mental health agencies, thereby establishing a stable network of mental health services. Finally, boards can take an active role in developing linkages between mental health agencies, or the network of agencies, and other human service networks. Specific types and examples of these three strategies are presented below.

Expanding Treatment Approaches

One of the most straightforward approaches to coordination is to build it into the therapeutic approach. Kahn, for example, has identified the provision of such functions as access, information, and advocacy as parallel to the socialization, developmental therapeutic, and rehabilitative functions of human services (1979, p. 27). Such approaches provide direct mental health services, as well as the necessary links with other services to help the client. For example, in the case of a catastrophe such as a train accident, both therapeutic mental health and human services linkage tasks would be included (Agranoff & Pattakos, 1979, pp. 21-22; Bourne, 1974, p. 668).

Therapeutic Mental Health
1. have people work through their grief
2. utilize crisis intervention technology for persons suffering from severe anxiety
3. establish ingroup processes
4. implement dyadic therapy models
5. utilize diagnostic technology

Human Service Linkage

1. link people to money
2. give insurance advice
3. provide transportation
4. set up problem-solving sessions
5. help persons find new jobs
6. run errands
7. link people to legal services
8. function as an advocate and expediter

This broader perspective to services does not exclude the normal services offered by the mental health program but expands them in order to help clients solve their problems.

Also of increasing importance is the need for the mental health center to develop relationships with the health care sector. The individual physician and the general hospital have long been prominent, but there is an increasing need to include other care givers, such as nurse practitioners, physician extenders, and health institutions such as neighborhood health centers and health maintenance organizations. A recent study of mental health centers found few examples of CMHC and medical providers working together (U.S. Dept. of HEW, 1979).

Coordination with Other Mental Health Agencies

One direction that agencies must look to is other mental health programs. For example, a youth mental health services network developed in Tacoma, Washington includes the following (Fields, 1978): a youth services bureau, which refers young persons to services within and outside the system; a counseling and tutoring project for youth encountering difficulties in a school setting; a children's hospital health center for crisis assessment and short-term hospitalization; a voluntary children's service home builders program designed to keep families intact during periods of crisis by providing professional staff to work with the family in the home; an emergency foster home program; a mental health center children's service, including family, group, and individual counseling; and a system operations manager based in the mental health center. Interagency networks like this one have developed all over the country in recent years.

Long (1974, pp. 23-24) has suggested that the elements of such a coordinated model include:

1. General intake and assessment of client's problems.
2. Knowledge of service facilities.
3. Responsibility for referring clients.

4. Responsibility for a formal contract between clients, system managers, and programs.
5. Responsibility for evaluating the quality of the service rendered to the client.
6. Follow-up to obtain feedback on both client service and agency effectiveness.
7. Responsibility for administering funds for the operation of the coordinative system.
8. Responsibility for researching areas of unmet needs and gaps in the service delivery system.

Datel and Murphy (1975, p. 37) add that a governance structure is essential, which not only evaluates the effectiveness of the model but unfreezes barriers to effective service, institutionalizes policy changes, and develops innovative funding and administration.

Service networks can also include a variety of helpers. First, mental health "gatekeepers" are persons outside both mental health professions and human services agencies whose occupational roles give them special leverage or put them on the scene at points of crisis in people's lives. Some obvious roles are physicians, nurses, teachers, attorneys, police, and firemen. Less obvious roles are barbers, bartenders, astrologers, and fortune tellers. These persons are a part of the helping network, being the most frequent referral agents to agencies.

Second are persons who have special talents and interests in the area of helping or counseling, regardless of occupational background. Some individuals function as sources of "therapeutic" support and service to friends, relatives, and associates. While these persons function in helping roles, we know little in any systematic way about how they operate, make contacts, and provide their service. It might be useful to integrate these people into more structured helping relationships by developing cooperative relationships with formal mental health workers.

A third group is the professional workers and service agencies outside mental health but part of the human service agency array. Included here are several types of agencies, including income maintenance, social services, child welfare, employment and training, public health, vocational rehabilitation, aging, and many others. Agencies need to be in contact with mental health programs when their clients need to be linked to mental health services. The development of these relationships between human services agencies will be covered in the next section.

Building Human Services Linkages

The development of "systems" among the vast array of human services that have emerged in the past two decades of program growth is a subject of increased importance. The number of Department of Health, Education and Welfare (DHEW) programs alone exceeds 300. In addition, there are non-DHEW federal programs in employment and training, veteran's assistance, criminal justice, housing, and food and nutrition-related services. In addition, there are state and local government programs, as well as voluntary (nonprofit) and for-profit programs. The best estimates place the number of individual human services programs between 500 and 600. The growth of these programs has led to problems in excessive program independence, fragmentation, duplication, inaccessibility, and ineffectiveness in service delivery, and to difficulties in evaluation.

The course of action that has been undertaken to deal with these problems has been labeled "human services integration." Actually, this term loosely identifies a great number of coordinative activities that attempt to achieve some coherence and understanding in the array of services. Agranoff and Pattakos (1979, pp. 9-10) identified services integration activity along four dimensions: (1) a broadened service delivery approach, where providers approach the client as a person with complex needs, ensuring through such means as case management, information, and referral that those needs are met; (2) an attempt to create "program linkages," where independent agencies coordinate, working toward a comprehensive multiagency service delivery system; (3) the efforts of governmental units to pull together the strands of various programs within the intergovernmental system, developing policies that cut across programs; and (4) the creation of new organizations or "umbrellas" that encompass a number of human services in order to support improved policy management, program linkages, and services delivery. It should come as no surprise that mental health and mental disability related programs have been at the core of these efforts to integrate services. Integration is both consistent with the new approaches to mental health treatment and necessary to accomplishing its aims. At the same time, mental health programs are essential to support the work of other types of human services. Some brief examples of coordinative activities between the services will be suggested.

Informal contacts. The most basic integrative relationships are informal contacts between agency personnel. Generally, as a staff member in one agency comes to understand that the client's needs are broader than the responses his or her agency can supply, contacts are made with staff in other agencies. Many of these relationships, such as those between mental health and welfare, vocational rehabilitation, child welfare, and employment and training, are never formalized.

Interagency agreements. The next logical step is for two or more agencies to enter into an agreement to coordinate. Generally this occurs when agency transactions to solve problems are regular, but the contacts can be ad hoc or irregular, too. A common form of agreement might take place when vocational rehabilitation, employment, and training agencies accept referrals of mentally disabled clients from the mental health center.

Program linkage systems. Often, related problems among agencies lead to the development of a "human service system." For example, mental health and developmental disability systems have been expanded to encompass children's services, vocational rehabilitation, special education, youth services, and aging. These systems engage in such activities as interagency staffings, shared service agreements, joint case management systems, cooperative information systems, and joint planning and evaluation systems. Some consortia have developed one-stop or colocated multiservice centers, where a large number of agencies operate under the same roof.

Single area bodies. Other services in addition to mental health have considered developing cooperative systems. Single purpose planning and coordinating bodies include child care councils (4Cs), senior citizen councils, rehabilitation councils, youth services networks, health systems agencies, criminal justice planning councils, and CETA manpower planning councils.

Community service councils. For over a century, private charitable organizations have been involved in coordination. The most familiar example is the United Way movement, which began with efforts to coordinate fund raising and reduce duplication of effort. United Way and similar organizations are becoming increasingly involved in the planning and evaluation of services. As these agencies have begun to receive public funds, they are joining in public-private partnerships for planning and coordination of services. There are also many general community development organizations, such as The Woodlawn Organization (TWO) in Chicago. These "community councils" identify needs, secure resources, plan new programs, evaluate existing programs, and coordinate total service efforts.

Policy management activities. Regional and state planning agencies, as well as city, county, and state government human service offices, increasingly attempt to broadly (that is, across many individual programs with a problem or target population focus) assess needs, set priorities, make resource allocations, foster a particular course of action, and monitor the outcomes for the jurisdiction. Mental health planning and program development will increasingly have to interact with these relatively new activities.

Umbrella agencies. States and some cities and counties in the past decade have combined their human services units into new departments, called Departments of Human Resources (DHR). Twenty-eight states have combined public welfare and at least two other human services into a DHR. Mental health is almost always part of the umbrella. Although these large agencies are formed for diverse purposes and are quite dissimilar in operation (Agranoff, 1977), they all attempt to develop improved coordination between programs.

TACTICS IN FACILITATING COORDINATION

The variety of possible strategies for fostering interagency linkage and coordination provides a framework within which boards can consider alternative actions. The conditions that facilitate coordination and the linkages in common practice have been described above, but specific tactics for boards are presented here. It should be clear at this point that there are no simple rules for generating coordination. Any reasonable set of suggestions must be cast in the context of contingencies, since the complexity of the interagency network and the costs to agencies of the accommodations they must make affect the success of efforts to establish linkages. With this qualification, we suggest the following tactics for facilitating coordination.

The first set of suggestions involves assessment of the current state of coordination in the service system. These activities are most conveniently performed by the staff.

Compile an inventory of the mental health and related resources in the local community.

Catalog the resources in the community that are informally part of the mental health system (for example, physicians, clergy, teachers, and so forth) and gauge their contribution to treatment and community support.

Identify social supports for psychiatric clients that other formal community organizations could provide and the possible interactions among the organizations—as, for example, in the area of deinstitutionalization.

Investigate the current common patterns of interaction among mental health agencies. Determine the kinds of linkages that now exist.

Investigate the current state of resource dependency among mental health agencies, including the basic network of referrals, shared resources, contracts, and so on.

Determine the current conflicts and animosities among the agencies.

Establish a process evaluation research project to identify the major effects of the current service network in producing gaps and/or unnecessary duplication in service. Even a partial study may produce a basis for action.

Determine what specific resources agencies have devoted to interagency relations and linkages. Identify client advocates who refer clients to other services and follow-up care, for example, or agency staff assigned to interagency planning.

Determine how current regulations might be used directly or indirectly to encourage or support coordination efforts.

Note agency objections to linkage and coordination. Use these data to overcome resistance.

When possible, join in evaluations by other agencies to investigate the need for coordination and local impediments to it, with the possibility of developing a formal network.

The second set of suggestions involves the board in an active or adjudicative role in the evolution of coordination among service agencies.

The board may establish a task force to bring selected staff into a face-to-face forum to identify interdependencies and work out linkages.

If informal interagency agreements are functioning satisfactorily, the board may do more harm than good by insisting that the relations be formalized or made more elaborate. If there are problems in the conduct of linkages, if conditions change, or if key linkage personnel move (a common event), the board's assistance in devising new linkages may be helpful, but again the form of linkage should not outstrip its purpose.

Intervention by the board may be useful in negotiations over coordination. The board may intervene by providing help to parties to find innovative accommodations.

The third set of suggestions regarding the development of linkage and coordination involves investigating resources available for joint programs or planning.

The board may help mental health agencies work out the details for financing shared personnel, services, or physical facilities.

Board members or staff can examine federal and state program announcements for demonstration project funds for local service coordination.

Board members can serve on boards, task forces, or advisory councils of other local mental health and human service agencies to help identify new funding sources and influence coordination with mental health.

A fourth and final set of possible actions involves an education role for the board.

Boards can act as information clearinghouses for mental health agencies, providing information on local services and personnel resources, examples of linkage programs in other communities, and information on support programs for coordination.

Boards may assist in the development in in-service training programs that examine community support systems and the potential forms of interagency coordination.

Boards must view these tactics within a larger context of local objectives, needs, and resources. Though it is clear that the coordination of services and operations is an increasingly necessary response to newly recognized treatment needs and the growing scarcity of resources, a variety of approaches to linkage and coordination are possible. These approaches are not necessarily interchangeable in terms of the degree or type of coordination they establish. Thus, the critical and very difficult task boards face is to devise workable mechanisms for coordination that fit the particular configuration of local needs and resources.

REFERENCES

Agranoff, R. Human services administration: Service delivery, service integration and training. In T. Mikulecky (Ed.), Human Services Integration. Washington, D.C.: American Society for Public Administration, 1974.

Agranoff, R. Political constraints on the mental health budgetary process. Journal of Mental Health Administration, 1975, 4, 38-57.

Agranoff, R. (Ed.). Coping with the demand for change within human services administration. Washington, D.C.: American Society for Public Administration, 1977.

Agranoff, R., & Pattakos, A. N. Dimensions of services integration: Service delivery, program linkages, policy management, and organizational structure. Rockville, Md.: Project SHARE Monograph Series, 1979.

Benson, J. The interorganizational network as a political economy. Administrative Science Quarterly, 1975, 20, 229-249.

Bourne, P. G. Human resources: A new approach to the dilemmas of community psychiatry. American Journal of Psychiatry, 1974, 131, 666-669.

Burgess, M. A., Nelson, R. H., & Wallhaus, R. Network analysis as a method for the evaluation of service delivery systems. Community Mental Health Journal, 1974, 10, 337-344.

Datel, W. E., & Murphy, J. G. A service integrating model for deinstitutionalization. Administration in Mental Health, 1975, 3, 35-45.

Emory, F. E., & Trist, E. L. The causal texture of organizational environments. Human Relations, 1965, 18, 21-32.

Fields, S. Growing up and stretching out: Mental health services for youth. Innovations, 1978, 5, 2-15.

General Accounting Office. Returning the mentally disabled to the community: Government needs to do more. Washington, D.C.: U.S. Government Printing Office, 1977.

Hall, R., et al. Patterns of interorganizational relationships. Administrative Science Quarterly, 1977, 5, 563-601.

Ilfeld, F. W., & Lindeman, E. Professional and community: Pathways toward trust. American Journal of Psychiatry, 1971, 128, 75-81.

Joint Commission on Accreditation of Hospitals. Standards for services for developmentally disabled individuals. Chicago: JCAH, 1978.

Kahn, A. J. Social policy and social services. New York: Random House, 1979.

Kaplan, H. M., & Bohr, H. Change in the mental health field. Community Mental Health Journal, 1976, 12, 244-251.

Long, N. A model for coordinating human services. Administration in Mental Health, 1974, 2, 21-27.

Lytwak, E., & Hylton, L. Interorganizational analysis: A hypothesis on coordinating agencies. Administrative Science Quarterly, 1962, 6, 395-420.

Lytwak, E., & Rothman, J. Towards the theory and practice of coordination between formal organizations. In W. Rosengren and M. Lefton (Eds.), Organizations and Clients: Essays in the Sociology of Service. Columbus, Ohio: Charles E. Merrill, 1970.

Metcalfe, L. Policy making in turbulent environments. In K. Hanf and F. Scharph (Eds.), Interorganizational Policy Making: Limits to Coordination and Central Control. Beverly Hills, Cal.: Sage Publications, 1978.

Meyers, W. R., Grisell, J., Gollin, A., Papernow, P., Hutcheson, B., and Serlin, E. Methods of measuring citizen board accomplishment in mental health and retardation. Community Mental Health Journal, 1972, 8, 313-320.

O'Brien, G. Interorganizational relations: Perspectives for the mental health administrator. In S. Feldman (Ed.), The Administration of Mental Health Services. Springfield, Ill.: Thomas, 1971.

Pondy, L. Toward a theory of internal resource allocation. In J. Livingston and S. Gunn (Eds.), Accounting for Social Goals. New York: Harper & Row, 1974.

President's Commission on Mental Health and Mental Illness. Report to the President. Washington, D.C.: U.S. Government Printing Office, 1978.

Schmidt, S., & Kochan, T. Interorganizational relations: Patterns and motivations. Administrative Science Quarterly, 1977, 22, 220-234.

Turner, J. C., & Dean, B. A new NIMH program promotes community support systems. Innovations, 1978, 5, 16-17.

U.S. Department of Health, Education and Welfare. A service delivery assessment on community mental health centers. Boston: Region 1 Office, DHEW, 1979.

Wamsley, G., & Zald, M. The political economy of public organizations. Bloomington: Indiana University Press, 1976.

Warren, R. L. Mental health planning and model cities: "Hamlet" or "Hellzapoppin." Community Mental Health Journal, 1971, 7, 39-49.

IV
SPECIAL POPULATIONS

Because society as a whole and mental health professionals in particular have failed to respond to the diverse needs of a multi-ethnic, multiracial society, federal guidelines have emphasized availability, accessibility, and acceptability of mental health services. Strict adherence to a disease model of causation and treatment exacerbated this failure by ignoring or denying the importance of environmental, social, and political influences on the incidence and prevalence of mental disorders. As a consequence, clinicians with these views tended to be insensitive to the values and beliefs patients held about mental health care. They were also likely to be blind to the manner in which their own prejudices affected the choice and course of intervention.

One would assume then that the mental health professionals described above would be most successful with people most similar in background to themselves. Conversely, the most dissimilar clients would receive the poorest service. Indeed, the literature has characterized the best candidates for psychotherapy as young, upper-middle class, verbal, intelligent, and only slightly disturbed. The greatest therapeutic failures have occurred with the poor, minorities, or severely disturbed. A classic work published in 1958 by Hollingshead and Redlich, Social Class and Mental Illness, alerted professionals and policy makers to biases in service delivery. The authors offered evidence that socioeconomic status was related to diagnosis, psychiatrist choice of intervention, and prevalence of treated mental disorders. Subsequent studies by other investigators have extended these findings to include the variables of race, sex, and age.

The purpose of this Part is to acquaint the reader with the special problems and concerns of those major subpopulations that have been underserved or misrepresented by mental health agencies and private practitioners. Several groups are analyzed in terms of making services more accessible, available, and appropriate to them while taking into account their cultural values, social structures, and specific needs. Each group raises unique problems in service delivery that should be addressed by planners and clinicians.

Bestman is critical of mental health in general and community mental health in particular for making blacks the targets of discrimination. She claims that the caregivers are either uninformed or intolerant of the culture and lifestyle of blacks. This results in

313

biased interventions, including overuse of medication, hospitalization, and more severe diagnostic categorization. Blacks are also underrepresented in the mental health manpower pool, and when employed are hired at the clerical or paraprofessional level. Overcoming these prejudices will be difficult, for black Americans do not trust public agencies. They rely on alternate sources for help in the form of family, folk healers, and religious figures.

Bestman concludes that if community mental health truly wants to provide effective services, it must build on the strengths of blacks—kinship networks, strong religious ties, adaptability in family roles, and an achievement orientation. More black staff must be hired, and centers must become more geographically accessible either by providing transportation or establishing "mini-centers."

Services for children were not officially acknowledged as a CMHC responsibility until the 1975 Amendments. Unique considerations for children's programs include an emphasis upon chronological age and support resources, for instance, significant others and community institutions. These services are more costly than those for adults because they demand staff with more specialized training, more joint planning with other service systems, and a greater variety of placement settings. Behar describes essential elements in children's services, the diagnostic process, and referral networks.

In discussing the chronically mentally ill, Cutler points out that the resources they require are the same as those for the normal population. The difference lies in their inability to obtain them. Intervention should encompass basic living skills, social skills, occupational training, and therapeutic intervention. The use of case managers is crucial to successful outcomes for this population. Cutler draws a paradigm for a service support network for the long-term patient.

The fastest growing ethnic group in the United States is Hispanic Americans. Gonzales states that the community model for Hispanic mental health services is far superior to that of the medical or criminal justice model. Prominent elements in designing services are education, socioeconomic status, language, family, and degree of acculturation and biculturalism. Historically, community institutions, schools, courts, and social service agencies have not been attuned to these elements. CMHCs can affect positive change through ties to these institutions, as well as by altering their staffing and financing patterns to fit the needs of Hispanics.

Demographic statistics indicate that the average American is growing older. With a growing number of senior citizens, manpower and financial resources should be directed toward programs for them. Yet Kahn indicates that CMHCs are responding in the opposite direction, giving a disproportionate emphasis to younger and healthier clients. Depression and dementia are the principal mental disorders in the aged. Through their commitment to a defined population within a geographic area, CMHCs are particularly suited for working with older adults. Minimal disruption of daily routine is important to the population, as is family support in therapeutic interventions.

The mentally retarded are no different from anyone else in terms of the prevalence and severity of emotional disorders. They experience the same feelings; and, in fact, most are emotionally stable. Their disorders are, in any case, reversible irrespective of their intellectual abilities. Rowitz informs us that the major difficulty in working with mentally retarded persons with emotional disorders is that no integration between the system that primarily serves the retarded and the mental health system exists. Professionals in the former system often ignore emotional problems, while professionals in the latter frequently refuse to work with the retarded. Since almost all of the current types of interventions can be applied to the mentally retarded, only certain forms of insight psychotherapy would be inappropriate.

It is the utmost irony that the population group that makes the greatest use of mental health services is underserved. Yet women, by virtue of a discriminatory mental health system, have too often been victims of maltreatment rather than recipients of quality care. Russo and VandenBos argue that while revolutionary changes have occurred in the role of women in contemporary society, sex-role stereotyping has been a common occurrence among mental health professionals. Some typical problems of women, wife-battering and substance abuse, are virtually ignored, while others, phobias and conversion hysterias, are disproportionately treated. Providers neglect important ancillary services that are essential if women are to use the center: transportation, baby-sitting, and temporary residence. Russo and VandenBos point out that women are underrepresented as administrators, staff, and board members. They note that eliminating sex bias and sex-role stereotyping in mental health will help to alleviate these conditions in the society at large.

20

BLACKS AND MENTAL HEALTH SERVICES
Evalina Bestman

INTRODUCTION

The community mental health center movement of the past few decades has advocated a comprehensive network of mental health services for all of the population of a designated geographical area commonly referred to as a catchment area. In some instances, some black mental health professionals believed that this approach of community-based services might prove to be a corrective factor in eliminating or minimizing the enormous disparities between psychiatric treatment for white and black Americans.

Blacks have been painfully aware of the dual system of mental health services within American society. This duality has had grave consequences for black communities, because the populations at greatest risk are denied access to appropriate treatment designed to help individuals recover from mental illness with the ability and skills to function in positive ways within the community. Combined with this is the reality that blacks, because of the very nature of their status in American society (victims of racism, the majority of whom are poor and working class) will have to depend on public health and mental health delivery systems. Again, it appears that groups at greatest risk and who can least afford private care are the groups that receive less. Blacks continue to be largely poor and the target of discriminatory acts even in mental health systems.

Failure is the only way to rate performance of community mental health centers and their overall role in addressing the mental health needs of the black community. The community mental health center movement has been and continues to be reflective of institutional racism that predominates in American society. One can always cite exceptions to the rule; however, the centers, in most instances, have not been responsive to minority groups. Because of racist attitudes at all levels of administration—national, regional, state, and local—the number of black staff and clients is not representative of the populations of the catchment areas. Thus, community mental health centers and the mental health movement continue to be dominated by white middle-class-oriented individuals.

With this as a given, it has been difficult, for a number of reasons, to establish programs that meet the needs of blacks. (1) Attitudes, beliefs, expectations, and values are in conflict, because their cultural roots do not have a Western European origin. (2) There is extensive ignorance of the lifestyles, beliefs, values, customs, and so on of blacks on the part of the American majority. (3) Often, where such knowledge does exist, the beliefs and practices of black Americans are rejected or are viewed as inferior to the majority's beliefs and practices. An example of this is seen in the concept of delayed gratification. In white middle-class America, an individual who is able to delay gratifying his needs is viewed as exhibiting "good mental health behaviors." In the 1960s, in the War on Poverty program in Miami, all sorts of crises developed because the white power structure had scheduled monthly salary payments. The blacks were demanding weekly or biweekly payments because they knew that federal grant dollars can be unreliable. In fact, they had not been paid for some months, while Congress played politics in refunding or continuation funding of social programs. In this instance, it needs to be added that the whites, in discussing the problem, viewed as irresponsible those people whom they perceived as not being able to budget monies on a monthly basis.

Traditionally, blacks served by the community mental health centers are by and large provided inpatient, aftercare, and drug abuse services. The aftercare services more often than not utilize chemotherapy as their only therapeutic modality. Black staff, where present, are hired largely for paraprofessional, clerical, and other minor supportive staff positions, such as janitorial services. Traditionally, children and outpatient services are blatantly geared to nonblack populations.

In a meeting of over 1,000 black leaders representing over 300 organizations and millions of constituents, the National Black Agenda for the 80s was formalized. They recommended:

Reform the current mental health system to provide mental health services to Blacks who have historically been deprived of these services even though the Black population experiences a disproportionate number of societal pressures which provoke mental health problems.

Gear inpatient Black-oriented programs toward education for the prevention of alcoholism.

Support prevention of drug abuse and the treatment of victims of drug abuse by increased funding to Black-oriented drug treatment programs. [Joint Center for Political Studies, 1980]

The Special Populations Subpanel on the Mental Health of Black Americans for the President's Commission on Mental Health (1979) concluded that the two major problems in American society affecting the mental health functioning of black Americans are racism and poverty. The subpanel's report emphasizes the deleterious effects of black life in America and in fact postulates that these factors contribute to the etiology of mental illness within the black communities. Additionally, the subpanel's findings demonstrated that racism operates as a major impediment to the delivery of quality mental health services to black Americans.

The impact of racism in American society has received great national attention. A Task Force of the Joint Commission on Mental Health of Children (1970) stated:

Racism is the number one public health problem facing America today. The conscious and unconscious attitudes of superiority which permit and demand that a majority oppress a minority are a clear and present danger to the mental health of all children and their parents. . .

The racist attitudes of America which cause and perpetuate tension, are patently a most compelling health hazard. Its destructive effects severely cripple the growth and development of millions of our citizens, young and old alike. Yearly, it directly and indirectly causes more fatalities, disabilities and economic loss than any other single factor.

DEMOGRAPHIC CHARACTERISTICS

The latest census data of 1974 revealed that 24 million black Americans reside within the United States. However, the major organizations within the black community such as the National Association for the Advancement of Colored People (NAACP), the Urban League, and various sororities and fraternities believe that blacks have been undercounted in the census by as much as 10 million. Black males have a median age of 21, and black females have a

median age of 24. In terms of life expectancy, at birth, blacks are
expected to live for 67.0 years as compared to 72.7 for whites, although those blacks achieving age 70 tend to have a longer life span
than whites. Death due to homicide, tuberculosis, hypertension,
heart disease, syphilis, diabetes, genital cancer, strokes, pneu-
monia, cirrhosis of the liver, and genital, digestive, and respira-
tory cancers are greater for blacks than for whites.

There has been a steady migration of blacks from rural areas
to inner cities. The result is that black populations are concentrated in the large metropolitan urban areas such as New York,
Chicago, Los Angeles, Atlanta, Houston, Baltimore, Washington,
D.C., and so forth. The majority of black rural populations are
located throughout the southeastern region of the United States.

Blacks are disproportionately represented on the lower end
of the socioeconomic scale. Thirty-one percent of black Americans
as compared to 9 percent of whites are living in poverty. Inflation
has created a bleaker existence for black communities. Unemployment and underemployment have affected blacks the most. The
inner cities, where the majority of black Americans reside, are in
worse shape economically in 1980 than they were a decade ago. The
rate of unemployment has doubled since 1969, to 13 percent (as compared to 6 percent for whites), and the number of unemployed blacks
has nearly tripled, to 1.4 million. The rates run devastatingly high
among black teenagers—approximately 40 percent.

During 1974, 35 percent of all black families had a female
head, as compared to 11 percent of white families. Forty-four percent of black "female headed" households had incomes below the
U.S. poverty level. Median income was less than half that of black
households with a male head, and considerably less than that of
white families having a female head.

The educational achievements of blacks are also lower than
those of whites. As of 1970, 62 percent of white urban populations
had completed high school, as compared to 39 percent of the blacks.

Overall, the demographic analysis of the black community
presents a picture of a people living in large, densely populated
urban areas, and subsisting on poverty incomes. Housing is sub-
standard, and educational opportunities are generally poor. The
implications for mental health are significant; in fact, blacks tend
to suffer from illnesses and diseases that thrive in highly stressful
environments.

MENTAL HEALTH PROBLEMS

Historically, it has been assumed by the psychiatric community that blacks are inclined to display pathological behaviors with

resulting psychoses. The lay black community consequently associates mental health with the most disabling forms of mental illness.

Blacks are likely to be evaluated as more severely disturbed than whites. Whites have a greater chance of being diagnosed with depressive disorders or psychoneuroses, while blacks are more likely to be diagnosed as schizophrenics. Blacks are disproportionately diagnosed as schizophrenic, with a very poor prognosis for recovery. It is interesting to note that the psychiatric community assumed that blacks did not experience stresses that would result in symptoms of depression or anxiety. Until very recently, psychiatrists were in fact taught that blacks did not get depressed.

Dr. Richard Dudley (1979), a black physician, outlined in his paper for the President's Commission on Mental Health explanations for the assumption that "clinical depression was non-existent among Blacks." (1) When blacks are clinically depressed, feelings of guilt and suicidal trends are less evident, while somatic complaints are more likely to predominate. (2) The reason for lower suicide rates among blacks is assumed to be the fact that black adults, by virtue of cultural norms and childrearing practices, are less likely to internalize hostility. (3) Blacks are believed to be too irresponsible and happy-go-lucky to become depressed.

Black mental health professionals have questioned the utilization of models of mental health advocated by the traditional mental health professions within the black community. As a result, research on the mental health needs of blacks has been designed and conducted by black researchers. Black psychologists, social workers, and psychiatrists have taken the position that individual functioning must be viewed within a cultural, social, political, and economic context. Even more important, they have advocated that mental health problems of black people are not due in most instances to intrapsychic deficiencies, as whites want blacks to believe.

The mental health of blacks cannot be assessed in a vacuum. The assessment must be conducted within a cultural and social context. When making assessments of mental functioning, mental health professionals must take into account the perspective of the group to which the individual belongs.

It is imperative that the evaluation of mental health services be conducted from within a determinate cultural framework. Studies have shown the relationships between culture and mental disorder (Linton, 1956; Giordano & Giordano, 1976). Cultures within the United States differ not only in adaptive strategies and stress points, but in basic conceptions of the etiology and classification of psychopathology, in modes of behavioral deviance (including differential symptomatology), and in perceptions of appropriate remedies (Lefley & Bestman, in press). The boundaries of mental health should then be extended to deal with some of the social and physical realities of being black in America (PCMH, 1978).

Many mental health problems are in fact a consequence of societal ills. Blacks experience alienation, depression, anger, rage, and fear as a result of poverty and the individual and institutional discrimination of which they are victims. Poverty and racism resulting in malnutrition, inadequate housing, poor schooling, and insufficient and inappropriate health and social services cause terrible emotional and mental damage.

Consequently, black mental health problems include conditions involving significant psychological and emotional distress that does not fit neatly into customary categories of mental disorder. There are problems and hazards faced by members of the black group for whom social and environmental conditions pose added burdens. Despite this fact, there is no psychiatric category for individuals displaying behavioral symptoms that result from racial victimization.

Still taking into account societal issues, Wilcox (1973) has postulated that the mental health status of blacks is largely reactionary. In essence, blacks react to the conditions of racism fostered by America's white society. When blacks fail to conform to the norms of the white culture, they are evaluated as social and mental deviants.

There are some epidemiological considerations in addressing black mental health issues. Extensive research has been aimed at investigating racial differences in diagnosing mental disorders. Fried (1975) concluded that blacks have higher rates of mental illness than whites. However, most other research in this area is inconclusive. See and Miller (1973) stated:

> as research comparing Black and White incidence and prevalence of serious mental disorder accumulated, it became clear that few certain epidemiological patterns could be identified. Since no recent study has attempted to determine true prevalence or incidence, it is still not known whether Blacks and Whites have similar or different rates of serious mental disorders.

It is known from the epidemiological data that there is a differential in mental hospital admission rates. In 1970, blacks exceeded whites in mental institutions by 52 percent (Milazzo-Sayre, 1977). Per 100,000 population, there were 214.2 white males as compared to 444.5 blacks and other nonwhite males, and 111.2 white females as compared to 212.0 black and other nonwhite females.

Black males show the highest rates of mental disorder from state hospital data. Blacks are admitted for custodial care in mental institutions somewhat sooner than whites. Black admissions to mental institutions are less likely to be voluntary and less likely to be initiated by a spouse or offspring. Blacks are more than eight times as likely to become institutionalized for drug addiction as whites, and death from alcoholism is three times more common among blacks than whites (Staples, 1976; Levitan et al., 1975).

Regarding the differential admission rates, it is important to remember that criteria for admission to public mental health institutions are determined primarily by white psychiatrists and secondarily by other white mental health professionals. The negative basic assumptions—myths and stereotypes that are held and put into action by the orthodox mental health system—contribute to the disproportionate admission rate for blacks.

With respect to treatment, a number of studies are available that demonstrate patterns of differential and unequal treatment provided black and white patients in the mental health system. Nonwhite patients are more likely to receive arbitrary diagnosis based on limited or ambiguous symptoms (De Hoyos & De Hoyos, 1965); are less often accepted for psychotherapy; are more often assigned to inexperienced therapists; are seen for shorter periods of time; and more often receive either supportive or custodial care, or drugs alone (Gross & Herbert, 1969; Hunt, 1962; Yamamoto, James, & Palley, 1968).

BARRIERS TO EFFECTIVE MENTAL
HEALTH SERVICES

As cited earlier, black Americans are underrepresented in the service population of the community mental health centers throughout the United States. There are numerous barriers that prevent blacks from utilizing mental health centers. Often, when the utilization rate of blacks is discussed, mental health professionals make the mistake of placing the blame on black Americans for not aggressively seeking out mental health services. More attention should focus on the center's failure to deliver effective and culturally appropriate services and, consequently, its failure to attract black clientele.

It must be recognized that one of the major barriers to the utilization of community mental health centers by black Americans is the conflict in value systems. The majority of individuals trained as mental health professionals are white. They bring their life experiences to bear in the evaluation and treatment of black clients.

The majority, and in most instances all, of the staff members of various mental health facilities are ignorant of black culture, including health practices, values, belief systems, definition and role of family, and so on. The values, stereotypes, and biases of the service provider often serve as impediments to accurate diagnosis and subsequent establishment of treatment plans. In fact, behavior often viewed as deviant by nonblacks may very well be "normal" behavior for the black community. An example of this is seen in the common phrase "A black who ain't paranoid is crazy." In a racist society, claims of oppressive, discriminating acts are very real, but are often labeled as paranoid by mental health professionals. Then, too, blacks have different attitudes toward caretaking responsibilities for family and community members experiencing problems. When it becomes apparent that all options outlined by the group fail to aid the individual in resuming a normal level of functioning, then they resort to the other formal systems of care.

Some of the options that may be considered by blacks are: (1) Self and family treatment, where home remedies and advice are solicited from friends and relatives, and medications are shared. (2) Cultural treatment, which is typically administered by folk healers, sometimes with supernatural significance. The intent is to determine whether the illness is caused by evil spirits. If needed, appropriate ceremonies are performed to rid the body and mind of such spirits. (3) Religious treatment, which involves contact with religious leaders for the purpose of determining whether one is being punished because of the commission of sinful acts or, in some cases, if one is possessed by evil spirits (Charles, 1979; Bestman, 1979).

The responses of black Americans to individuals having emotional or mental problems are determined to a great extent by what the members of the family, friends, or community residents view as causal factors. For example, if a child's behavior is believed to be caused by evil spirits, then the family will seek to involve the church or traditional folk healers such as rootworkers.

Rootwork has been defined as "a highly organized system of beliefs shared by Blacks who were raised in the Southeastern United States or who retain close ties there with family and friends" (Wintrob, 1972, p. 54). Its central concept is the belief that misfortune and illness can be caused as well as cured by magical means. Although it has been said that its beliefs and practices are derived from West African sources, Haitian Vodun, and European witchcraft, the influence of Protestantism is also very much in evidence within the practitioners' shops. Bibles, crosses, and prayers are incorporated into most of the healing rituals.

Why the use of traditional or folk healers rather than mental health professionals?

1. The former are usually of a similar ethnic background.
2. They are nonjudgmental.
3. They prescribe a treatment plan that can be understood by the client and is aimed at achieving specific goals.
4. They accept the fact that external forces affect and influence behavior.
5. They refrain from labeling individuals, who are therefore not stigmatized.
6. They operate in the individual's language and belief system.
7. Cost is minimal, and no bill collectors or credit collection agencies are likely to be involved.
8. Treatment is short-term in nature, and oriented toward problem solving. It is not concerned about the past history of the individual.

There is another myth about the black community's ability to take care of its own. Underutilization of health and mental health resources has had a tremendous toll on the survival of black communities. Societal and environmental stressors—primarily racism—have rendered many black Americans dysfunctional and distrustful of health care systems. Of course, the present systems discourage early intervention in mental health care. It appears that unless blacks demonstrate symptoms that can be diagnosed as classically psychotic by the mental health establishment, the legitimacy of the black as experiencing mental health problems is questioned. The tragedy is that many Americans ignore the realities of these factors and come up with simplistic explanations—that black Americans are unemployed because they are lazy, in jail because they are born criminals, illiterate because they are inherently unintelligent, ill because they are unsanitary or ignorant.

In fact, the black community is not very tolerant of dysfunctional individuals who fail to conform to standards of behavior established by the black community itself. When behavior approaches a level that is not consistent with established expectations, family members seek help from traditional healers within the community, the church, and/or the traditional mental health system. For most blacks, unfortunately, involvement with the mental health delivery system results in hospitalization.

The stress on individualism in American society is contrary to the cultural-value practices of black Americans. Their strength is in group membership, belonging to a family, church, organization, and community or neighborhood. For reasons of tradition and of basic survival in an oppressive society, blacks place great emphasis on unity and sharing, and they encourage cooperative ventures and support each other politically, emotionally, and economically.

The distrust of the mental health system is pervasive within the black community. Middle-class blacks view the system as another way that the government uses to collect data on their personal lives. In a racist society, if a white vice-presidential candidate is crucified for having undergone mental health treatment, then those blacks holding responsible professional/administrative positions will naturally believe that knowledge of their involvement with the system can supply employers with ammunition for termination or denial of promotion. They believe that material and information is not confidential, even when it does not affect a matter of life or death. The use of information to discredit them on the job and in the community is of primary concern. Thus, there is also suspicion of the mental health providers, who are largely white.

Additionally, chemotherapy and psychosurgery are viewed by the black community as ways the keepers of a racist society have decided to keep individuals from being intellectually curious and exercising their rights to free speech and political involvement.

Linguistic barriers also exist. There is, of course, much controversy within the black community concerning "Black English." Nevertheless, it is agreed that black Americans do share a common style of communication that involves the use of certain words, expressions, phrases, and body and hand movements. Many words used in black dialect are not understood by whites. For example, a white therapist approaching a black adolescent client would begin the conversation with: "Hello! How are you?" A black therapist may simply begin with "What it is, Brother?" Body and hand movements are also used a great deal in talking. People will naturally avoid utilizing an agency where staff cannot communicate with them. With mental health care, the client's emotional condition may deteriorate because of the trauma that he experiences in not being able to communicate his symptoms or concerns, and thus not being able to receive appropriate care.

Some agency directors who have sought to address these issues have indicated that the strong prevailing ethnocentric attitudes serve as barriers. Even when some providers are educated about the culture, their inherent belief in the superiority and "rightness" of white America's way of life prevents them from accepting and fully understanding different ways of behaving and different value systems.

Another major barrier to the utilization of mental health centers by black individuals is the racial and/or ethnic background of the mental health provider. When the client and practitioner are of the same race or socioeconomic background, or have similar life-styles, language, and value systems, there is a greater probability that the client will utilize the center. This has been demonstrated in the University of Miami–Jackson Memorial Medical Center's Community Mental Health Center in Miami, Florida, which has community-based ethnic teams (black American, Bahamian, Cuban, Haitian, and Puerto Rican). The teams are staffed with mental health professionals of the same or similar background as the populations served. The client population of the center corresponds with the catchment area census data. Thus, the utilization pattern by minority group members of the center is highly correlated with having staff of the same or similar racial and/or ethnic background of the client population.

MENTAL HEALTH PROGRAMS FOR THE BLACK COMMUNITY

Programs designed for the black community need to take many things into consideration if mental health professionals are truly concerned about meeting the mental health needs of blacks. The services must be designed most of all to build on the strengths of black people.

Historically, services and programs at mental health centers have not been developed from a transcultural perspective. They are outgrowths of experiences with and observation of Western European cultures. It is extremely important that centers serving black populations establish services and treatment plans that emerge from a knowledge base of the culture, lifestyles, belief systems, health practices, and language of the people. Basic to this is definition of terminologies. A case in point is the prevailing definition of family usually referred to as immediate family constellation (nuclear family) comprised of mother, father, and children. Because black families/households often consist of other family members, such as aunts, uncles, cousins, grandparents, and godchildren, the anthropological and sociological literature describes blacks as having an "extended" family system. This label is foreign to most blacks and does not represent what a family is in the black community. In essence, a family cannot be conceived of as separate and apart from all relatives (relatives are part of—not an extension of—a family unit).

A rather simple but most threatening act by most mental health centers is the hiring of black staff at all levels. The issues of rapport building, identification, and role modeling are important in the treatment and prevention of mental illness. Communication barriers will also be minimized. Black practitioners are more sensitive to behaviors and symptoms that can be evaluated as legitimately pathological in terms of black intrapsychic and social functioning. Thus, the common diagnostic errors and ineffectual treatment may be eliminated.

It is important as well that the representation of blacks in the mental health professions be increased for the additional issue of trust. Blacks are aware of dual standards of treatment and the abuse and neglect of their health and mental health needs by white professionals. The visibility of black practitioners and their active involvement provides the black populace with the impression that the center may indeed be serious about serving their community.

One major problem is that blacks are underrepresented in the mental health professions. It is estimated that 350-500 black physicians are psychiatrists. In a 1973-74 survey of residents in psychiatry, 1.7 percent were black. In 1977, 4 percent of the American Psychological Association membership was black. In 1975, 12.4 percent of the students in graduate schools of social work were black. According to enrollment data for baccalaureate nursing programs in 1962-63, 8.5 percent were blacks (Cannon & Locke, 1977). The major black institutions, such as Atlanta University System, Meharry Medical School, Howard University, Florida Agricultural and Mechanical College, North Carolina Agricultural and Technical College, Tuskegee Institute, and Norfolk State College, serve as excellent resources for the training of black mental health professionals.

Not enough attention is devoted to the location of facilities. If a center is not located within the community where clients reside, the need for transportation is not given priority funding. Indeed, in a recent application for a conversion grant for transitional housing submitted to the National Institute for Mental Health, the cost of purchasing a van for transporting clients to day treatment programs, job training sites, and so forth, was included. Staff reviewing the application indicated that the van was not an allowable expense. Yet it is apparent that one of the reasons for the underutilization of services is the high cost—and in some instances unavailability—of public transportation.

It is preferable that mini mental health centers be located throughout the catchment area so that services can be decentralized. The "mini centers," which are often storefront clinics, are neighborhood-based and easily accessible. The members of the community will identify with a facility that is visible in their neighborhoods. For example, locating services in one of the apartments of a local housing project will in all likelihood be received positively by the residents of the project.

A comprehensive assessment of the needs of the community should be conducted by black researchers. All program development should evolve from the needs identified by members of the black community. There will be a need for innovative prevention, early intervention, and consultation and education. Extensive outreach should be an essential part of the center's program. Because of the stigma attached to the term "mental health," the center will never get blacks to respond to its services if the staff does not make every effort to go where the people are—homes, churches, and schools.

The philosophy of the center must be consistent with the life and history of the people to whom services are directed. To this end, programs within the black community cannot operate in a vacuum and ignore the roles that environment and society play in the lives of blacks. Programming must focus on the environmental and societal factors that impinge on the individual functioning in a mentally healthy manner. This is a far different perspective from the current assumption that children who are having problems in school have to learn how to adjust to the school to solve their problems. For minority children, the centers should look at how schools can change to accommodate the children. The literature abounds with documentation that schools across this country operate out of a white middle-class-oriented system. Yet the tendency is to harass children into believing that something is wrong with them. Why does this attitude prevail? One can attribute it to the training and indoctrination of mental health personnel. Another factor is the prevailing definition of reimbursable mental health treatment.

Finally, community mental health centers will never be effective in the black community unless they operate as agents for social action or change (Pierce, 1972). Black Americans are in a struggle for survival in the United States politically and economically. If centers do not address the basic social needs of black people, in addition to the usual mental health problems, then their existence within the black community is essentially irrelevant.

REFERENCES

Bestman, E. W. Cultural, linguistic and social barriers in providing health services to Haitian refugees. Paper presented at Dade County Conference on Haitian Refugees, Miami, Florida, December 1979.

Bestman, E. W., Lefley, H. P., & Scott, C. S. Culturally appropriate interventions: Paradigms and pitfalls. Paper presented

at the 53rd Annual Meeting of the American Orthopsychiatric
Association, Atlanta, Georgia, March, 1976.

Cannon, M. S., & Locke, B. Z. Being black is detrimental to one's
mental health: Myth or reality. Phylon, December, 1977.

Charles, C. Anthropological considerations on barriers affecting
delivery of health care services to Haitian refugees in South
Florida. Paper presented at Dade County Conference on Haitian
Refugees, Miami, Florida, December, 1979.

De Hoyos, A., & De Hoyos, G. Symptomatology differentials between Negro and White schizophrenics. International Journal of
Social Psychiatry, 1965, 11, 245-255.

Dudley, R. Racism and mental health: An overview. Paper prepared for Subpanel on Mental Health of Black Americans, President's Commission on Mental Health. December, 1977.

Fried, M. Social differences in mental health. In J. Kosa & I. K.
Zola (Eds.), Poverty and Health. Cambridge, Mass.: Harvard
University Press, 1975.

Giordano, J., & Giordano, G. P. Ethnicity and community mental
health. Community Mental Health Review, 1976, 1, 1-14.

Gross, H., & Herbert, M. The effect of race and sex on variation
of diagnosis and disposition in a psychiatric emergency room.
Journal of Nervous and Mental Disease, 1969, 148, 638-642.

Hunt, R. Occupational status in the disposition of cases in a child
guidance clinic. International Journal of Social Psychology, 1962,
8, 199-210.

Joint Center for Political Studies. The national black agenda for
the '80's: Richmond conference recommendations. Washington,
D.C., 1980.

Lefley, H., & Bestman, E. W. Community mental health and
minorities: A multi-ethnic approach. In S. Sue & T. Moore
(Eds.), Community Mental Health in a Pluralistic Society. New
York: Human Sciences Press, in press.

Levitan, S. A., Johnston, W. B., & Taggart, R. Minorities in the
United States: Problems, progress and prospects. Washington,
D.C.: Public Affairs Press, 1975.

Linton, R. Culture and mental disorder. Springfield, Ill.: Charles C. Thomas, 1956.

Milazzo-Sayre, L. Admission rates to state and county psychiatric hospitals by age, sex, and race, United States, 1975. NIMH Mental Health Statistical Note No. 140, Department of Health, Education and Welfare Publication # (ADM) 78-158. Washington, D.C.: Superintendent of Documents, U.S. Government Printing Office, November 1977.

Pierce, W. The comprehensive community mental health programs and the black community. In R. Jones (Ed.), Black Psychology. New York: Harper and Row, 1972.

President's Commission on Mental Health (PCMH). Report of the Special Populations Subpanel on the Mental Health of Black Americans. Washington, D.C.: Superintendent of Documents, U.S. Government Printing Office, 1978.

See, J. J., & Miller, K. S. Mental health. In K. S. Miller & R. M. Dreger (Eds.), Comparative Studies of Blacks and Whites in the United States. New York: Seminar Press, 1973.

Staples, R. Introduction to Black Sociology. New York: McGraw-Hill, 1976.

U.S. Bureau of the Census. Female family heads. Current Populations Reports, Series P23, No. 50. Washington, D.C.: Superintendent of Documents, U.S. Government Printing Office, 1974.

U.S. Bureau of the Census. The social and economic status of the black population in the United States, 1974. Current Population Reports, Series P23, No. 54. Washington, D.C.: Superintendent of Documents, U.S. Government Printing Office, 1975.

Wilcox, P. Positive mental health in the black community: The black liberation movement. In C. V. Willie, B. M. Kramer, & B. S. Brown (Eds.), Racism and Mental Health. Pittsburgh, Pa.: University of Pittsburgh Press, 1973.

Wintrob, R. Hexes, roots, snake eggs? M.D. vs. occult. Medical Opinion, 1972, 1, 54-61.

Yamamoto, J., Dixon, F., & Bloombaum, M. White therapists and Negro patients. Journal of National Medical Association, 1972, 64, 312-316.

21

CHILDREN'S SERVICES
Lenore B. Behar

The community mental health movement began with a focus on providing mental health services for adults close to home in order to prevent institutionalization. It was not until the late 1960s and early 1970s that the community mental health centers (CMHCs) began to address the needs of children. Initially, the rationale was to offer primary prevention services to assist children in growing into emotionally healthy adults. However, more recently, secondary and tertiary services have also been undertaken in response to the current needs of children, their families, and communities. What kinds of services to offer is a complex problem, for a CMHC has the obligation of considering not only a variety of diagnostic and treatment services for children but also prevention services as well. Whether one chooses to regard children's services from an economic or humanitarian point of view, they clearly hold an important place in the full complement of community mental health services. However, because of the special nature of children, the delivery of such services has its unique requirements and problems.

THE UNIQUENESS OF CHILDREN'S PROGRAMS

Age Group Problems

Much growth and development is accomplished in 18 years. A 12-year-old child is very different from a two-year-old child, far more dissimilar than two adults with a ten-year age difference. The two-year-old obviously does not possess the cognitive, verbal, or physical development to participate at the same level with the

331

12-year-old. Services are developed with the differences in age
groups in mind. Generally, three divisions are appropriate for
children between birth and 18: preschool; 6 to 12; and 13 to 18.
Naturally, the physical size and psychological maturity of each
child is taken into consideration, for some 14-year-olds are more
like 16-year-olds, while others are more like 12-year-olds.

Ecological Considerations

Another way in which children's services differ from those
for adults is a recognition that in order to make significant changes
in a child's life, the child's ecological system must be considered.
An ecological system encompasses the significant people who directly affect the child, including parents, siblings, friends, teachers,
pediatrician, probation officer, and scout leader. Unlike adults,
children cannot readily leave areas of their lives that contribute to
their problems. Communication must be developed with relevant
people in the child's ecological system, so that they may understand
the child and help to bring about needed change.

No set of guidelines exists to cover the treatment of all children; each situation must be negotiated and planned for individually.
Because of the necessity of working with a number of people, children's mental health services take more time per individual client
and, therefore, are more costly. Money problems are inherent in
children's services because state allocations, parents' fees, or
third-party reimbursements usually cover only direct services,
while the necessary services to parents, teachers, and others are
funded from other sources. Unless these ancillary services are
provided, the impact of the direct services to the child is greatly
diminished.

Specialization of Staff and Treatment

Children's mental health is a field of specialization requiring
special training in delivery and supervision. Accurate diagnosis requires a special understanding of cognitive, speech, physical, and
emotional development. Children have very different treatment
needs as well. Special techniques have to be used with many children because they are not able to participate in counseling sessions
or "talking therapy." Typically, those professionals who understand adolescents and work effectively with them may not be skillful
in understanding the developmental and psychological problems of a
three-year-old. An important warning is that children are not little

adults; consequently, they need different services and different understanding.

Joint Planning

One of the greatest needs in this field is that of joint planning with other service systems that have responsibility for children—the educational, the juvenile justice, and the child welfare systems. When concentrating on only one client, each of these systems can collaborate with the others. However, when it comes to overall planning for system linkages, there is usually less interagency cooperation. This results in duplication of services and waste of public funds. Unfortunately, there is no clear delineation of responsibility, making it impossible to enforce a blanket statement such as "all residential treatment programs will be operated by the mental health system."

Depending upon local interpretation, local funding, and availability of staff, a residential treatment program may be operated successfully by any of the systems as long as there is appropriate input from mental health professionals. On the other hand, a special education class for emotionally disturbed children could be operated as a day treatment program by a mental health center rather than by a school. The important issue is not who runs the program, but that two similar and competing programs should not be operated by different agencies when other badly needed services are being overlooked. Perhaps the most flexible approach to joint planning is that it is the mental health center's responsibility to make sure that high quality psychological services are available in the community, while it is the school board's responsibility to make sure that high quality education is being provided by local schools. Such division of responsibility and assurance of quality are usually the result of direct operation of programs.

KINDS OF SERVICES NEEDED

The Intensity and Restrictiveness Continuum

Community mental health center services for children comprise both direct and preventive services. In considering direct services, one can view the range of possible services as a continuum of care in terms of intensity and restrictiveness. Intensity describes how much of the child's day is directed toward working on the child's problem. In weekly outpatient services approximately one hour per week is devoted to direct work by child and therapist on the child's problems. In an intensive treatment program, such as that found in psychiatric hospitals, there is an effort during almost all of the child's waking hours to address the child's treatment needs, whether through a supervised evening recreation program or a structured daytime classroom situation. Restrictiveness refers to freedom of movement and choice about daily activities. A child who is receiving weekly outpatient services has few therapeutic restrictions on what he or she does during the rest of the week, while a child living in a hospital has a narrower band of choices in association with peers, reading materials, or foods.

The purpose of the continuum of care is twofold. It is important to maintain the flexibility to move from one level of intensity to another. For example, a child who is receiving services on a weekly outpatient basis may not respond and may need to move into full day treatment. A seriously disturbed child may be receiving intensive hospital treatment but may be able to move to a halfway house. The second reason for continuum of care is that children should not have to settle for more or less intensive treatment than they need because the middle pieces are missing.

The Disability Continuum

Children with some kinds of psychological problems do not mix well with children having other types of problems, either because the treatment programs needed for these two groups are quite different or because the groups of children are incompatible. Children who are articulate, insight-oriented, and willing to examine their feelings, motivations, and behaviors require treatment different from that for children who have limited intelligence, brain damage, or poor impulse control. The first group would do well in a traditional, psychotherapeutic environment, while the second group would benefit more from psychoeducational and psychosocial rehabilitation. The second group is considered chronically impaired and needs a long-term, graduated program to learn how to get along in society. The first group might be considered remediable, while the second group has continual treatment needs.

Viewing the mental health needs of children in terms of age group and type of disability is a factor that may not be present in planning services for other populations. Figure 21.1 presents the array of services needed for age and disability groups. It also illustrates which agencies refer children to mental health centers, a topic to which we now turn.

FIGURE 21.1

Community Mental Health Services for Children

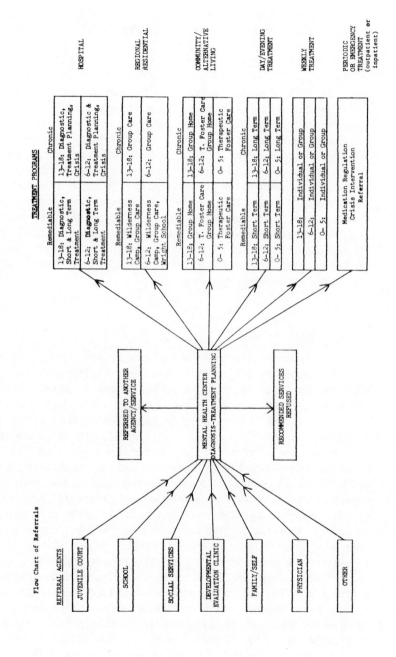

335

REFERRALS

A request for service or referral for a child, except in the case of older adolescents, is usually made by someone else. An adult, sometimes a representative of another service system, may come to believe that a child has a problem that could be helped at the center. If the child's parents have legal responsibility, however, the state usually requires that the parents either make the contact with the center or sign a consent form allowing the other agency to refer. In most communities, the CMHC staff visits or calls other agencies to explain services available at the center and procedures for referral. The importance of explaining the referral process to other agencies cannot be overemphasized, for it is often the failure to convey this information that leads to frustration and the subsequent accusation that the center is unresponsive to community needs. The center should clarify to the referring agent and to the family what services will be provided, at what cost, and within what time frame. More than for any other client group, it is vital to be responsive not only to the children but also to their parents and other service systems.

DIAGNOSIS

The initial step with children, as with all other client groups, is to determine the nature of the problem, whether subsequent services are needed, and, if so, what kind. The diagnostic evaluation includes the usual professional assessment techniques, for example, interviews, observations, psychological testing, and information gathered from other sources. The child's family gives a historical perspective and a picture of the current living situation. Other information is collected from those who know the child well, including teachers, court counselor, health care provider, and other concerned adults. Clearly, permission must be granted by the family or legal guardian to obtain such information. Although in most states children do not need to give their consent, it is helpful to explain to them what is being done on their behalf and why.

Once the diagnostic assessment has been completed, the outcome is shared with the family and other significant people with the permission of parents or guardian. It is at this point that a decision is made about the necessity for further action, either at the center or in another context. Possibly, a decision would be made that a child does not need a treatment program offered by the center, but that a therapeutic intervention could be carried out in the child's classroom. In such a situation, it becomes crucial for the diagnostician to convey findings to the teacher.

The diagnostic service provided by the center is the hub of all
services for the child: plans for treatment are developed; critical
decisions are made by other agencies; and the child and family decide whether they will participate in the recommended program. If
the center fails to communicate adequately with the family at this
point, the family may refuse recommended services. Unfortunately,
many families are labeled "resistant" because these steps have not
been taken to help them understand the recommendations.

TREATMENT PROGRAMS

The types of treatment programs that a mental health center
should have available for children are presented in Figure 21.1.
They can be offered directly by the center, by contracts with private
providers, through joint arrangements with other agencies, through
collaborative arrangements with neighboring mental health centers,
or by participation in a state-wide mental health system (the usual
manner of obtaining state hospital services). Some of the treatment
programs listed in Figure 21.1 are better known than others, so a
few comments about them are in order.

Periodic or Emergency Treatment

Periodic or emergency services should be available on both
an outpatient and inpatient basis. They are frequently provided to
"walk-ins" during clinic or after hours. It is extremely important—
yet it rarely happens—that a specialist in children's services handles
emergency situations. Practitioners who are not familiar with the
psychology of children frequently recommend more drastic solutions
than are actually needed. An adolescent who has become enraged
and violent may be admitted to the hospital, although a judiciously
handled discussion might be sufficient to calm him down. The use
of medication for children is a tricky business and demands the careful understanding of one accustomed to dealing with such matters.

Individual or Group Therapy

Individual or group therapy on an outpatient basis has been the
core of traditional children's services since the beginning of the
child guidance movement. Therapy is usually provided on a weekly
basis and depends on the age of the child. For young children,
therapy takes the form of play group, activity group, or individual

play therapy, while for older children it has the character of adult-like talking or recreational therapy. The therapy may be short- or long-term, ranging from three months to over a year in duration.

Parent Services

Parent services must be provided on a regular basis. The traditional approach is a therapy or collaborative hour for the parents either on an individual or group basis. However, other modes of working with parents are being tried, including parent education groups and parent support groups. These approaches focus on helping the parent to learn how to help his or her child rather than on treatment of the parent's problems. These approaches are particularly necessary in cases where the child is chronically impaired—for example, in cases of autism—because the parent must learn to deal with the child as well as to cope with his or her own feelings.

Services to parents of very young children may also include educational approaches to helping parents understand how children develop, so that their expectations are not unrealistic. When younger children are treated individually or in a group, parents may observe the treatment sessions, and the therapist can serve as a model for their future interactions with the child. For older adolescents there may be a choice not to involve the parents, especially if a major goal is to help the child live independently of a difficult family situation.

Day and Evening Services

For many CMHCs, day or evening services are relatively new ventures. With the current emphasis on building in an educational component for treatment programs that keep the child out of school, it has become necessary to develop separate programs for different age groups. Most typically, day treatment programs are for children who are too disturbed to function within the special education classes of the public schools. Joint efforts between schools and mental health centers can permit children to spend a part of their time in one program and part in the other, to the extent that they can manage successfully in both situations. The financial advantage of collaborative efforts cannot be overlooked, as the schools may be able to provide teachers, materials, and transportation. It is not unusual to have the day treatment component of the mental health center provided in the public schools. This arrangement is a more intensive and restrictive program than a special education class, which, in most cases, has a stronger academic emphasis.

Day treatment programs for adolescents and preschool children may have an indirect relationship to the public schools. For the adolescents who dropped out of school because of severity of impairment, poor grades, or negative attitudes toward school, vocational skills may be acquired through other agencies, such as vocational rehabilitation, technical schools, and community colleges. The focus of day treatment for adolescents who are not responsive to formal educational activities is on developing social and community living skills. Treatment for the preschool child may be given in the form of a therapeutic preschool or nursery. Collaboration with the public school system is geared to preparing the child for entry into that system by working with teachers and other personnel to understand the child's needs. Additionally, for some disturbed preschool children, the possibility of shared time in a public kindergarten and a therapeutic preschool program represents an important step toward mainstreaming.

Some day treatment programs also continue into the late afternoon and evening. As unusual as day treatment programs are, evening programs are rarer. They can be particularly effective for the adolescent who needs supervision after school in the context of a therapeutic environment. Although from outward appearances, evening treatment programs parallel recreational rather than educational programs, a significant therapeutic impact can be made through supervised peer group interaction, group therapy, and individual treatment.

Residential Services

It is a difficult professional decision to move a child out of a home situation for the purposes of treatment. There are two major reasons for such a move: (1) when the child's disturbance is serious enough to warrant a 24-hour program, or (2) when the relationship between the child and parents or guardians becomes so disintegrated that a moratorium is needed. These are not easy criteria to discern, and unless the child represents a serious danger to himself or to others, such a decision is made only after long-term contact. Usually, a less intensive mode of treatment is tried first to see if there are sufficient ingredients present for a less restrictive program to work.

There are two living arrangements that are preferred alternatives to full-time residential treatment. The child may live in a "group home" or "therapeutic (foster) home" in which he or she attends school rather than receiving educational services within the treatment program. The difference between a group home and a therapeutic foster home depends on the number of other children placed in that treatment setting. A group home involves four to ten children, while a therapeutic home involves one to three children. In both instances, a therapeutic couple, teaching parents, house parents, or therapeutic foster parents, as they are alternatively called, are parent substitutes and supervise the children just as natural parents would do. Typically, children with the more treatable disorders participate on a relatively short-term basis of nine months or less, while those with chronic impairment require longer care. For some chronically impaired children, group home living may be a lifelong experience.

Intensive, 24-hour residential services in which all aspects of treatment are provided on site may be operated by a CMHC, although such programs are sometimes operated on a regional basis serving several catchment areas. They may be run by the state, by a consortium of mental health centers, or by a private organization from whom services are purchased. Such programs vary in treatment orientation and include models of reeducation, psychosocial rehabilitation, and wilderness camping. The most intensive of all residential programs are found in hospital settings.

In any residential treatment program, the focus must be on helping the child and changing his or her home environment, so that the two may be reintegrated as soon as possible. Without this focus, institutionalization becomes more likely as years go by. Some children run a greater risk of institutionalization than others because, although they respond very well to the structure of an institutional setting, their problems reoccur when they return to normal life situations. These children should be moved into less restrictive settings, such as halfway houses, group homes, or other residential centers, so that their contact with normal community living is increased. Another problem of residential programs is the risk of poor quality care or even abuse. In recent years, litigation has prompted development of more safeguards than in the past.

Residential care is expensive and the more intensive it is, the more expensive it becomes. Because children's services are almost always more expensive, budget cuts can be devastating to their quality. Therapeutic environments must certainly be better than the environment from which the child was taken. Programs must be monitored carefully, particularly the larger programs where staff works on a shift/rotational basis and individuals are less likely to be held personally accountable.

Preventive Services

Another important function of the community mental health center is prevention. One might construe all children's programs to be preventive, but, in another sense, there must be services for children and families to prevent mental health problems in the children themselves. The earliest stages of prevention occur in family planning and prenatal care since most professionals believe that the first step to good mental health is being a wanted and healthy child. Family planning and family life education have recently been directed toward teenagers and young adults, so that they can make intelligent choices about whether to have a child. Mental health professionals can help young adults understand their motivation for wanting to get pregnant and, in that way, help to ensure that pregnancies are truly a part of conscious planning.

The professional has the opportunity to help prepare an expectant mother and father for the psychological changes in themselves and in their relationship after the child's birth. It is important, too, to help parents-to-be gain understanding of the emotional needs of their newborn. Additional information about the development of the child should be shared, so that new parents can develop reasonable expectations.

Screening at an early age identifies deviations from normal development. By the time children are three or four years old, problems in psychological and emotional development can be identified. It is at this stage that early intervention can prevent more serious problems. Many mental health centers offer parent education, and some centers even have a "tot line" that allows parents and others responsible for the care of children to call in with questions about childrearing. Counseling sessions to parents who have taken the wrong track in childrearing can be quite helpful. Direct services may also be delivered to the child in the context of a normal day care center or nursery school by assisting the child care worker in using new strategies in the classroom. In more serious situations, a therapeutic preschool should be available for the child to attend.

Quality day care services for preschool children have been advocated as a healthy place for children when parents are out of the home. The success of Head Start has contributed significantly to the belief that good day care is beneficial and nondestructive of the family system. The mental health professional can train and consult with teachers so that they may foster healthy emotional development in the children.

Throughout childhood and adolescence, children move through school, recreational, and social systems that have a strong bearing on how they view themselves. In all of these systems, it is important that those responsible for children understand how to foster their mental health. It is the professional's duty to assist in the training of these people, so that they may perform maximally in their roles.

Consultation to public schools is an important effort on the part of mental health centers. Such consultation can be used for teacher training or for spotting children in trouble. Mental health consultation can also be used to strengthen parent education programs. Many schools offer a mental health component from the earliest grades in the form of guidance counselors. In communities where guidance counselors are part of the school system, a mental health professional can "back-stop" that person with consultation and referrals.

Another way in which to view preventive mental health services is to consider crisis points in the life of a child. A crisis may occur when the child enters school and experiences stress or when a special disposition is being considered. Such dispositions might involve placement in a special class, movement into foster care, or involvement with the judicial system. At these times, a professional can give information, clarify issues, and help the decision maker to consider alternatives. Other crisis points in a child's life may be of a different sort, related to the death of a parent or the separation or divorce of parents. Special support should be available to children experiencing such crises, so that they can better deal with their reactions in the healthiest way possible.

CONCLUSION

The delivery of mental health services to children is at a crossroad. In the early days of child guidance, diagnosis and treatment were given to those who came for help. At this point, mental health providers are expected to extend services beyond those who request them. Schools, courts, and child welfare agencies are becoming aware of the mental health needs of their children. These agencies can greatly benefit from the sharing of knowledge and skills of the mental health professional. A reasonable approach to addressing children's problems is for the mental health center to engage in joint planning with these systems. A true continuum of care for children, ranging from prevention to the most intensive treatment, requires the manpower and expertise of all service systems providing for children. The development of a complete array of services is also dependent on the sharing of resources.

Despite a broadening of interest and responsibility on the part of CMHCs for the care and treatment of children, there are still areas for which effective techniques are not available. Research and evaluation are needed to determine what approaches might be useful for some of the more resistant disorders of childhood, such as childhood schizophrenia. The use of medication needs additional study since not much is known about its effectiveness nor about its long-range side effects.

It has become increasingly important to document program effectiveness. Replication of programs should be based on examination of successful models, but examination of models that have failed is also important so that the same mistakes will not be repeated. In this era of accountability, public funds must be put to the best use. More important than fiscal accountability, however, is the obligation to the children and their families. We must do the best possible job in first helping them to be healthy and happy children, so that they may grow into healthy and happy adults.

SUGGESTED READINGS

Joint Commission on Mental Health of Children. New York: Harper and Row, 1970.

The President's Commission on Mental Health: A Report to the President. Papers on the mental health of American families in volumes I and III. Washington, D.C.: U.S. Government Printing Office, 1978.

22

THE CHRONICALLY MENTALLY ILL
David L. Cutler

INTRODUCTION

Throughout history, perhaps no other group of people has been so ambivalently regarded as the chronically mentally ill. These people were often confined to prisons, escorted to the edge of town to fend for themselves, or beaten until they quieted down or died. They were burned in the Inquisition as witches, chained to stocks by the Greeks, Romans, and early Americans, and placed involuntarily in large untherapeutic mental institutions in the nineteenth and twentieth centuries throughout the world (Arieti, 1974).

The early nineteenth century was characterized by a brief renaissance of hope during the so-called "moral treatment" era. Men like Pliny Earle, who was superintendent of the state hospital at Northampton, Massachusetts, and John Gault at the Eastern Virginia Lunatic Asylum, who adopted the foster home plan for long-term patients, were highly successful in restoring many persons to active community life (Caplan & Caplan, 1969). But the great crusade of Dorothea Dix, which resulted in large numbers of state institutions being built, was for the most part not accompanied by an adequate number of visionary administrators. As a result, the state hospital movement broke down rather rapidly in the latter part of the century to a collection of untherapeutic custodial care institutions. The psychiatric belief of the time was that schizophrenia was an incurable illness that led progressively to profound dementia. The result was the dehumanizing experience of institutionalization, described in "A Bushel of Shoes" (Brooks, 1969), as patients were converted into "career" mental patients.

344

The current community mental health movement can be regarded as a reaction to the custodial care era. Its earliest manifestations were the works of Adolf Meyer and William James at the turn of the twentieth century. These men, along with Clifford Beers, a former patient who wrote about his hospital experience (Beers, 1939), are regarded as the originators of the mental hygiene movement. Meyer believed that human beings were in constant balance with their environment and that emotional distress was in part a reaction to a clustering of overwhelming stressful environmental life events. Mental illness was, therefore, a significant breakdown of a person's ability to adapt to stress. Meyer insisted that people could be educated to adapt to stresses and prevent the onset of severe mental illness. Moreover, this kind of knowledge was teachable to parents who could help their children avoid the tribulations of mental illness. Meyer's efforts to gain support for these ideas turned out to be both the beginning of the child guidance movement and the roots of the community mental health movement.

The 1920s and 1930s saw the development of the child guidance clinics throughout the country, but it was not until the mid-1950s that the community mental health movement actually had its modern beginnings. Several factors were instrumental in facilitating the rapid movement of chronically mentally ill people from the hospital to the community. In 1955, there was a peak population of over half a million patients in state hospitals in this country. In that same year, antipsychotic medications were introduced into standard hospital psychiatric treatment, markedly reducing incapacitating symptoms. Many were able to leave the institutions (Bloom, 1977). In addition to the revolution in psychopharmacology came a revolution in social treatment. The therapeutic community movement, an outgrowth of the treatment of soldiers in World War II, began to gain impetus and establish itself as a major modality (Jones, 1953).

Another important development occurred in state hospital administrative structure. Services were organized on a regional basis so that persons from a given geographic area were housed in one particular unit. Staff at the hospital were then able to develop consistent working relationships with service agencies and providers in the community to which the person was to be released. Professional expertise now existed in the community, paving the way for readjustment to community life. This configuration extended the role of hospitals to reducing recidivism.

A third parallel development occurred in 1955, when Congress appointed the Joint Commission on Mental Health and Mental Illness. It was charged with examining the state of mental health care in the country. The results of its investigation, reported to President Kennedy in 1961, suggested the need for community-based treatment for long-term patients. The Community Mental Health Centers Act of 1963 provided for the construction of federally funded mental health centers throughout the country, and the Amendments of 1965 appropriated funds for staffing.

Although the past two decades have witnessed rapid establishment and development of community mental health programs, until very recently mental health professionals have not received sufficient training in skills needed to organize and manage community support systems for the chronically mentally disabled person. Consequently, many well-staffed comprehensive community mental health programs have in effect failed to meet the needs of this historically neglected population (Talbot, 1979).

In the remainder of this chapter we will attempt to describe the characteristics of chronically mentally ill persons, the needs they have for long-term community survival, and some strategies for rehabilitation.

DEFINITION OF CHRONIC MENTAL ILLNESS

The chronically mentally ill population is comprised roughly of three groups: deinstitutionalized individuals, "revolving door" persons who go in and out of hospitals, and individuals with chronic disability who are not hospitalized. There are programs specifically developed for each of these groups. For example, the LINC program (Terwilliger & Johnson, 1976) is a remotivational care program for institutionalized patients. It helps long-term back ward patient groups in quasi-families of five move first to an apartment complex on the hospital grounds and later to a house in the community. While maintaining their long-term ties to each other, the members of the group are systematically trained in daily living skills and eventually returned to the community to function as a social unit in their own homes. Between 1974 and 1979 more than 80 persons hospitalized an average of 25 years have been retrained, discharged, and remain in the community.

By contrast, the PACT program in Madison, Wisconsin, specifically focuses on the revolving door patient (Stein, Test, & Marks, 1975). This program picks up patients in the midst of acute psychotic episodes from the time they arrive in the emergency room of the local hospital. It escorts them back into the community, and provides treatment and training in community living in the natural environment. It, too, has been highly successful.

The chronically mentally ill usually carry a diagnosis of schizophrenia, but may also have manic depressive disease, organic brain syndrome, or a variety of addiction conditions and personality disorders. Recent estimates indicate that there are roughly 900,000 schizophrenic persons under the care of the community, of whom about half have been hospitalized at least once (Minkoff, 1978). Since the incidence of schizophrenia in the U.S. population has ranged from .043 to .069 percent over the last 25 years (Day & Semrad, 1978), the fraction of the population defined as schizophrenic during each year (prevalence) is between .23 and .47 percent. This yields between 500,000 and 1 million persons in need of treatment on an annual basis. Currently, the total estimate of cost of the treatment of schizophrenia in the United States is $14 billion annually (Minkoff, 1978).

CHARACTERISTICS OF THE CHRONICALLY DISABLED

In order to plan treatment strategies in a systematic way, it is convenient to group the characteristics of chronically disabled persons into the various environmental spheres in which these strategies are carried out. I will therefore utilize the following five functional area components: personal, social, productive activities, recreational, and ability to get services.

In terms of personal functioning, the chronically disabled person exhibits a wide variety of bizarre, disturbing symptoms and behaviors. Such persons often hear voices, believe that others are attempting to harm them, feel that they are being controlled by outside forces, and experience incoherent or extremely speeding thoughts. These symptoms create a tremendous handicap for the individual, in addition to the reactions they cause in others. Since organizing thinking and carrying thought sequences to a logical conclusion is impaired, the chronically disabled person will tend to have difficulty even in coping with the basic necessities of daily living. Judgment and impulse control become distorted and unpredictable. The capacity to hold a job is lost, and therefore also the capacity to earn money. In addition, there are invariably problems in generalizing from one learning situation to another, so that what is learned while in the hospital may be worthless once the patient returns to the community. This particular characteristic becomes a key issue when attempting to design programs. It requires that rehabilitation efforts be conducted in vivo, that is, in the environment in which the patient is to use them.

In the social-interpersonal area, the chronically disabled exhibit great problems. Relations with other people are often severely strained by what is experienced as extreme dependency and idiosyncratic behaviors. Lacking self-confidence in social situations, the chronically disabled may often respond to minimum stress by brief episodes of increased symptomatology or acting out behaviors. This interferes with meeting their own needs and with the rights of others around them.

With respect to recreational activities, chronically disabled persons are often highly deficient in the capacity to seek out and enjoy leisure time activities. They often fear interpersonal contacts and usually expect to fail. Ambitious attempts to "mainstream" disabled persons into leisure activities with "normals" often result in loss of self-esteem. Generally, they will avoid these situations unless other chronically disabled persons are present and take part.

Productive activities are markedly limited. There is a great deal of difficulty in concentrating for more than a few minutes, let alone for the eight hours a day, 40 hours a week it takes to maintain a job. Without extensive retraining and graduated work rehabilitation, it is usually unrealistic to expect more than uncomplicated, time-limited volunteer work.

Finally, the manner in which chronic patients engage the services sector is crucial to organizing their mental health programs. These persons, although highly dependent on medication to relieve thought disorders, often refuse chemotherapy. Even if they accept medicine, they frequently forget to take it. Generally, motivation is lacking to attach themselves to workers in mental health agencies. Without a strong effort on the part of the agencies, these patients will slip through the cracks in the program and not receive the services they need. The extensive and serious impairments in the various life spheres identified simply are not treatable in short-term situations. Rather, they require a long-term sustained contact with a service system that is assertive and persistent in its outreach activities on an indefinite basis.

NEEDS OF THE CHRONIC PATIENT

All of us require food, shelter, work, recreation, and rewarding social interactions. We can usually fulfill these needs without formal assistance and without developing symptoms. Chronic patients cannot. If someone else does not provide food, they may not eat. If a place to live is not offered, they may sleep on a sidewalk. Chronic patients usually lack the determination to negotiate red tape, even to get a welfare check, social security, or disability insurance. If someone doesn't organize a leisure activity program for them, they won't have much fun. Ultimately, if someone doesn't reach out, such patients will have no friends and may retreat to an inner world of unreality.

In short, chronic patients lack what Mary Ann Test (1979) has called "network cement." They simply do not stick themselves to other people. On the contrary, they have a tendency to avoid others except for those who share the same living quarters. It is important that those who are designated to make up a support services network for the chronic patient be highly attuned to this fact. The process of assuring that the long-term patient has an adequate support network is now known as case management and is a key function to meeting the needs of the chronic patient. The goal of case management is to assure that long-term patients are enmeshed in a social support system that can be designed in the least restrictive environment. Case management may occur in the state hospital or it may occur in the community. The case manager assesses the patient's problems, plans an array of services and supports, links the patient to the various services, and advocates for the various services to be delivered. The case manager then organizes a monitoring system to assure that this support network works in a continuous and collaborative manner on a long-term basis.

SUPPORT NETWORKS FOR LONG-TERM PATIENTS

In order to develop a unified approach to case management, it is important to be familiar with some of the recent literature and theory concerning the nature of support networks. Caplan (1974) has described the function of support systems as a refuge or sanctuary to which the individual may return for rest and recuperation in between his sorties into the stressful environment. Boisevan (1974) characterized the structure of personal support networks in terms of concentric zones. In the personal zone are close relatives and intimate friends; intimate zone 1 includes other relatives and friends with whom there is frequent contact; intimate zone 2 comprises relatives and friends with whom there is infrequent contact; and in the nominal zone, there is no direct contact, but potential connections with other zones.

Collins and Pancoast (1976) have written on the nature of natural helping networks and have characterized them in terms of density, geographic proximity, and the existence of natural helping persons whom they identify as "central figures." These natural helpers do not have to be told when someone is in trouble. They find out and see to it that the person is linked to someone who can provide the necessary assistance.

Pattison, DeFrancisco, Wood, Frazier, and Crowder (1975) report that emotionally healthy individuals live in a functional psychosocial kinship system of 25 to 30 persons upon whom they are interdependent for affective and instrumental support. They indicate that psychotic individuals are part of a very small social matrix consisting of approximately four to six persons upon whom they are profoundly dependent. Cutler (1979) described the need to "build a new permanent family-like group" for chronically mentally ill persons who have exhausted their natural networks and who do not have the necessary numbers of persons in their individual support systems with which to share the dependency.

However, most importantly, recent literature has shown that in order to withstand stressful life events people require a highly segmented rather than a highly dense social network. For example, Hirsh (1980) studied coping mechanisms of widows and determined that those who had support systems that contained a high degree of integration between family members, friends, and work associates did not do as well as those who had networks with clear boundaries between the family, social, and work segments.

For the purpose of working with long-term chronically mentally ill patients, we make the assumption that as adults they too require a functional segmented support network of 20 to 30 individuals upon whom they can be interdependent rather than just dependent. In addition, the network should provide both support and opportunity, and its members should derive from many "walks of life"—relatives, ex-patients, work associates, and service providers, to name but a few. It is useful to associate the various network segments with functional components relating to basic needs for community survival for the long-term patient. The assumption is that the long-term chronically mentally ill person cannot form an adequate segmented support network. It is, therefore, incumbent upon the case manager to aid that person in the development of such a network. In order to do so, it is helpful to develop a schema for evaluating the structure and function of the network that does exist and point out missing or weak segments and links. Figure 22.1 identifies segments by both their intimacy and their functionality. Individual participants in a particular segment are listed according to functional roles they may play with respect to the identified patient.

Personal Segment

This is the segment that most immediately surrounds the individual. It consists of spouse, parents, children, roommates, and others who share the same roof. For a long-term patient, these individuals provide both affective and instrumental support—that is, they provide emotional support, and they do things for the individual. Within this schema, intervention is oriented toward the attainment

FIGURE 22.1

Augmented Folk and Service Support Network for the Long-Term Patient

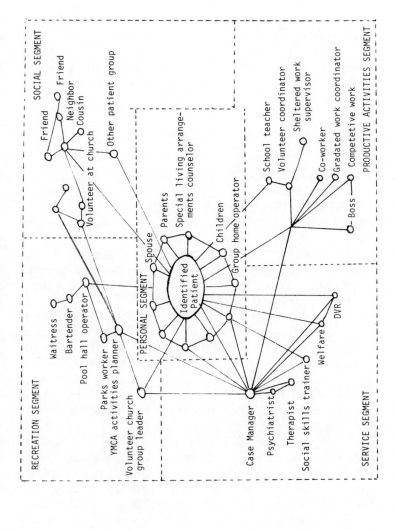

of more personal independence by encouraging the development of basic living skills, for example, personal hygiene, food preparation, transportation, shopping, budgeting, and tidiness. Although the members of this most intimate network segment may not have the skills or the inclination to teach such things, it is important for the case manager to understand that these people are the major reinforcers of these kinds of behavior. They have the greatest amount of daily contact with the person, and their expectations have a profound effect upon whether or not the person carries out the activities or depends upon someone else to do them. These people should therefore be contacted by the case manager and involved in the planning for training in such basic skills of daily living that the patient may receive.

Social Segment

Persons in this segment are friends, neighbors, school mates, and more distant relatives. Most long-term patients have lost most of the individuals from this segment of their natural support systems. Developmentally, it is within this group that much of the growth in the area of interpersonal skills occurs. Members of this segment can also provide affective support that is separate from and not as ambivalently regarded as that from the personal segment. The function of the case manager is to plug the long-term patient into a new network of friends.

Augmented folk networks, such as those described by Cutler and Beigel (1978), are operated by church or civic groups. They are designed and developed for social and interpersonal support, but may play a variety of other functions. Most long-term patients need the provision of a support network first before they will begin to learn new skills. The socialization or friendship level is almost as important as the personal level and in fact may often be called upon to substitute for it.

Within the friendship crucible a mixture of activities takes place that allows long-term patients an opportunity to look outside themselves and their personal networks for ideas and skills. Needless to say, these augmented folk networks will not form and develop without the help of the case manager in a community action-organization framework (Cutler, 1979). Community people can be urged to become involved with long-term patients as volunteers in an organized way via civic or church groups, and then must receive training and consultation in order to support that activity.

Recreational Segment

This segment may be a part of the social segment or a part of the productive activities segment. Long-term patients have a profound capacity not to enjoy themselves. They will not spontaneously arrange enjoyable activities, so the case manager must constantly work on maintaining ties with local programs and projects. When placed in such situations, patients will often initially not appear to appreciate the experience. This network segment must be in place for several months before personnel will be able to discern that a patient has become involved. Recreation-oriented organizations such as the YMCA, health clubs, parks and recreations programs in cities, and other public service-oriented activity groups are examples of this sort of network segment. Case managers need to consult with staff of these programs to desensitize them to the idiosyncracies of chronic patients and their slow progress.

Productive Activities Segment

This segment is usually at the periphery of a chronic patient's existence. Though they may talk and act grandiosely and unrealistically about future education and jobs, many long-term patients do not feel they can be productive. Nonetheless, a planned program to integrate them into meaningful activities should be considered and eventually developed by the case manager. These activities usually mean work activities, but can be volunteer activities, or even a consumer education program to get a GED or college credit. Some community voluntary action centers have organized specialized programs in which long-term patients are placed in a setting commensurate with their current interpersonal abilities and work skill levels. Patients can spend a few hours a day volunteering for routine activities. In these situations they begin to develop the self-control and lengthened attention spans necessary for their next step, which might be sheltered work for pay or vocational training. The productive activities segment is extremely important, since all individuals have a need for meaning in their lives. It doesn't matter exactly where on the production continuum a person is, so long as that person is proceeding in a direction commensurate with realistic goals. Case managers must be sensitive not to set overly high or low expectations for their clients. Sometimes it takes a good deal of time to assess at what level a person must begin. Progress occurs slowly, over a period of months or even years to graduated employment, part-time employment, and in some cases competitive employment.

Programs like the Fairweather Lodge (Fairweather, Sanders, Maynard, & Cressler, 1969) and Fountain House (Beard, 1978) have
demonstrated this kind of result. Functional work may take the
place of the recreation segment or the social segment if the person
is involved enough in the work. However, the other segments are
important and should also be encouraged.

Services Segment

Traditionally, mental health workers have tended to regard
themselves as having to be mother-father-sister-brother-cousin-
uncle-work-associate-friend-and-neighbor to the long-term patient.
However, case manager-therapists must learn to share this burden
with other segments of the natural environment. In addition, they
must spread the service burden over their various service colleagues.
A service segment for the long-term patient is usually made up of a
therapist, a welfare worker, a psychiatrist, a vocational rehabilitation worker, and persons managing or administering recreational
and socialization programs. A variety of emergency therapists, day
program therapists, outpatient therapists, aftercare therapists, and
hospital workers may also play a role at some time in the service
delivery to a long-term patient (Lamb, 1976). It is important for
these service providers to interact with each other in as open a manner as possible, so as to provide an uninterrupted flow of services.
In addition, service segments of the network should link to the other
segments through the case manager. Generally, it is most practical
and resource efficient for case management responsibility to belong
to one of the "therapists" or service providers in the mental health
center.

The Joint Commission on Accreditation of Hospitals standards
requires planning-linking conferences whenever the patient is changing treatment and also at certain turning points in treatment. Those
conferences should include the patient, the case manager, family
members, friends, and other service providers. Methods for conducting such meetings resemble social network intervention as described by Cutler and Madore (1980).

SERVICES TO THE CHRONICALLY
MENTALLY ILL PERSON

Mental health programs must provide an extensive and coordinated spectrum of services in order for chronic patients to
adapt to the community. Stein, Test, and Marks (1975) have shown

that chronic patients can be maintained outside the hospital less expensively than in the hospital. Their patients were more likely to become involved in working situations and maintain a better quality of life when provided with an array of services and work rehabilitation options. In a study entitled "Community Support Systems for the Long-Term Patient" (1979), Stein and others describe some of those elements and, in particular, focus on how to effect continuity of care.

Another comprehensive model, the Balanced Service System, can be used in organizing services for the chronically mentally disordered. The overall goal of this model is to reduce mental disabilities and their adverse effects. Three types of service environment are identified: Protective (hospital), supportive (clinic), and natural (private home or work situations). Also identified are eight different service functions: (1) identification, (2) stabilization, (3) growth, (4) sustenance, (5) case management, (6) prevention, (7) general health, and (8) ancillary. Service functions that are most relevant to the chronically mentally ill populations are identification, crisis stabilization, growth, sustenance, and case management. These service activities are to be provided in the least restrictive environment in order to evaluate and build on the assets and disabilities of the patient/client. For the long-term patient, the model assumes that "cure" is not realistic and allows for permanent or indefinite membership in the system.

In summary, the support needs of the chronically mentally ill person are dependent upon the combination of specific service and support functions organized by the case manager and delivered by professional and natural providers in helping networks in the community. Without this hand-in-hand relationship between professionals and natural providers, the chronically mentally ill person would be abandoned in the community.

THE ROLE OF BOARDS

Advisory and governing boards can have a strong impact on the development of both service segments and augmented folk network segments of the support systems for chronic patients. They can advocate with mental health management, other boards, political groups, church groups, legislators, and the service providers to ensure that the mental health service delivery system is effective. Boards can broaden their understanding and effectiveness by taking part in some of the natural network provider activities themselves.

It is important for boards to take an active leadership role in the planning and negotiating of the services, as well as in the natural network segment of the system. Their own rich personal networks, as well as their energy and skills, can often make the difference between the success or failure of a community-based program. When boards are able to plan and implement services to the chronically mentally ill, they can experience the remarkable progress that is possible. The risk for board members in terms of frustration is significant, but the rewards are even greater, for the recipients are those who would otherwise lead unproductive and unhappy lives. The satisfaction that one experiences when improvement occurs, particularly with those formerly regarded as hopeless, is enough to make the time and effort seem very well spent.

REFERENCES

Arieti, S. (Ed.). American handbook of psychiatry (2nd ed.). New York: Basic Books, 1974.

Beard, J. H. The rehabilitation services of Fountain House. In L. I. Stein & M. A. Test (Eds.), Alternatives to Mental Hospital Treatment. New York: Plenum Press, 1978, pp. 201-209.

Beers, C. A mind that found itself. New York: Doubleday, 1939.

Bloom, B. Community mental health: A general introduction. Monterey, Calif.: Brooks/Cole Publishers, 1977.

Boissevan, J. Friends of friends: Networks, manipulators, and coalitions. New York: St. Martin's Press, 1974.

Brooks, D. K. A bushel of shoes. Hospital and Community Psychiatry, 1969, 371-375.

Caplan, G. Support systems in mental health: Lectures on concept development. New York: Human Sciences Press, 1974.

Caplan, R., & Caplan, G. History of psychiatry in the 19th century. New York: Basic Books, 1969.

Collins, A., & Pancoast, D. Natural helping networks. Washington, D.C.: National Association of Social Workers, 1976.

Cutler, D. Volunteer support networks for chronic patients: New directions for mental health services. Community Support Systems for the Long-Term Patient, 1979, 2, 67-74.

Cutler, D., & Beigel, A. A church-based program of community activities for chronic patients. Journal of Hospital and Community Psychiatry, 1978, 29, 497-501.

Cutler, D., & Madore, E. Community-family network therapy in a rural setting. Community Mental Health Journal, 1980, 16(2), 28-34.

Day, M., & Semrad, A. Chapter II. In A. M. Nicolai, Jr. (Ed.), The Harvard Guide to Modern Psychiatry. Cambridge, Mass.: Harvard University Press, 1978.

Fairweather, G. W., Sanders, D. H., Maynard, H., & Cressler, D. L. Community life for the mentally ill: An alternative to institutional care. Chicago: Aldine, 1969.

Hirsh, B. J. National support systems and coping with major life changes. American Journal of Community Psychology, April 1980, 8, 153-166.

Joint Commission on Accreditation of Hospitals. Principles for Accreditation of Community Mental Health Service Programs. Chicago, 1979.

Jones, M. The therapeutic community. New York: Basic Books, 1953.

Lamb, H. R. Community survival for long-term patients. New York: Jossey-Bass, 1976.

Minkoff, K. A map of chronic mental patients. In J. A. Talbott (Ed.), Chronic Mental Patients: Problem Solutions and Recommendations for Public Policy. Washington, D.C.: Ad Hoc Committee on Chronic Mental Patients of the American Psychiatric Association, 1978.

Pattison, E. M., DeFrancisco, D., Wood, P., Frazier, H., & Crowder, J. A. Psychosocial kinship model for family therapy. American Journal of Psychiatry, 1975, 132, 1246-1251.

Stein, L. I. (Ed.). Community support systems for the long-term patient: New directions for mental health services. New York: Jossey-Bass, 1979.

Stein, L. I., Test, M. A., & Marks, A. Alternatives to the hospital: A controlled study. American Journal of Psychiatry, May 1975, 132, 515-522.

Talbott, J. H. Deinstitutionalization: Avoiding the disasters of the past. Hospital and Community Psychiatry, 1979, 30(9), 621-624.

Terwilliger, W., & Johnson, R. H. Placement of long-term patients into autonomous community living situations: The LINC program. Unpublished manuscript, 1976.

Test, M. A. Continuity of care and case management in community treatment. Paper presented at the National Conference on Creating a Community Support System for the Long-Term Patient, Madison, Wisconsin, May 1979.

23

HISPANIC-AMERICANS AND
MENTAL HEALTH SERVICES
Josué R. Gonzalez

In preparing this work, I was struck by the urgency of the topic. Social agencies are now faced with offering adequate, appropriate, and accessible mental health services for millions of persons who share a common Hispanic heritage and language. Unfortunately, these same agencies are often ill-prepared to meet their societal obligations. Indeed, the history of their response to Hispanic Americans has been poor. Three behavioral scientists, writing in the American Psychologist, declared that

> In the United States, the Spanish-speaking/surnamed population receives mental health care of a different kind, of a lower quality, and a lesser proportion than any other ethnically identifiable population. Demographers consistently agree that ethnic minority group members who are poor receive less health care than the rest of the population. Studies confirm the demographic findings; in fact, some indicate that the problem may be more serious in mental health care. [Padilla, Ruiz, & Alvarez, 1975]

It is the purpose of this chapter to examine various factors contributing to the kinds of mental health care offered Hispanic Americans. The presentation centers on three topics: (1) demographic characteristics of Hispanics; (2) special attributes of Hispanic Americans influencing mental health programs; and (3) issues for agencies working with Hispanic Americans.

DEMOGRAPHIC CHARACTERISTICS OF
HISPANIC AMERICANS

Hispanic Americans constitute the nation's fastest growing
ethnic group, and they are expected to become the nation's largest
ethnic group in the coming decade (Macias, 1977). The 1975 Current
Population Reports estimated that 11.2 million Hispanics resided
in the United States. These figures have been widely criticized as
grossly undercounting the actual number. In its report to the President's Commission on Mental Health, the Special Populations Sub-
Task Panel on Mental Health of Hispanic Americans estimated that,
in fact, 23 million Hispanics currently live in the United States.

Geographically, there are three major concentrations of Hispanics. The greatest number are those of Mexican heritage; they
are located in the Southwestern states of Texas, Arizona, New
Mexico, Colorado, and California, with smaller numbers in other
states, notably, Illinois, Michigan, and New York. Those Puerto
Ricans who leave their island migrate primarily to New York State.
Cuban Americans are concentrated in Florida.

The U.S. Bureau of the Census estimated in its 1975 report
that 59 percent of all Hispanics were of Mexican descent, 16 percent
were Puerto Ricans, 7 percent were of Central and South American
origin, and 6 percent were Cuban Americans. The remaining 12
percent were identified as "others" (including Filipinos).

Poverty is the single major problem facing Hispanics. Census
Department figures reported by Dieppa and Montiel (1978) reveal
that Hispanic income level is lower than that of the general population, with median family income being $4,964. Puerto Ricans earn
much less than Cubans and Mexican Americans.

The low educational achievement that accompanies poverty is
also present with Hispanics. The same study indicated that Hispanics were markedly lower in their educational attainment than the
remainder of the population. Mexican Americans in the 25-34 age
group had a median of 10.8 years of school, while Puerto Ricans
completed a median of 9.9 years. Cubans were exceptional in at-
taining a median of 12.4 years.

A large, young population is also characteristic of Hispanics.
Mexican Americans were reported to have a median age of 17.8
years, Puerto Ricans, 18.3 years, and Cubans, 28.4 years, as
compared to the median age of 28 for the rest of the population. The
median age of 17.8 years for Mexican Americans indicates that more
than half the Mexican-American population in this country are not
old enough to vote and, thus, have no voice at the polls.

Language is another major factor for Hispanics. The same
study indicated that 72 percent of Mexican Americans sampled stated

that Spanish was their mother tongue, while 95 percent of the Cubans responding answered similarly. Forty-seven percent of the Mexican Americans stated they spoke Spanish at home, while 72 percent of the Puerto Ricans and 87 percent of the Cubans said they too spoke Spanish at home.

Dieppa and Montiel concluded that the future prospects for Hispanics in the United States appeared bleak for the following reasons. Mexican Americans and Puerto Ricans (who account for 71 percent of the Hispanic population) constitute the youngest population in the country, with a median age of about 18 years, and have one of the lowest levels of education. This low level of education relegates Hispanics to menial, low-paying jobs that result in conditions of poverty and familial stress. Problems occurring with these conditions are poor health, malnutrition, mental illness, delinquency, school dropouts, family breakdown, and other socioeconomic ills that perpetuate the cycle of poverty. Present social policies at the national and state level continue to be predicated for the most part according to a "universal" perspective that precludes the development of "selective" policies and specialized programs designed to relate to the particular needs, problems, and potentials of Hispanic families (p. 7).

Hispanics, then, form a unique grouping of individuals who have been largely, and, in some cases, systematically excluded from needed attention from social service agencies. Perhaps poverty and language factors have been the most formidable barriers that agencies have helped to perpetuate.

THE APPLICABILITY OF SOCIAL SERVICE
MODELS TO HISPANIC AMERICANS

A community agency always selects an operational model which it then implements. The model is not always chosen as the result of serious deliberations. However, it is crucial in determining what the important issues are for the agency, client, and community, as well as in determining the locus and extent of the intervention. The models—community, medical, and criminal justice—are presented here in terms of their applicability to Hispanic-American mental health needs.

THE COMMUNITY MODEL IN HISPANIC
MENTAL HEALTH SERVICES

The community model stresses the existence of an individual as a member of a series of social systems, that is, the family, neighborhood, and community. The individual's role is that of an active participant working to resolve difficulties within the appropriate system. To be eligible for services in this model, the participant must declare a need for a service. The objective of the intervention is the reordering or restructuring of community resources to remedy the self-declared deficit.

Several prominent factors are considered in the implementation of a community model, including education, socioeconomic status, language usage, degree of acculturation and biculturalism, and the role of the family. These factors are considered in the interaction of community, participant, and agency worker.

The Education Factor

The educational system exists as the major community socializing institution. Until recently the use of Spanish was forbidden in local classrooms at the risk of corporal punishment or expulsion. This policy was enforced even when the child spoke only Spanish and could not understand lessons in English. The message was clear—that the child's Spanish heritage was inferior to that of the Anglo majority. The purpose of the educational system was to teach Hispanic-American children to conform to the larger society's values.

The result of such pressures was to present the Hispanic-American child with several unattractive alternatives. One was to accept Anglo values while discarding his heritage. This choice usually led to feelings of inferiority, low self-esteem, and depression. At times, these feelings were mobilized into antisocial acts as a way of protesting against the educational system. Another alternative was to reject the Anglo values and preserve the Hispanic heritage. This choice, however, usually labeled the child as a deviate and resulted in the individual's dropping out of school. These severe academic demands were likely to produce profound emotional disturbances. The ultimate irony was that the school systems that engendered these difficulties in their students would inevitably "blame the victims" for their failures, claiming that they were lazy or incapable of learning.

As a result of such pressures, children often formed gangs that claimed their primary allegiance. Gangs provided opportunities to express displeasure at being forced to accept foreign values and different behavior patterns. Social service agencies that sought to intervene with the gang members, rather than the group as a whole, were doomed to failure. Similarly ill-fated were attempts to modify a gang member's behavior without addressing community problems that led to the gang's formation.

To illustrate, many agencies attempt to reduce the incidence of paint and glue sniffing in Hispanic gangs. Such efforts are meaningless and meet with a poor response unless the issue of sniffing is seen as a larger community problem. Children are frustrated by a dying educational system marked by low operating funds and poor bilingual resources. The community faces the pressures created by poverty conditions and family units that may be deteriorating.

The Socioeconomic Factor

Hollingshead and Redlich (1958) proposed that the incidence, diagnosis, and treatment of mental illness were closely related to social class. They found that the lower the social class, the greater the number of individuals seeking mental health services, the poorer the prognosis, and the lower the level of treatment received. Historically, Spanish-speaking people have endured high rates of unemployment, have been underpaid for their work, and have had a disproportionate share of people living below the poverty level (U.S. Department of Labor, 1970).

These factors seemingly place the Hispanic American at high risk for mental illness. Other indices, such as rates of migration and acculturation, also contribute to high risk (Brody, 1969; Mostwin, 1976). Accordingly, one would expect Hispanics to make frequent use of mental health services.

The literature, however, generally shows that Hispanic Americans underutilize those services (Jaco, 1959; Karno & Edgerton, 1969; Padilla, Carlos, & Keefe, 1976). Reasons proposed to explain this fact include a strong family support system, which reduced the need for traditional services, and a longstanding distrust of community agencies.

Trevino (1979) examined the relationship between the ethnicity of clients and staff at various community mental health centers in Texas. The data indicated that no underutilization occurred when utilization rates were compared to general population figures. Trevino found that those centers with a low number of Mexican-American staff had expected utilization levels, while those centers with large numbers of Mexican-American staff demonstrated a moderately greater utilization rate. He also found that those centers with a low number of Mexican-American administrators were underutilized by Mexican Americans, while those with a large number of Mexican-American administrators were overutilized.

Language Factors

Assessment and treatment of Hispanic-Americans' mental health has been criticized as being based on inadequate concepts. Accordingly, many variables have been proposed as influencing the proper evaluation of their psychopathology.

The assessment and treatment procedure is a complex interaction involving the manner in which patients present themselves to an evaluator and the evaluator's perceptions and interpretation of that information. Hispanic Americans present themselves in various ways depending on such variables as mood, language used by the interviewer, and degree of client acculturation.

Concern has been raised that the Spanish used by Mexican Americans may be misunderstood by professionals not familiar with Spanish language customs (Edgerton & Karno, 1971; Kiev, 1968; Martinez & Martin, 1966; Padilla, Ruiz, & Alvarez, 1975; Ramirez, 1972; Torrey, 1970). Edgerton and Karno (1971) surveyed over 400 Los Angeles barrio residents in a study of Mexican-American attitudes toward mental illness. The data indicated that their responses in English were different from those in Spanish. The best predictor of responses was the language spoken during the interview. The responses may have differed from English to Spanish because respondents presented themselves and their values in a different fashion when speaking another language. Behavioral, language, and value cues might also have differed between English and Spanish respondents.

DelCastillo (1970) claimed that his patients showed more signs of severe psychopathology when interviewed in their primary language (Spanish) than when interviewed in English. He concluded that clients are more comfortable in expressing themselves in their native language, and, therefore, reveal more of themselves. Using a second language, he claimed, also resulted in filtering the content. Speakers were "simply more on guard," and presented themselves in more socially acceptable ways.

Marcos, Urcuyo, Kesselman, and Alpert (1973) conducted a systematic evaluation of the language problem. The schizophrenic patients were interviewed in English and Spanish. Statistically significant differences were obtained between the English and Spanish interviews for scales dealing with somatic concerns, anxiety, emotional withdrawal, tension, mannerisms and posturing, depressive mood, hostility, and an overall pathology score. The results were interpreted as demonstrating that Spanish-American schizophrenic patients demonstrated more psychopathology when interviewed in English than in Spanish.

In a replication of the Marcos study, I discovered that there were marked differences between English and Spanish interviews, even though the patients were fluently bilingual (Gonzalez, in press). The results were interpreted as supporting DelCastillo's contention that bilingual patients demonstrated more psychopathology when speaking in Spanish than in English. This study also supported the growing body of literature which proposes that professionals working with bilingual clients will receive different impressions based on the language of the interview.

Acculturation/Biculturalism

Acculturation refers to the process whereby an individual incorporates the values, beliefs, and mores of another cultural group. The process can be a function of an individual's decision to adopt the values of another culture, or the result of society's forcing these values on all of its members.

The acculturation process is one in which tension, stress, and conflict are inevitable. Modifying one's values to those of another group typically results in psychological distress. A prominent assumption of acculturation is that the primary set of values was deficient, and that those who taught and believed in the "old" values must have been naive, mistaken, or foolish. Thus, children may learn that their cultural heritage is not good enough and that they must learn a better system. Much familial stress and fighting accompany decisions to shift value systems.

It is not uncommon, for example, for families to be so divided on the issue of acculturation that they form factions centering on their respective beliefs. Within large extended families, such splits may be evidenced by noticing that the children have English names, such as "John," rather than the Spanish, "Juan." Other differences may arise in the manner families order themselves. In traditional Hispanic families, the older generations direct the younger, and the males direct the females. Younger, acculturated family members may rebel at the thought of having their elders play such an important part in their lives. Generational differences can be quite acute, especially when paired with the adoption of competing belief systems.

A recent alternative is that of biculturalism. This concept refers to a process by which an individual chooses to live within the cognitive framework provided by two cultures. Hispanic Americans can, for example, maintain their ethnic heritage at home, yet be aware of and act in accordance with Anglo values at work.

Hispanic Americans have long been pressured to acculturate to the values of the Anglo society. Such stress has been observed in mental health clinics as resulting in feelings of depression, anger, or alienation. A community model would emphasize the importance of stressing a bicultural adaptation to external pressures.

Family Support Systems

Early research on Hispanic Americans stressed the extended family as a major support system. Tuck's (1946) work on Mexican Americans in San Bernardino, Griffith's (1948) study of Mexican-American youth, and other research efforts (Clark, 1959; Madsen, 1961, 1964; Rubel, 1966) have all emphasized the strength of the extended family in helping an individual cope more effectively with stress.

Keefe, Padilla, and Carlos (1978) gathered data on family ties and mental health over a three-year period. Their data indicated that Mexican Americans were likely to have more relatives living in their community than Anglos had. Mexican-American family groups were also more likely than Anglos to span three or more generations. A major difference between Mexican-American and Anglo families was that Anglos were more likely to turn to extrafamilial resources for help and support, while Mexican Americans relied more on their extended family.

Much has been made of the tremendous strength that Hispanic-American families offer their members. I have witnessed many staff meetings in which cases were referred to the family unit for treatment under the assumption that the extended family could rehabilitate a disturbed member. Caution must be used, however, in expecting the family to provide optimal care. The family is not a panacea and cannot remedy all problems. In some cases, referring to a family is the agency's way of "dumping" a particular case. This is especially common when problems are clearly community based, such as difficulties with educational policies or problems arising from low socioeconomic conditions.

Curanderismo

A traditional form of mental health care within the Mexican-American community has been the use of curanderos. Curanderos are practitioners of curanderismo, a belief system used to explain intrapsychic and interpersonal difficulties. Accordingly, curanderismo may be considered a specific type of personality theory.

The two most common conditions, mal ojo, and susto, are the result of disturbed interpersonal relations. The curandero remedies the condition by working very closely with the disturbed individual, seeking to restore the balance of the person's being. The cause of the malady and the steps taken to remove the affliction are carefully discussed. In such a fashion, the individual is encouraged to resume his typical interactions with his family, neighbors, and community.

Curanderismo exists because it works. It serves a specific purpose, that of ordering natural phenomena in a way that makes life understandable and, therefore, manageable. Persons who utilize curanderos do so because their world has become disordered and they are no longer coping adequately in it. Through his use of ritual and religion, the curandero brings peace and harmony to the individual. He accomplishes this by strengthening and fortifying individual defenses rather than by uncovering and interpreting unconscious motivations.

Curanderismo plays an important cultural role, with its heritage in Indian tradition, medieval Spanish beliefs, and religious influences. However, it would be a mistake to ascribe too much importance to this issue. In my experience, those who use curanderos are more likely to be either elderly citizens or very traditional immigrants. The others tend to be individuals who use a curandero because of family insistence.

THE MEDICAL MODEL IN HISPANIC MENTAL HEALTH SERVICES

The medical model is the most pervasive method of describing intrapersonal problems. In this model, an individual declares himself/herself to be a patient, suffering from a disease that can be diagnosed and remedied only through the intervention of a professional. The patient is not held to be at fault for his disorder, since he is assumed to suffer from a disease over which he has no control. Treatment usually consists of a series of visits during which the expert actively seeks to achieve a resolution of the patient's problem.

The medical model, as traditionally used in community mental health centers, has long been under attack as inapplicable to the needs of Hispanic Americans. As Lugo (1975) stated:

> It is not enough to bring mental health centers to the
> barrios and staff them with Spanish-speaking Chicago
> mental health practitioners or for the barrio community

to give input to or control mental health centers in the
barrios if the net result is nothing more than substitu-
tion of brown faces for white, and Spanish for English.
The changes needed are far more basic than provision
of mental health services by Chicano practitioners who
can speak Spanish to their clients. . . . Until recently,
researchers studying the lack of use of mental health
facilities by Chicanos concluded that Chicanos could not
afford to pay the required fees, facilities were too distant and uninviting, and the language factor mitigated
against their use. No one looked at the irrelevancy of
the methods of diagnosis and treatment. [p. 9]

THE CRIMINAL JUSTICE MODEL IN HISPANIC
MENTAL HEALTH SERVICES

Many problems encountered by Hispanic Americans are frequently resolved through a legal model. In this perspective, a
public organization declares an individual to be an offender of the
community's mores. The transgression is resolved through the
court system, with the goal being the maintenance of the existing
social order. The disruption is viewed as being totally under the
control of the offender who is to be punished for the protection of
the rights of the larger society.

The mental health needs of Hispanic Americans have to a
large degree been addressed through the legal system. Community
problems, such as an educational system that regularly produces
dropouts, can be resolved by imprisoning the community's adolescents rather than by addressing the educational system. The
alienation of people who cannot obtain jobs can be dealt with through
the selective incarceration of the most vocal community critics
rather than by creating job training programs or alternative community action programs.

AGENCY ISSUES IN WORKING WITH
HISPANIC AMERICANS

Issues concerning mental health agencies generally focus on
three areas: accessibility, availability, and appropriateness of the
services delivered to special populations with special needs. While
the definition of need varies with the model the agency chooses to
use, the themes are applicable regardless of the model selected.

Accessibility of service refers to the difficulty prospective participants encounter in using the agency's services. Such physical realities as the availability of adequate transportation services, proximity to the service site, and rate of fees are strong determinants of an individual's participation in a treatment plan. Accessibility also refers to whether necessary services are offered at times that are convenient for the community, or whether the center insists that crises occur between the hours of 8 A.M. and 5 P.M. Another concern is whether the community is aware of the services offered by that agency. If not, the services may be said to be inaccessible or even nonexistent.

Once the person reaches the agency, availability of service becomes prominent. Simply, are the services that are offered generally available to the community? If so, are they reflective of those needs declared by the target population? It is important that the center staff and board actively work with their community to assess local conditions.

Appropriateness of services refers to providing trained personnel who can work with an individual in the language of his/her choice, and who can respond in a manner acceptable to that individual.

In addition to accessibility, availability, and appropriateness, seven other major problem areas must be considered in the implementation of a mental health service delivery system. These are not intended to comprise a comprehensive roster, but are issues that must be addressed in delivering mental health services to Hispanic Americans.

Financing

It is common knowledge that monies are increasingly hard to obtain and that pressure for fiscal accountability is mounting from many areas. Such pressures should result in board members asking themselves the following questions:

How are the dollars allocated with respect to Hispanic programs? The major index of center involvement is the percentage of the total budget allocated for such programs.

How are the decisions made about distribution of monies? Openness in decision making should be a major concern for the board.

Are Hispanics involved in resolving the financial questions that directly affect them?

Has the Hispanic community been approached for financial support of the agency?

Staffing

While the board or director may set general policy, the staff acts as the final interpreter of such policies. Accordingly, the following questions may be asked:

How reflective of the community is the staff?
How does an agency recruit its staff, especially minority staff members?
Who is hired and who is not? Who makes those decisions? Perhaps a more accurate description is to ask who is fired first when monies are tight.
Once staff, especially minority staff, are hired, what steps are used to keep them?

Training

An area often overlooked is that of the training of personnel. This is often interpreted as training only certain staff members, but adequate training refers to all agency staff from receptionists to administrators.

What is the relationship between community agencies and the schools that provide the training for their staff?
How extensive are the inservice training sessions, and how reflective are they of the problems typically encountered by the center's staff in working with Hispanic Americans?

Policy Direction

The following questions may be asked:

Does a long-term policy exist for the delivery of adequate, appropriate, and available mental health services for Hispanic Americans?
Who has input to the plan?

Planning and Evaluation

Evaluation efforts are sometimes low priority issues at centers. Yet, how a center evaluates and interprets its interventions with Hispanics is of critical importance in determining the adequacy of the efforts.

Without regular surveys, can an agency be aware of the needs of the minority community?

How are programs monitored?

Do the evaluators possess the clinical skills necessary to assess properly those issues relevant to Hispanic Americans?

Linkages

It is necessary to examine to what extent an agency interacts with other social systems in the area as a way of assessing the scope of the interventions.

What formal and informal relationships exist between the community agency and other community institutions, such as schools, police, churches, health department, and so on?

Is sanction given to staff to work with staff from other agencies in order to coordinate intervention plans?

Are efforts made to assess which systems are utilized by the Hispanic community so contact may be established?

Prevention

The primary assumption of prevention programs is that environmental stress can increase the incidence of mental disorders. Strong prevention efforts then address the reduction of external stress in order to minimize the need for mental health services.

What percentage of the budget is reserved for preventive programs?

Does the agency recognize as a primary goal the identification of major stress sources in the community?

Are members of the Hispanic community involved in addressing these areas which produce major stress reactions?

CONCLUSION

Hispanic Americans constitute a large, rapidly growing segment of the population. Mexican Americans, Puerto Ricans, and Cuban Americans are the major groupings under the Hispanic rubric. Hispanics are generally younger, poorer, and have a lower level of educational achievement than the rest of the population. The majority must struggle to survive under hostile living situations.

Reactions from social service agencies toward Hispanics have typically been either to ignore or to condescend. Hispanics present special needs, different language, strong customs and heritage, and the pressure of living under constant poverty, which must be addressed by any agency seeking to provide services. Problem areas faced by agencies working with Mexican Americans in particular were discussed.

Hispanic Americans are rapidly making their needs known to community agencies. The communication, however, requires an informed response. Hopefully, interaction will result in more adequate, appropriate, and available services for an important segment of this country's population. Local agencies could then be instrumental in improving the quality of life for millions of Hispanic Americans.

REFERENCES

Brody, E. B. Migration and adaptation: The nature of the problem. American Behavioral Scientist, 1969, 13, 5-13.

Clark, M. Health in the Mexican-American culture. Berkeley: University of California Press, 1959.

DelCastillo, J. C. The influence of language upon symptomatology in foreign-born patients. American Journal of Psychiatry, 1970, 40, 240-241.

Dieppa, I., & Montiel, M. Hispanic families: An exploration. In M. Montiel (Ed.), Hispanic Families. Washington, D.C.: National Coalition of Hispanic Mental Health and Human Services Organizations, 1978.

Edgerton, R. B., & Karno, M. Mexican-American bilingualism and the perception of mental illness. Archives of General Psychiatry, 1971, 24, 286-290.

Gonzalez, J. R. Language factors in the presentation of self. Psychiatric Annals, in press.

Griffith, B. American me. Boston: Houghton-Mifflin, 1948.

Hollingshead, A. B., & Redlich, F. C. Social class and mental illness: A community study. New York: John Wiley, 1958.

Jaco, E. G. Mental health of the Spanish Americans in Texas. In M. F. Opler (Ed.), Culture and mental health: Cross-cultural studies. New York: Macmillan, 1959.

Karno, M., & Edgerton, R. B. Perceptions of mental illness in a Mexican-American community. Archives of General Psychiatry, 1969, 20, 233-238.

Keefe, S. E., Padilla, A. M., & Carlos, M. L. Emotional support systems in two cultures: A comparison of Mexican Americans and Anglo Americans. Los Angeles, Spanish Speaking Mental Health Research Center, UCLA, Occasional Paper No. 7, 1978.

Kiev, A. Curanderismo: Mexican-American folk psychiatry. New York: Free Press of Glencoe, 1968.

Lugo, E. The urban barrio. In R. Duran (Ed.), Salubridad Chicana: Su preservacíon y mantenimiento. (The Chicano plan for mental health). Washington, D.C.: U.S. Government Printing Office, 1975.

Macias, R. F. U.S. Hispanics in 2000 A.D.—Projecting the number. Agenda, 1977, 7(3), 16-20.

Madsen, W. Society and health in the Lower Rio Grande Valley. Austin: Hogg Foundation for Mental Health, 1961.

Madsen, W. The Mexican Americans of South Texas. New York: Holt, Rinehart, & Winston, 1964.

Marcos, L. R., Urcuyo, L., Kesselman, M., & Alpert, M. The language barrier in evaluating Spanish-American patients. Archives of General Psychiatry, 1973, 29, 655-659.

Martinez, C., & Martin, H. Folk diseases among urban Mexican Americans. Journal of the American Medical Association, 1966, 196(2), 147-150.

Mostwin, D. Uprootment and anxiety. International Journal of Mental Health, 1976, 5(2), 103-116.

Padilla, A. M., Carlos, M. L., & Keefe, S. E. Mental health utilization by Mexican Americans. Monograph number three of the Spanish-speaking mental health research center, 1976.

Padilla, A. M., Ruiz, R. A., & Alvarez, R. Community mental health services for the Spanish-speaking/surnamed population. American Psychologist, 1975, 30, 892-905.

Ramirez, M. Towards cultural democracy in mental health: The case of the Mexican American. Revista Interamericana de Psicologia, 1972, 6, 42-50.

Report to the President's Commission on Mental Health from the Special Populations Sub-Task Panel on Mental Health of Hispanic-Americans. Reprinted by the Spanish Speaking Mental Health Research Center, UCLA, 1978.

Rubel, A. J. Across the tracks: Mexican Americans in a Texas city. Austin: University of Texas Press, 1966.

Torrey, E. F. The irrelevancy of traditional mental health services for urban Mexican Americans. American Journal of Orthopsychiatry, 1970, 40, 240-241.

Trevino, F. M. The utilization of community mental health services by Mexican Americans as a function of institutional staffing characteristics. Unpublished doctoral dissertation, University of Texas Medical Branch at Galveston, 1979.

Tuck, R. Not with the first: Mexican Americans in a southwest city. New York: Harcourt, Brace, & Co., 1946.

United States Bureau of the Census. Current population reports: Persons of Spanish origin in the United States, March, 1975. Washington, D.C.: United States Government Printing Office, 1976.

United States Department of Labor. Report on the manpower needs of Spanish-speaking Americans. Washington, D.C.: United States Department of Labor, 1970.

24

SERVICES FOR OLDER ADULTS
Robert L. Kahn

Despite the great urgency of services for the aged, community
mental health centers in this country have been very disappointing
in meeting this need. Not only have the CMHCs manifested a disproportionate emphasis on the treatment of younger persons, but
with the passage of years they have shown a consistent trend toward
even younger and healthier clients. This paradoxical state of affairs is all the more questionable considering that there have been
operating examples of successful mental health programs for the
elderly, both in this country and abroad. In this chapter I will try
to formulate some of the major problems and principles in developing services for older adults. These principles cannot be applied
mechanically, but depend for implementation on current administrative, financial, and legal constraints, as well as on the particular
resources and characteristics of the individual CMHC.

THE MENTALLY ILL AGED: WHO THEY ARE

Before discussing services it is necessary to consider the
specific qualities of the elderly psychiatric population that could determine the kinds of services needed.

The Chronic Patient

It is not enough to classify a patient just on the basis of his
chronological age. There are considerable differences, for example
between those elderly persons who developed a chronic major mental illness early in life but lived to an old age, and those persons

who developed a mental disorder for the first time after they had grown old. The chronic patients are most commonly schizophrenics, with many years of custodial institutionalization behind them. These patients had been discharged in great numbers from the state hospitals as part of the deinstitutionalization program. It was assumed that patients would somehow be better off in small "community facilities" rather than in large mental hospitals. Although the program has always been controversial, it is generally regarded as a failure. Some have blamed this on the lack of adequate community programs to provide alternative services. Others have regarded this group of chronic schizophrenics as the most difficult to manage of all client groups. Not only have they suffered a major psychotic disorder for many years, but they have become socially isolated and incompetent through their separation from ordinary social interactions and responsibilities. Deinstitutionalization has also been regarded as producing a traumatic dislocation from an environment that may have become "home" to the patients and therefore one in which they were more comfortable. It is likely that in the future these chronic schizophrenics can be best treated in the hospital, although there will be less prolonged institutionalization to create the problem in the first place.

The chronic schizophrenic, chronically institutionalized patients are more likely to resemble younger chronic schizophrenics than psychiatric patients with disorders of old age. It would make more sense to have an "after-care" or "deinstitutionalization" clinic that handled such patients regardless of age. The service concepts described in this chapter are primarily intended for those persons developing mental disorders for the first time in later life.

Mental Disorders of Old Age

The principal mental disorders among the elderly are depression and dementia. Depression is a mental disorder characterized by such feelings as discouragement, helplessness, and hopelessness, and by difficulties in such functions as eating and sleeping. Some depressive complaints may be found in about 20-25 percent of the elderly population, but is severe in about 10-15 percent. In middle age and in the sixth and seventh decades, depression is more likely to affect women; after age 80 the rate for men is higher. At all ages the suicide rate is higher for men; for women there is an actual decline after middle age, but for men the suicide rate constantly increases.

Many epidemiologic studies have shown that about 5 percent of all persons 65 years of age and older suffer from dementia or intellectual impairment due to organic brain disease, with another 10 percent having some mild disorder. The rate increases with age.

Dementia, of which the most common form is the senile or Alzheimer's type, is a progressive deteriorating disease, starting slowly but ultimately affecting all intellectual functions and the ability to perform the acts of everyday living. It is necessary to distinguish dementia, which is due to diseases of the nervous system, from normal changes due to aging. "Senility" is not a regular outcome of growing old. By virtue of all the things that have occurred in their lifetime and because of the lapse of time, old persons may seem to have a poor memory when they are actually functioning normally. Because of the stereotypes of older people, they themselves are more likely to think that they have poor memory. However, decline in speed of response has been reported as the most consistent normal change with age.

Altered brain function, with impaired intellectual functioning, disorientation, and psychotic behavior, can develop rapidly in some elderly persons due to the secondary effects of physical disease or the toxic effects of drugs administered for medical purposes. These conditions are important to recognize because they are often reversible.

PRINCIPLES OF INTERVENTION

General Statement

Many persons with mental disorders of old age could be well treated in conventional systems of medical and mental health care. But the community mental health center based in a catchment area with a defined population has a great potential for treating many of the special problems of the elderly.

What distinguishes the aged mentally ill from younger persons is the increasing level of complexity involved in dealing with them. Elderly psychiatric patients tend also to have medical and social problems, making it extremely difficult to work out the integration of the various resources. Who is the primary care giver and who is secondary? There may be jurisdictional disputes, with agencies or services fighting for the right either to care for or to exclude a particular client or patient. Persons with very similar sorts of mental problems may end up at a social agency, a medical clinic, or a mental health center depending on factors other than specific mental symptoms.

Let us consider some of the specific complexity problems noted in depression in later life. It has been observed that while younger persons are likely to express their depression in the form of psychological complaints, the elderly increasingly express their feelings in the form of preoccupation with bodily functions, such as delusions of having cancer. This somatic concern has been termed "masked depression" because the patient's depressive symptoms are less open or explicit, although many clues to his feelings may still be present. Since these persons and their families see themselves as having a medical rather than a mental health problem, they will seek out the family doctor or other medical assistance. Many of these persons may refuse mental health referral even when assured of their physical health. The association between physical condition and depression is also very strong because the presence of physical illness is the most prominent external precipitating factor leading to depression in the elderly. Such patients may require continuing active general health care, along with treatment for their depression. The medications that are prescribed for such patients for treating their medical condition may represent contraindications for use of antidepressive drugs that have been found to be so helpful. In any case, there is a difficult problem in coordinating the medical care.

Dementia is the mental disorder that has been most difficult to manage in the formal mental health system. In part, this is due to the negative expectations that most mental health professionals have toward patients with organic brain impairment. But there is actually considerable area for positive involvement. The basic principle is that even in dementia psychological factors play an important role in determining the severity of the behavioral symptoms. These patients perform more poorly under conditions of stress, such as dislocation, and in the face of environments with limited stimulation and opportunity for autonomy such as found in most custodial institutions. The majority of dementia patients have been reported as showing marked depressive manifestations as well. Since depression affects intellectual performance even in younger persons, treatment of the depressive features may lead to improved mental performance. Even such symptoms as wandering or incontinence may have a major emotional component and therefore be subject to psychological modification.

Although dementia is a chronic, progressive disorder, the treatment goals should be oriented to prevention, secondary and tertiary. This approach emphasizes limiting the severity of the mental impairment and the long-term consequences of the disease. One of the basic characteristics of this kind of prevention is early intervention, which is believed to offer the best possibilities for providing the most successful management. Early intervention with the family can be particularly effective. It has been found that,

rather than "dumping" their sick elderly into institutions, families
are very protective and may go to extreme lengths to avoid institutionalization. At the same time, it has been observed that elderly
mentally disordered persons are a severe burden on the family.
Once the burden becomes overwhelming, the family may then make
an irrevocable decision to extrude the sick person. Early intervention working with the family, however, may prevent the critical
point from being reached, enabling the patient to be maintained in
the community.

SPECIFIC PRINCIPLES

Guaranteed Commitment

In order to provide more than token service for the mentally
ill aged, it is necessary to establish an atmosphere of confidence in
which the CMHC can be seen as genuinely interested in old persons
and as concerned for their interests and for the problems encountered by their families and helpers. The totality of the program and
the commitment of the personnel will determine whether or not the
confidence exists. But the basic ingredients should include: (1) having someone always available for telephone consultation with general
practitioners and family members, and (2) having a range of clinical
services, including ambulatory as well as inpatient services, with
the guarantee that the service the patient needs can always be provided. It is also necessary to demonstrate to the old people and
the community that the staff's interest is not to rush patients off to
an institution.

Naturally, a service commitment will lead to an increase in
the number of elderly referrals. However, certain kinds of service
requests will be reduced. As an example, intensive involvement as
in institutionalization will be decreased. Knowing that services are
available when needed will act as a powerfully supportive factor for
managing the aged in the community.

Minimal Intervention

This is perhaps the most elusive principle to grasp, since it
seems to run counter to prevailing views on provision of services.
It is based on the recognition that while those with emotional disorders may be harmfully neglected by too few treatment resources,
they may also be harmed by too extensive intervention. The harm is
caused by infantilizing clients, depriving them of autonomous func-

tioning and responsibility, separating them from the informal social support network, and teaching them how to play the role of a sick person.

One of the early experiences that led to this concept was derived from military psychiatry during recent wars. It was found that men who developed acute psychiatric disturbances in combat had a far greater recovery rate if they were removed from their outfits for just a few days and then returned to duty, rather than being removed from the combat zone to large medical facilities. It was believed that the men did better because they had the support of their buddies in the outfit and had a chance to reestablish their own adaptive resources.

The most obvious component of this principle is to minimize disruption. As much as possible the elderly person should be dealt with in his usual neighborhood and family setting. It has been repeatedly shown that one of the severest stresses for the aged is dislocation of any kind. Moving the person from home to hospital or from institution to institution may add stress and produce a more deteriorated mental picture than would otherwise be shown. It is likely that much of the impairment and apathy observed in older persons in institutions is an indirect reflection of the noxious effects of being institutionalized rather than the direct consequences of the mental disorder itself.

It is desirable to keep the old person in his own home and community setting as much as possible. Two specific services that may have a powerful impact on minimizing disruption are home evaluation and care, and day care. By seeing patients in their own homes, mental health personnel can make a more accurate assessment of the resources available to their patients, and also communicate the message that the treatment is oriented toward the home. The home care may be the primary intervention, or it may be used for aftercare following hospitalization.

Day care has become an increasingly useful service in meeting the needs of older persons. The type of day care can be varied, functioning as part of a hospital for the treatment of persons with greater degrees of physical care requirements, or as part of a social agency, or primarily as a mental health facility. Studies of younger subjects have shown that treating the patient in day care leads to better long-term results than 24-hour hospitalization. Numerous observations of elderly patients have shown that even persons with dementia can be kept out of long-term institutional care by the use of day care facilities. Although providing mostly group interactions, the day care programs are so helpful because they provide (1) a structured social experience for persons living alone; (2) support for families that are caring for the older person but, because of other commitments such as working, need some help during the day; (3) opportunity for good nutrition; and (4) supervision of medication.

Time-Limited Treatment

Day care facilities are an excellent example of minimization through limitation of time involved. Depending on the individual needs, a patient may spend from one to six days in day care. (The general principle is that the least amount of time necessary should be used for treatment.) Time considerations should also be prominent in considering 24-hour care systems. An institution does not have a harmful effect on an old person just because it is an institution. It is the social-psychological context in which the institutionalization is seen as a rejection or abandonment that is harmful. If the patient feels cut off from his family and community, the institution is regarded as a terminal placement and the negative reactions set in. Accordingly, it is desirable to minimize the stressful impact by using time-limited institutionalization. If, for example, the patient, his family, and the intervention staff all know that four weeks is the expected duration, they will act consistently with that expectation. Of course, in those instances where more inpatient time is needed, the arrangement can be preserved for an additional period.

Holiday Relief

A basic principle of minimal intervention is that a little help judiciously provided may prevent the development of the need for more intensive intervention. One such technique that has been successfully employed has been termed "holiday" or "respite" relief, in which chronically ill persons who are being maintained by their families at home are hospitalized by appointment for a week or two just to permit the family to enjoy a vacation. Without the support of the week or two of relief, the family members may need to protect themselves by permanently institutionalizing the patient.

"Overdosing"

As we have just described, intervention can be excessive if it creates too much of a disruption in terms of length or setting of treatments. A more complicated and subtle form of excessive treatment has been called "overdosing." In such a situation, help may be administered on a piecemeal basis that is apparently a legitimate response to individual deficiencies, but which has a total negative impact, such as increasing mental deterioration or causing earlier death. It has been reported, for example, that having specialists such as social workers or nurses caring for persons with dementia may paradoxically result in higher death rates. This effect seems to be produced in part by the infantilization that occurs when other people are planning too much of one's life. Also a caring person is often likely to put an old person in an institution which, in itself, is associated with greater mortality. There is even a theory concerning institutional care and "social invisibility," according to which the fate of people with mental impairment will vary with the presence or absence of family, friends, or caring persons in their environment. The latter, out of concern for the older person, may take steps that lead to his or her institutionalization. In contrast, if a person is socially "invisible," there may be nobody around who cares enough to pay attention to his troubles and so he gets by in the community. Paradoxically, this may turn out to add to his longevity. Since it will frequently be difficult to decide whether intervention is appropriate or excessive, it is best to keep the situation flexible, so that the patient himself can make a choice or withdraw from a service once begun. Even within the context of a needed intervention, it must be realized that excessive fostering of dependency can have negative consequences.

Indirect Intervention

In many instances the elderly patient can best be treated indirectly, by working with a member of his family. Family members may have anxieties about the client's behavior and doubt their own adequacy at management. They need to acquire more understanding of the nature of the mental condition and how to cope with the behavioral changes. Improving their outlook and demonstrating to them that there is concern for their problems as well as those of the client can have a salutary effect on both of them.

CONTINUITY OF CARE

Too often, because of the complex factors involved with geriatric patients, there is difficulty in coordinating the component services. The patient may have needs that must, either simultaneously or over time, be dealt with by several agencies differing in staff, intake criteria, and treatment philosophy. It has been reported that best results are encountered when there is continuity of care, in which there is both a limited number and a constancy of personnel who deal with the patient. The CMHC may have the opportunity to take the initiative in setting up cooperative arrangements with related agencies, so that some key person may be designated as the coordinating agent no matter where the patient is physically located. It is certainly extremely difficult to achieve continuity of care, but it remains an ideal for which we must strive.

SUMMARY

Some of the major problems and principles involved in providing services for older adults in CMHCs were discussed. It was pointed out that there is a major difference in programs required for the chronically ill who happen to have grown old, and those persons who developed a mental illness for the first time in old age. Older persons present more complex problems, requiring the interaction and coordination of mental, physical, and social care. Dementia affects only a small proportion of the elderly, but has been most difficult for the mental health professions to deal with because of preconceptions concerning functional and organic disorders. It was indicated that there is usually a significant emotional component in dementia and that treatment of this component may have substantial effects on behavior. Realistic goals for dementia should be secondary and tertiary prevention, minimizing both the severity and consequences of the impairment. The basic principles in providing service for the aged are guaranteed commitment, minimal intervention in all aspects, and continuity of care.

REFERENCES

Butler, R. N., & Lewis, M. I. Aging and mental health: Positive psychological approaches. St. Louis: C. V. Mosby, 1973.

Frankfather, D. The aged in the community: Managing senility and deviance. New York: Praeger, 1977.

Glasscote, R. M., Gudeman, J. E., & Miles, D. G. Creative mental health services for the elderly. Washington, D. C.: American Psychiatric Association, 1977.

Kahn, R. L. The mental health system and the future aged. Gerontologist, 1975, 15(2), 24-31.

25

MENTAL HEALTH SERVICES FOR
THE MENTALLY RETARDED INDIVIDUAL
Louis Rowitz

Mental health service delivery in the United States does not equitably provide services to all who need help. The President's Commission on Mental Health (1978) has documented this statement throughout a series of four volumes. The contributors reported that there are many groups in our population who are unserved, underserved, or inappropriately served. The reasons given include financial barriers, lack of access, lack of specialized care, and discrimination because of age, sex, race, cultural background, or type of disability.

One of the major disability groups not adequately served by the mental health field is the mentally retarded and their families. The President's Commission noted that a primary diagnosis of mental retardation does not preclude the existence of mental illness. The Commission went on to explain that mentally ill, mentally retarded persons have fallen through the cracks of the mental health and mental retardation service systems partly because of a number of interlocking differences between caregivers and their agencies. Mental health practitioners seem to accept the myth that mentally retarded clients do not profit from psychotherapeutic intervention; they are uninformed about mental retardation and the needs of these clients and their families. Mentally retarded persons with psychiatric problems tend to be shifted back and forth between mental health, mental retardation, and correctional systems. And, there is a paucity of local community intervention programs for mentally ill, mentally retarded individuals.

The Task Panel on Mental Retardation of the President's Commission on Mental Health suggested four basic premises about the mental health problems of the mentally retarded: (1) mental illness

384

and mental retardation are distinct and separate problems; (2) the great majority of mentally retarded are not mentally ill; (3) mentally retarded people experience the same spectrum of feelings as people without mental retardation; and (4) emotional disorders are reversible irrespective of intellectual abilities.

This chapter looks at several dimensions of the problem of mental health services for mentally retarded clients and their families. First, the problem of mental disability is reviewed, defining differences between mental illness and mental retardation. Then follows a discussion of mental retardation as a diagnostic and classification problem. Next is an exposition of the issues associated with service delivery for mentally retarded persons with psychiatric impairments, and a description of available psychotherapeutic interventions. Finally, the chapter concludes with some recommendations for the future.

MENTAL ILLNESS AND MENTAL RETARDATION

The concepts of mental illness and mental retardation are often confused because both are frequently considered mental disabilities. The 1980 edition of A Psychiatric Glossary, published by the American Psychiatric Association, defines "disability" as "deprivation of intellectual or emotional capacity or fitness," and it quotes the federal government's definition of "disability" as "inability to engage in any substantial gainful activity by reason of any medically determinable physical or mental impairment which can be expected to last or has lasted for a continuous period of not less than twelve full months." (p. 30)

Part of the difficulty in distinguishing between mental illness and mental retardation is the similarity between the two categories. Milgram (1972) pointed out that mental illness and mental retardation as major diagnostic groups are comprised of heterogeneous populations. However, the behavioral characteristics of those assigned either diagnostic label are quite diverse. The diagnosis of mental illness (especially schizophrenia) and the diagnosis of mental retardation are very unreliable, and the diagnostic labels do not provide an adequate determination of the behavioral patterns associated with them. Milgram noted that the fields of mental health and mental retardation are marked by a dualistic diagnostic system that distinguishes disorders that are biomedical from those that are sociocultural in etiology. Moreover, both fields have shifted from an emphasis on complete recovery to alleviation of maladaptive symptoms. Butterfield (1967) points out that institutionalization for mental illness or mental retardation has a negative effect on the individual, which may aggravate the original problem.

Even though there are similarities between mental illness and mental retardation, the differences are also quite clear-cut. The American Psychiatric Association (1980) defined mental illness or mental disorder as:

> An illness with psychologic or behavioral manifestations and/or impairment in functioning due to a social, psychologic, genetic, physical/chemical, or biologic disturbance. The disorder is not limited to relations between the person and society. The illness is characterized by symptoms and/or impairment in functioning. [p. 89]

The same organization adopts the definition of mental retardation used by the American Association of Mental Deficiency:

> Mental retardation refers to significantly subaverage general intellectual functioning existing concurrently with deficits in adaptive behavior, and manifested during the developmental period. [p. 5]

Thus, mental illness and mental retardation refer to different clinical entities. Mental retardation relates to abnormal behavior associated with defects in intellectual capacity and limitations in the ability to adapt to community living situations. On the other hand, mental illness refers to psychological and behavioral problems demonstrated through inappropriate, unrealistic, and irrational behavior (Kurtz, 1977). Another important distinction is that the majority of the mentally ill possess normal intelligence. Kurtz notes that mental illness is usually defined as treatable, with an eventual disappearance of symptoms being possible, while treatment for mental retardation is usually seen as a way to help alleviate or remediate some of the problems. Mentally retarded people do not become intellectually normal.

On the question of the disappearance of symptoms for the mentally retarded, there is an immediate complication. Many cases of mild mental retardation (often called educable mental retardation by the schools) are defined within the school system. These children are often considered retarded the six hours a day that they attend school. For the remainder of the day, they are considered normal within their home environments and they can lose the mental retardation label when they leave school in late adolescence (Rowitz, in press-b).

Another interesting distinction between mental illness and mental retardation is the appearance of a life cycle difference. On the one hand, mental retardation is often seen as referring to children, regardless of the age of the disabled person. Mental illness, on the other hand, is often seen as referring primarily to adults, although some discussion is given to childhood disorders and disorders of old age (PCMH, 1978).

MENTAL RETARDATION: DIAGNOSIS AND CLASSIFICATION

The definition of mental retardation offered by the American Association on Mental Deficiency in effect presents only one dimension of the diagnostic and classification system presented by that same association. The diagnostic manual (Grossman, 1977) states that both biomedical and behavioral classification systems should be used for mental retardation. The biomedical diagnostic system separates individuals on the basis of etiology or presumed etiology, and the manual gives the following justifications for its use: (1) mental retardation is "a manifestation of some underlying disease process or medical condition" (p. 8); (2) the biomedical classification scheme was developed so that it would be acceptable to medical personnel of various specializations; (3) attempts were made to keep the AAMD biomedical classification scheme consistent with other medical classification systems; and (4) the biomedical classification system is set up for use by residential facilities, clinics, and other facilities that deal with mentally retarded clients.

The AAMD definition of mental retardation is based on the behavioral system of classification rather than on the biomedical system. The behavioral system evaluates individuals on the basis of degree of impairment in functioning. According to this system, the individual must show impairment in both measured intelligence and adaptive behavior. Moreover, the definition of mental retardation lacks any reference to etiology. Intellectual functioning is assessed by the use of a standardized intelligence test, such as the Stanford-Binet or Wechsler Scales. The obtained intelligence quotient is then translated into a system of levels of mental retardation: mild, moderate, severe, and profound. The same levels are used on the second dimension of the behavioral system, which is called adaptive behavior, although there is not much agreement on the measures of adaptive behavior to be used in the diagnostic system. Moreover, the individual must be retarded in both intellectual functioning and adaptive behavior functioning to be considered retarded under this system.

The two diagnostic systems are quite cumbersome in that a child may be labeled by the biomedical system alone; he may be

labeled by the behavioral system alone; he may be labeled retarded
by the intellectual functioning criterion without the adaptive behavior
criterion; or he may finally be labeled all three ways, depending on
the service provider (Rowitz, 1974b). Regardless of the method of
diagnosis, a review of the literature of mental retardation shows
many biases in the labeling of children. In summary, some of these
research findings are as follows (Rowitz, 1974a). Minority children
are overrepresented among those labeled with minimal retardation.
Most children labeled with minimal retardation come from low socioeconomic homes. There is a big proportion of social disruption in
families with high-level retarded children. Children who are behavior problems in school are more likely to be labeled retarded
than children who are better behaved. In fact, the school is the primary labeling agency for mildly retarded persons. The incidence of
diagnosed mental retardation is highest in the school-age years and
much lower in the preschool and adult years. There is a prepon-
derance of labeled retarded males in comparison to retarded females.
A recent study reports that the original identifiers of mental retardation for a large urban retardation clinic population were primarily
medical rather than nonmedical sources (Rowitz, in press-a).

Other classification schemes also exist in mental retardation.
MacMillan (1977) points out that special educators currently classify
children into three broad categories: educable mentally retarded
(EMR), children with IQs between about 50-55 to 75 on a standardized
IQ test; trainable mentally retarded (TMR), children with IQs be-
tween 25-35 up to 50-55; profoundly mentally retarded, children with
IQs below 35.

This classification scheme does not use adaptive behavior
scales and appears resistant to the incorporation of these types of
measures in determining mental retardation. The British classify
their children into groups according to the services required: subnormal and severely subnormal (MacMillan, 1977). The subnormal
usually require special education, training, and sometimes medical
care. They have IQs of about 50 or below and usually require custodial services. Rutter (1971) has specifically questioned the usefulness of an adaptive behavior dimension in classification and argued that social adaptation is a meaningless term because it ignores
subcultural considerations and social circumstances within which
adaptation is to take place. Rutter's arguments are relevant to both
the British and American classification systems.

The complexities inherent in diagnosis and classification in
mental retardation become even more intricate when we superim-
pose the problems of mental retardation with socioemotional disorder. The American Association of Mental Retardation manual
(Grossman, 1977) refers diagnosticians to the American Psychiatric

Association diagnostic manual when a psychiatric impairment accompanies mental retardation.

Before concluding this section, it is important to discuss briefly the concept of developmental disability. This is an administrative designation used by the federal government, and now also by state and local providers, to refer to an individual with substantial developmental problems manifested during the first 22 years of life. Prior to the change in developmental disabilities legislation in 1978 (P.L. 95-602), a developmentally disabled person was defined as an individual with mental retardation, cerebral palsy, epilepsy, autism, or dyslexia manifested during the developmental period prior to age 18. The 1978 revisions have complicated the picture of who will be considered developmentally disabled under the law. It seems that mental retardation and the other disabilities mentioned are still included under P.L. 95-602, but that other disability groups will also be included. Not only do we find professional groups establishing diagnostic and classification systems, but we also find federal, state, and local legislation setting up additional methods of classifying disabled individuals.

SERVICES FOR THE MENTALLY RETARDED
POPULATION WITH PSYCHOLOGICAL IMPAIRMENTS

Since World War II, there has been an increasing movement toward developing community services for the mentally ill and the mentally retarded. A community impetus was strongest in the mental health field first, in spite of the fact that mental retardation programs are a subsystem of mental health programs in many states. Community programs in mental retardation started almost a decade later than those in mental health. There has been much criticism of the assumption that mental health agencies were organized in such a way to offer comprehensive community programs for the mentally retarded population (Burton, 1971). Clinicians and administrators in mental health agencies were generally uninterested in the mental health problems of retarded populations.

The beginning of community mental retardation services occurred during the 1960s (Grossman & Rowitz, 1973). Many public school districts offered classes for the educable and trainable mentally handicapped, the impetus coming from state and federal legislation. Community residents have been resistant to having their taxes increased for special education, and they have been fearful of handicapped people living in their communities. Residents have also worried that a specialized living facility would lower property values and lead to more criminal activity. Thus, changes in approach to treatment and service have come about through external influence in the form of rules and regulations application from agencies outside the community.

Federal interest reached its culmination during the 1970s with the passage of the federal Education for all Handicapped Children Act (P.L. 94-142). MacMillan (1977) points out that certain basic rights were established by this law. First, the mentally retarded individual has the right to due process, which protects him from erroneous classification and labeling as well as from the denial of equal educational opportunities. The law also protects the individual from discriminatory testing in diagnosis and is meant to protect minority children. Third, it guarantees the right of handicapped persons to be placed in an educational setting that is the least restrictive environment. Finally, the Act states that handicapped persons must have individualized program plans, guaranteeing the accountability of educational institutions for their education.

The second aspect of the movement toward community services is specialized outpatient clinics for mentally retarded individuals (Grossman & Rowitz, 1973). Some problems have been noted with the clinic development. Service begins at the time an individual is admitted to the clinic and not at the time that the need for service is first identified. Also, the clinic tends to be based on a medical orientation. This can be an advantage in that many clinics try to incorporate a comprehensive team approach with the goal of improving the physical and psychological well-being of the mentally retarded individual. But it can be a disadvantage, too, as when the clinic is seen as a stopgap measure prior to institutionalization. The clinics' shift away from institutionalization toward community support has occurred during the 1970s. They have, however, remained primarily a medical rather than an educational or nonmedical resource.

With deinstitutionalization and the general orientation toward community care, there are many individuals who are at a special risk of psychological and community adjustment difficulties because of their mental retardation (Hume, 1972). It is hard enough to live in society if one is normal, but the problems of community living are compounded even more if one is mentally handicapped. In a classic study on the adjustment of formerly institutionalized mentally retarded adults in the community, Edgerton (1967) discusses some of their problems. He finds that their adjustment is related to the availability of nonretarded benefactors rather than to any measured skill, attitude, training, or experience. Retarded individuals tend to deny their retardation and to pass as normal. It is clear from the study that psychological services intervention would have been quite beneficial for these people in their adaptation to community living.

Alternative living arrangements for the mentally retarded population have expanded greatly in the 1970s. However, these arrangements tend to duplicate those begun with the community mental health impetus—but then, availability has lagged behind those in the mental health field. Wood (1979) notes that the residential continuum for the mentally retarded ranges from most restrictive to least restrictive. He lists the following categories to show the variety of living situations:

1. nursing homes;
2. public institutions and ICF-MR facilities (interim care facilities);
3. clustered cottages or villages;
4. special purpose facilities located in the community;
5. large group homes (7-15 beds);
6. small group homes (4-6 beds);
7. two- or three-person alternative living arrangements;
8. surrogate family situation;
9. supported natural home and independent living.

As we move to the question of mental health care for the mentally retarded, a number of problems immediately enter the picture. Mental health systems have developed separately from and parallel to mental retardation systems. The service systems for other problem populations have also developed independently of mental health, for example, human service systems, correctional systems, and service systems for the aged. When a person enters one system, he is usually blocked from getting assistance from another. Thus, a mentally retarded individual being treated in the mental retardation sector finds it difficult to get help for psychological problems in the mental health sector. This latter point is discussed succinctly in a recent report of the President's Committee on Mental Retardation (1979).

> Being mentally retarded is bad enough; being mentally ill, too, makes it many times worse. It's not just that such double afflictions are difficult to treat. The sad but undeniable fact is that adequate treatment is extremely hard to come by; psychiatric professionals in the United States often refuse to work with mentally retarded persons; and mental retardation professionals often ignore deeper emotional disturbances which may be present in their clients. The result is that mentally retarded persons who suffer from psychiatric disturbances are frequently caught in the middle—a middle where all the needed services simply don't exist. [p. 63]

Wortis (1977) suggests some other reasons for problems associated with mental health service delivery for the mentally retarded. Since one part of the mental retardation system is in the medical area under the aegis of state mental health departments, and the other part of the service system is under the aegis of educational institutions in communities, much confusion arises over what is appropriate service. Public schools concentrate on educational diagnosis and class placement, and neglect the medical aspects of treatment. Psychological or social problems may or may not be handled in the school by counselors. Clinics and residential institutions may deal with medical problems, but they also undertake major educational responsibilities. Psychological or social problems are not dealt with to any great extent. Wortis also points out that mental health services, if provided in the mental retardation sectors, may be given by specialists other than psychiatrists. Hume (1972) further argues that mental health professionals will have to work through the mental retardation system as well as in concert with the parents in order to provide access to clients. A further argument can be given that the mental retardation service providers may have to develop contractual working agreements with mental health service providers to buy mental health care for the mentally retarded individual with psychological problems.

A number of guidelines have been developed on the principle that all people, regardless of disability, should have the freedom to use all services in society. These guidelines (summarized by Katz [1972]) also apply to the mentally retarded individual who needs services from the mental health sector.

The normalization principle states that every individual, handicapped or not, has the right to live as normal an existence as possible in a community. The mentally retarded person should have the chance to expand his capabilities in such a way as to learn socially appropriate ways of interaction. Mental health services should be available to all citizens of the community, and every retarded individual should have access to the full continuum of mental health services. It is important to provide coordination of services between the public and private sectors, as well as between different service delivery sectors: there should be a fixed point of referral, with some concern given for the continuity of care throughout the lifetime of the mentally retarded individual. All service sectors of the community should be involved in the planning, evaluation, and implementation of mental health services for the mentally retarded and other handicapped groups.

In terms of specific types of mental health services, both direct and indirect services will be needed (Hume, 1972). Direct mental health services include diagnostic evaluations, clinical interventions, psychiatric rehabilitations, and collaboration with non-psychiatric settings. Hume also suggests that similar services may be possible in nonpsychiatric service settings. Indirect services consist of education to community agencies, parents' groups, elected officials, administrators, and boards about mental retardation and the possibility of psychosocial problems among the mentally retarded. Indirect services also include mental health consultation to mental retardation service providers. Obviously, collaboration between service providers in the mental health and mental retardation sectors is necessary. Hume states that such a collaboration would be concerned with the determination of need for mental health services by the mentally retarded, priority-setting in meeting these needs, distribution of tasks through joint planning efforts, provision and methods of interagency and interprofessional collaboration where joint cases are involved, and program evaluation of these services.

Comprehensive community mental health centers (CMHCs) may well be the place for these programs for special problems. A recent NIMH report (1979) indicates that, for the year 1974, almost 4 percent of the additions to reporting CMHCs had been admitted with the primary diagnosis of mental retardation. The specific mental health problems of this population were not enumerated. Once we gain some knowledge about these mentally retarded users of CMHCs, it will be possible to develop special programs for them. Hume (1972) notes that these centers must be flexible and responsive to the mentally retarded and should develop special programs for them. It is possible for the CMHC to undertake direct service programs in the form of psychiatric, neurological, pediatric, and general medical services, as well as nonclinical services such as daycare, sheltered workshops, welfare counseling, guardianship management, and recreational and rehabilitation programs oriented to juveniles and adults. Hume makes the point that it will be necessary for mental health professionals to work closely with mental retardation professionals in these collaborative efforts. The major problem is that mental health providers have been extremely resistant to working with the mentally retarded or with the mental retardation service providers. Thus, mental health professionals will have to be trained to become aware of the special needs of all populations that might come knocking on their door.

THERAPEUTIC INTERVENTIONS

A large national study of over 400 deinstitutionalized mentally retarded people found that 13 percent of the sample reported psychological problems in addition to the problems associated with mental

retardation (Gollay, Freedman, Wyngaarden, & Kurtz, 1978).
Psychological problems were reported most frequently by older,
less retarded individuals. In addition, the authors found that social
and psychological counseling was received by about half the total
group at some time. The services were offered primarily by community agencies. Gollay and her associates argue that the greatest
unmet need comes from the mildly retarded population. The inter-
viewers in the study reported that there was, on the whole, an absence of psychological support services for retarded people with
behavioral problems.

The issue of the appropriate treatment interventions for mentally retarded, emotionally disturbed clients is complicated. Singh
(1972) discusses the two-sided arguments about whether psychotherapy is appropriate. Part of the difficulty is related to lack of
understanding of the personality of the mentally retarded, confusion
over the goals of psychotherapy, and applicability of psychotherapeutic techniques. Although modification may be necessary in techniques and therapist training, psychotherapy can be used with the
mentally retarded. The range of retardation and the extent of neurological handicaps may affect the degree to which psychotherapy can
be adapted for use with the retarded (Singh, 1972). People with less
severe forms of retardation have the most difficult problems of adjustment to community living and become frustrated by their intellectual deficits as they try to live in a way that they see intellectually
normal people live. These individuals seem to benefit most from
psychotherapeutic interventions. Those with severe biomedical
forms of mental retardation are less aware of their problems and
would appear to benefit less from psychotherapeutic interventions.
Behavior modification techniques have been found to be useful with
the more severe forms of retardation.

An incorrect assumption is that the mentally retarded are different in personality structure because of their handicaps. As they
differ in the etiology of their problems and the severity of their
handicaps, they also differ in types of personality. No single personality type is associated with mental retardation, and the range
of personality patterns as well as behavior disorders vary as much
in the mental retardation population as in the normal population
(Singh, 1972). It is possible to find schizophrenia, bed wetting,
sexual perversions, or sociopathic behavior in normal as well as
mentally retarded people. They have the same needs as the normal
populations, and they are both socialized to follow the norms and
values of their community.

On the issue of psychotherapeutic intervention, it is necessary
to look at different needs during different stages of the life cycle.
The mentally retarded need security, companionship, love, achieve-

ment, a sense of control, and independence (Katz, 1972). If their needs are unsatisfied, all sorts of community living failures can ensue and may lead to psychological problems for which treatment intervention will be necessary. The therapist must evaluate his client, regardless of intellectual ability, in terms of presenting problems and possible psychotherapeutic interventions. Leland and Smith (1972) show that psychological treatment techniques for mentally retarded children must be different from those for mentally retarded adults. Play therapy has been found to be useful, although this approach must also take level of disturbance and level of retardation into consideration. It may also be necessary to incorporate family therapy techniques in working with their families. Play activities in small groups may be used in conjunction with individual treatment (Moody, 1972). Group therapy methods can also be used effectively after a child reaches puberty.

For mentally retarded adolescents and adults, psychotherapy can work through problems and conflicts that prevent them from successfully adapting to their environment (Moody, 1972). The normalization treatment philosophy assumes that each individual should be allowed to reach his highest possible potential in the least restrictive environment. This means that psychotherapeutic techniques should probably be used to help individuals cope with the stresses of everyday life. Moody has commented that psychotherapy should be considered when a retarded person is showing emotional or behavioral symptoms that interfere with the ability to utilize intellectual, social, or vocational potential. Therapists should probably avoid focusing on insights and using reflective therapy, and concentrate instead on a very directive and structured approach. The treatment goal is to help the client find satisfactory methods of working out and minimizing conflicts. The therapist may also have to take a problem-solving approach and give specific instructions on behavior.

Group therapy is also helpful and may be used concurrently with other forms of individual or recreational therapy (Moody, 1972). The advantage of group therapy is that the mentally retarded individual has the opportunity to share experiences with others and learn methods of modifying social skills through the group process. Less verbal clients thrive in group therapy situations with more verbal group members (Moody, 1972). In fact, the less verbal client may do better in group therapy than in individual therapy, where verbal ability is much more important.

For the mental health professional working with mentally retarded clients, it is necessary to use collateral services along with psychotherapeutic techniques (Moody, 1972). It is important to use functional or performance assessments in working with the family of the retarded individual, and professionals should identify family and individual strengths and appropriate behaviors without a concern for finding the most appropriate diagnostic explanation for behavior. Professionals need to modify or develop new psychological treatment techniques. Psychodrama and sociodrama may be possible techniques to use with the mentally retarded.

A change in orientation is necessary. The mentally retarded in communities and institutions require psychological services to help them adjust to their environments: psychotherapy can be used for these people. CMHC administrators and boards must be convinced of the importance of reaching all population groups in their catchment area. Innovative treatment techniques should be encouraged, and continuing education for administrators, advisory boards, and professionals should be undertaken to expand treatment programs for their mentally retarded residents.

RECOMMENDATIONS

In summary, it is clear that the mental health service system has not been generally responsive to the needs of the mentally retarded. Community living entails many stresses, and the mental health care system must be responsive to all segments of the population, regardless of handicaps. The following recommendations can open the dialogue necessary to implement specialized mental health programs for the mentally retarded:

1. Specialized mental health service programs must be undertaken for people disabled by mental retardation.

2. Practitioners, administrators, and community mental health advisory boards must learn to distinguish between mental illness and mental retardation. The problems associated with these disorders are quite different. Moreover, each group is comprised of heterogeneous populations. Demographic differences within these populations must be differentiated from the demographic differences of people with other handicaps. When these differences are noted, practitioners and administrators can regard the mentally retarded with psychological problems as people with two major handicaps.

3. Specialized mental health services for the mentally retarded should be developed in the mental health service sector if possible. This means that mental health service providers may need special training to learn about mentally retarded individuals.

4. If the mental health system remains resistant to specialized mental health programs for the mentally retarded, then the mental retardation system must expand its network to include mental health specialists.

5. Specialized mental health information should be incorporated into continuing education programs for those professionals and paraprofessionals who do not normally undertake psychological interventions. For example, special educators and nurses working with the mentally retarded should be familiar with some psychological treatment interventions that are useful for mentally retarded clients.

6. Research and evaluation are needed for new treatment interventions or modification of existing interventions for the mentally retarded with psychological problems.

7. Special continuing education programs should be undertaken for board members and administrators concentrating on the psychological needs of special problem populations. Information on mental retardation is essential if they are to be responsive to the mentally retarded citizens in their community.

REFERENCES

American Psychiatric Association. A psychiatric glossary (5th ed.). Washington, D.C.: American Psychiatric Association, 1980.

Burton, T. A. Mental health clinic services to the retarded. Mental Retardation, 1971, 9(5), 38-41.

Butterfield, E. C. The role of environmental factors in the treatment of institutionalized mental retardates. In A. A. Baumeister (Ed.), Mental retardation: Appraisal, education and rehabilitation. Chicago: Aldine, 1967.

Edgerton, R. B. The cloak of competence. Berkeley: University of California Press, 1967.

Gollay, E., Freedman, R., Wyngaarden, M., & Kurtz, N. R. Coming back. Cambridge, Mass.: ABT Books, 1978.

Grossman, H. J. (Ed.). Manual on terminology and classification in mental retardation. Washington, D.C.: American Association on Mental Deficiency, 1977.

Grossman, H. J., & Rowitz, L. A community approach to services for the retarded. In R. K. Eyman, C. E. Meyers, & G. Tarjan (Eds.). Sociobehavioral studies in mental retardation. Washington, D.C.: American Association on Mental Deficiency Monograph Series, 1973.

Hume, P. B. Direct and indirect mental health services for the mentally retarded. In E. Katz (Ed.), Mental Health Services for the Mentally Retarded. Springfield, Ill.: Charles C. Thomas, 1972.

Katz, E. Introduction. In E. Katz (Ed.), Mental Health Services for the Mentally Retarded. Springfield, Ill.: Charles C. Thomas, 1972.

Kurtz, R. A. Social aspects of mental retardation. Lexington, Mass.: Lexington Books, 1977.

Leland, H., & Smith, D. E. Psychotherapeutic considerations with mentally retarded and developmentally disabled children. In E. Katz (Ed.), Mental Health Services for the Mentally Retarded. Springfield, Ill.: Charles C. Thomas, 1972.

MacMillan, D. L. Mental retardation in school and society. Boston: Little, Brown & Co., 1977.

Milgram, N. A. MR and mental illness: A proposal for conceptual unity. Mental Retardation, 1972, 10(6), 29-31.

Moody, C. Psychotherapy and mental retardation. In E. Katz (Ed.), Mental Health Services for the Mentally Retarded. Springfield, Ill.: Charles C. Thomas, 1972.

National Institute of Mental Health. The characteristics of persons served by the federally funded community mental health centers program, 1974. Washington, D.C.: Superintendent of Documents, 1979.

President's Commission on Mental Health. Washington, D.C.: Superintendent of Documents, 1978.

President's Committee on Mental Retardation. MR 78 Mental retardation: The leading edge. Washington, D.C.: U.S. Department of Health, Education and Welfare, 1979.

Rowitz, L. Social factors in mental retardation. Social Science and Medicine, 1974, 8, 405-412, (a).

Rowitz, L. Sociological perspective in labeling. American Journal of Mental Deficiency, 1974, 79, 265-267, (b).

Rowitz, L. Original identifiers of mental retardation in a clinic population. American Journal of Mental Deficiency, in press (a).

Rowitz, L. Present status of the labeling controversy in mental retardation. Mental Retardation, in press (b).

Rutter, M. L. Psychiatry. In J. Wortis (Ed.). Mental retardation: An annual review III. New York: Grune & Stratton, 1971.

Singh, R. K. J. Psychotherapy with behaviorally disturbed mentally retarded. In E. Katz (Ed.), Mental Health Services for the Mentally Retarded. Springfield, Ill.: Charles C. Thomas, 1972.

Wood, J. Residential services for older developmentally disabled persons. In P. J. Daniels (Ed.), Gerontological aspects of developmental disabilities: A state of the art. Omaha: University of Nebraska, 1979.

Wortis, J. The role of psychiatry in mental retardation services. In P. Mittler (Ed.), Research to Practice in Mental Retardation, Vol. 1. Baltimore: University Park Press, 1977.

26

WOMEN IN THE MENTAL HEALTH DELIVERY SYSTEM
Nancy Felipe Russo
Gary R. VandenBos

The President's Commission on Mental Health (PCMH) has found that "a substantial number of Americans do not have access to mental health care of high quality and at reasonable cost. For many, this is because of where they live; for others, it is because of who they are—their race, age, or sex; for still others, it is because of their particular disability or economic circumstances" (PCMH, 1978, p. vii). The Commission pointed out that traditionally trained practitioners are ill-prepared to deal with the problems of contemporary women; it was concerned "by the failure of mental health practitioners to recognize, understand, and empathize with the feelings of powerlessness, alienation, and frustration" that women express (PCMH, 1978, p. 7). The report of the PCMH's Subpanel on the Mental Health of Women (1978) explored the mental health problems of women in depth, underscoring the need for greater attention to women's issues in mental health training, research, and service delivery.

It is, indeed, a step forward for the designers of mental health services to recognize that women's service needs differ from those of men. Nonetheless, it must be remembered that women as a group are heterogeneous. The problems of minority women, handicapped women, young women, and aged women differ. All women, however, are directly or indirectly affected by sex role stereotyping and sex discrimination. The Subpanel underscored the powerlessness, dependency, and poverty associated with women's roles and the

---

The authors of this chapter would like to thank Yolanda Hooks, Carla Waltz, and Jane Winston for their assistance in the preparation of the manuscript.

devaluation of women's status as particularly destructive to women's mental health.

This chapter considers some changes in women's roles and identifies some of the ways sex bias and sex role stereotyping detract from the provision of services to women. It underscores the need for evaluation of their impact, setting out some training goals as strategies for change. Increasing the participation of women at all levels, as providers as well as policy makers, is viewed as a necessary condition for elimination of sex bias and sex role stereotyping in the mental health delivery system.

THE CHANGING ROLES OF WOMEN

Change in the stereotypes about men's and women's roles and family structure has not kept pace with the tremendous changes in women's family and work responsibilities (Smith, 1979). One dramatic change has been smaller family size and the completion of childbearing by most women in their early thirties. This change is associated with a remarkable decline in the proportion of women having more than three children. In 1965, the fertility rate of such women was 26.8 per thousand women, while in 1976 it was 7.3 per thousand. Consequently, the number of years of women's lives during which children are in school or have left home have increased substantially. The period during which preschool children are present averages about one-third of a typical married life span (Hofferth & Moore, 1979). The "empty nest syndrome" that has been identified for women embracing the traditional female role is but one outcome of this change. Housewives are particularly vulnerable to the effects of losing other roles (Bart & Grossman, 1978).

Childbearing and childrearing patterns are related to the work force participation of women, particularly married women and mothers. In less than a generation, the size of the female work force has more than doubled, with the major part of this change due to the behavior of married women. In 1947, less than one-third of all women could be found in the work force; in 1978, nearly half of all women were in the work force. In 1940, 15 percent of married women worked outside the home; in 1978, almost 50 percent of all married women worked outside the home.

The presence of young children in a household inhibits women's workforce participation, but not as much as one might expect. In 1978, over 40 percent of married women with children under age 6 were in the work force. Over 57 percent of such women with children ages 6-17 worked (Smith, 1979).

The powerlessness and poverty associated with women's status continue to have a detrimental impact on women's mental health

(Subpanel, 1978). The majority of women work because of economic need, but they are concentrated at the bottom of the occupational ladder in "women's jobs." Of the 40 million women in the work force, one-third are clerical workers. One-quarter work in domestic service, food service, education (excluding higher education), and health care (excluding physicians). Predominately female occupations are marked by low pay and limited opportunities for advancement. Within the same occupation, women often earn less than men. The median annual earnings of women who work full time are 60 percent of those of men. The earnings gap is greatest for minority women. Once in the labor force, women are more likely to experience unemployment than men.

In addition to the hours they devote to paid employment, married women also perform on the average an additional 27 hours of housework per week (Hofferth & Moore, 1979). Society's norms regarding sharing of household tasks is one reason for the overload. Although attitudes are changing, many women still hold the view that housework is the women's responsibility. This attitude varies by income level, age, and ethnic and racial background. For example, one study found that among black working-class couples, wives favored sharing tasks more than did husbands, while among Chicano couples husbands favored sharing tasks more than did wives (Hofferth & Moore, 1979).

The design of mental health services must reflect the fact that life circumstances contributing to disorders for men may not be the same as for women. For example, problem drinking is most often reported by unemployed persons of both sexes. However, employed women are not as likely as unemployed women to have drinking problems, while this difference is not the case for men. Further, married working women report higher rates of problem drinking than either single working women or housewives, while no such relationship occurs for men (Sandmaier, 1980). The mental health implications of the problems of working women, compared with those of men, are only beginning to be described and have not yet been addressed.

Sexual harassment is another of the recently publicized problems of working women. It is estimated that seven out of ten women experience sexual harassment on the job (Gordon, 1980). The dynamics of loss of self-esteem, anxiety, anger, and fear are similar to that seen in the rape victim (Hilberman, 1976), and the pattern of "blaming the victim" prevails on the part of society.

Child care continues to be a formidable problem for working women as well as for those unable to care for their children (chronically mentally ill, drug addicts, or alcoholics). Although total family size has been substantially reduced, 90 percent of adult women have or expect to have at least two children. Child care will become an increasingly important issue as the baby boom generation of the

1950s and early 1960s begins its peak childbearing years. In 1977, approximately 6.4 million children had working mothers; it is estimated that there will be approximately 10.5 million such children in 1990 (Moore & Hofferth, 1979).

Although the stereotypes about the effects of working mothers on children have fallen into scientific disrepute, they still persist along with guilt on the part of such mothers. It has been clearly established that a child's attachment to its mother and the child's general development are not impaired by a mother's working (Etaugh, 1974; Farran & Ramey, 1977). In fact, full-time homemakers do not spend most of their time in stimulating or in affectionate play with their children. The amount of such activity varies more with the educational level of the mother than with her employment status. Stereotyping has impeded the individual decision making that is needed for this highly personal issue. Whether or not the effects of day care will be viewed as positive, neutral, or negative depend on the mother, the father, the child, and the quality of alternatives available to them (Etaugh, 1974; Farren & Ramey, 1977; Hoffman, 1974; Portnoy & Simmons, 1978).

Concomitant with these changes in work and family roles of women has been the growth of families headed by women. Although these families constitute one-seventh of families in the United States, they include one-half of all families living in poverty. In the past ten years, the increase in the number of families living in poverty is due to the increase of the number of families with no adult male present. In 1930, the majority of such families were headed by widows. In 1975, the heads of such families were evenly distributed across all marital groups over age 25 (Gordon, 1979).

Minority women are overrepresented as heads of such households, and lack of access to child care has a great impact on them. In 1977, less than half of all black preschool children were living with both biological parents, compared with 87 percent of white preschool children. In 1977, 15 percent of all preschool children were living in female-headed families, but 10 percent of those families were white, as compared to 41 percent black (Moore & Hofferth, 1979).

These changes are occurring in the context of significant increases in life expectancy for women as compared to men. In 1930, white women surviving to age 20 could expect to live to 68.8 years of age. In 1976, such women could expect to live to 78.7 years of age (a 10-year increase). For black women, the comparable increase is even greater: from 57.2 years in 1930 to 71.6 years in 1976 (an 18-year increase). Increases for men have been substantially less: for white men, the figures are 66.0 to 71.6 years (a 6-year increase); for black men, 56.0 and 66.8 years (an 11-year increase). Thus, women live many more years after their children have left home and can expect to be widowed for a longer period of time (Gordon, 1979). The increased life expectancy also means that care for aged parents, which often falls to the woman, is an increasingly important issue.

These statistics highlight some of the changes in work and family roles that must be taken into account in the planning of mental health services. (A more complete picture of such changes can be found in The Subtle Revolution: Women at Work [Smith, 1979].)

Social change can itself be a source of stress, particularly when institutions are slow to recognize such change when it occurs. Society's failure to provide adequate child care services is a major contributor to the role overload of working women. The point of this discussion is not the stress associated with changing sex roles, however. The point is the need for mental health professionals to shed their own stereotypes and to develop an appreciation of the nature of women's changing roles and life circumstances. Knowing the facts is a step toward that goal. Failure to recognize the reality of the immense changes in work and family roles is one example of sex bias on the part of mental health service providers. But even if women's roles were not changing, the rigidity of traditional stereotypes would detract from delivery of services. As we will demonstrate, even women who chose traditional roles are harmed by stereotyping on the part of mental health professionals.

WOMEN'S NEEDS AND THE DESIGN AND DELIVERY OF MENTAL HEALTH SERVICES

Stereotyping has paradoxical effects. Women can be considered both underserved and overserved by mental health delivery systems. For disorders that are incongruent with society's idealized view of femininity and the proper role of women, such as alcoholism and illegal drug abuse, women's service needs have been hidden and ignored. Similarly ignored are problems that are congruent with society's devaluation of women, such as rape, wife-battering, and incest. Issues of access to service in these cases are paramount. For disorders congruent with sex role stereotypes, such as depression, conversion hysteria, and phobias, women show higher rates of service utilization than do men. Issues of appropriateness of services are central in such cases. And, there is concern that women's dependency on mental health services may be a problem in and of itself.

THE NEGLECT OF WOMEN'S NEEDS

Identification and treatment of disorders associated with a special stigma for women require a high level of expertise and sensitivity

that has been lacking on the part of mental health professionals.
Sandmaier (1980) describes how the stigma of alcoholism for women
means that persons around them contribute to their own tendency to
deny that they have a problem with alcohol. Physicians contribute to
the process of denial by avoiding confrontations with their clients.
A physician will listen to the alcohol-related symptoms of a woman
patient and then prescribe tranquilizers rather than refer her to an
alcoholism treatment program. This also adds to the greater incidence of polydrug abuse for women as compared with men (Sandmaier, 1980).

The stigma of being an alcoholic woman means that such women
have more guilt, anxiety, and depression than do alcoholic men.
They also have lower self-esteem and attempt suicide more often
than male alcoholics (Subpanel, 1978). Treatment settings that provide some protection from public exposure are more likely to report
higher proportions of female alcohol clients. In one study of alcoholic admissions to a wide range of treatment facilities, women
were found to comprise one-seventh of the patients at state and
county mental hospitals. In contrast, one-third of alcoholic patients
at private mental hospitals were found to be women (Sandmaier,
1980).

Although estimates of the percentage of females in the alcoholic
population range from 20 percent to 50 percent, less than 3 percent
of the treatment programs funded by the National Institute of Drug
Abuse and Alcoholism in 1976 were designed for women. Of a total
of 600 halfway houses for alcoholism in the country in that year,
only 30 (5 percent) were for women. Discussions of the problems of
alcoholism for women are often targeted toward the problems of the
wives of alcoholics, while the existence of female alcoholism is ignored (Homiller, 1977).

Substantial numbers of women with drinking problems are
found in every age bracket, socioeconomic class, racial and ethnic
group, region of the country, and employment situation. The image
of the alcoholic woman, however, vacillates between a lower-class
promiscuous woman and a middle-class housewife, with the housewife recently receiving more attention in the media. The few programs available in the mental health delivery system reflect the
stereotypes in their restriction of outreach and treatment efforts to
limited groups of women. If a woman happens to be very young,
single, nonwhite, poor, or not pregnant, her needs are likely to be
neglected. She simply does not fit the stereotypes (Sandmaier, 1980).

The problems of female drug addicts reflect a similar pattern
of neglect. Drug treatment facilities have been oriented toward the
needs of male addicts. Such programs continue to be targeted toward
the hard drug abuser (mostly male) and neglect the prescription drug

abuser (mostly female). As a result, the dropout rate of females in such programs is twice that of males, and women addicts seek treatment less often than men (Naierman, 1979).

The needs of institutionalized women have been similarly neglected. Consider the situation of women who have for some reason entered the criminal justice system. Small local jails, which represent 75 percent of the correctional facilities, are designed to house males. Since female prisoners generally represent less than 10 percent of the inmate population, it is considered economically impractical to develop separate treatment and rehabilitative programs for them. At the same time, many of these facilities will not allow coeducational programs. As a result, female prisoners who serve jail sentences in local correctional facilities, particularly in smaller towns and rural areas, frequently have no access to psychological services or to rehabilitation and educational programs.

Compounding the problems of chronically mentally ill women is the tendency to consider them genderless persons. According to this view, "the problems related to the illness are so massive that there just isn't time or energy to think much about them as women or men" (Test & Berlin, in press). Yet chronically mentally ill women are more likely to be sexually active than men. In one study, 59 percent of women versus 38 percent of men reported sexual intercourse in the previous months (Test & Berlin, in press). Although a substantial number of chronically mentally ill women have children, little is known about them as mothers.

The relative inaccessibility of birth control information and contraception, combined with the vulnerability of these women to rape and exploitative sexual relationships, suggests that the frequency of unwanted pregnancies among chronically mentally ill women may be substantial. Due to restrictions on Medicaid funding, legal abortion has been less likely to be an option for them than for women in general. Self-induced abortions are not uncommon among chronically mentally ill women, and many also experience the stress of unwanted childbearing, childrearing, and the trauma of adoption (Test & Berlin, in press).

ANCILLARY SERVICES: PREREQUISITES TO TREATMENT

The provision of ancillary services becomes particularly important for women, as their poverty and lack of control over resources in the family limit their ability to provide such services for themselves. Child care is a crucial ancillary service for women with responsibility for children. The traditional view of the role of mother means women who have problems that impair their ability to provide such services for themselves. Child care is a crucial ancillary service for women with responsibility for children. The traditional view of the role of mother means women who have problems that impair their ability to care for their children also must bear the guilt such impairment produces. When the problem has a stigma for women, as in the case of alcohol or illegal drug abuse, the woman usually blames herself. A major issue in therapy becomes how to forgive oneself for being a "bad mother." Since the treatment programs for such problems are oriented toward men and it is assumed that such men are not responsible for their children, child care is not offered. The lack of access to child care means that a woman becomes trapped in a system that gives her the responsibility for the care of children when she is unable to provide such care, and compounds her problem by reinforcing her view of herself as a "bad mother" for leaving them to seek help.

The projected demand for child care in the 1980s heightens the urgency of mental health planners to incorporate it into the design of mental health delivery systems. The difference that child care can make in women's service utilization rates underscores this need. In one residential drug treatment project, the ratio of men to women clients was 3 to 2. After offering residential services for both mothers and children, there was an increase of 33 percent in utilization by women clients. In another case, a satellite clinic in a multiservice outpatient alcohol project began providing babysitting. Utilization by women increased from 30 percent to over 50 percent (Naierman, 1979).

Transportation is another ancillary service of particular significance for women. Older women are less likely than older men to know how to drive, and women have less access to cars than do men (Erickson, 1977). Transportation services are particularly important in rural areas and other localities where public transportation is not a feasible option. Poor women may be denied access to care if they are unable to obtain low-cost transportation. The needs of the nonworking married women who may only have access to a family car in the evening may also be neglected if public transportation is not available.

Another ancillary service needed for women is housing. It cannot be assumed that women will have someone at home who will care for them, as is often assumed to be the case for men. Marital disruption may be more of a problem for women who need treatment. For example, men are more likely to leave their alcoholic spouses than are women, perhaps because women are socialized to care for those who depend on them (Sandmaier, 1980). Separation and divorce rates for chronically mentally ill women show a similar pattern (Cheadle, Freeman, & Korer, 1978; Segal & Aviram, 1978;

Test & Berlin, in press). In one study of the chronically mentally ill, 68 percent of the females had been married, as compared to 41 percent of the males. At the time of admission to the study, however, only 29 percent of the females were "currently married," as compared to 23 percent of the males (Test & Berlin, in press).

In summary, sex bias and sex role stereotyping have exacerbated the design problems of mental health policy makers in complex ways. It cannot be assumed that the etiology of a particular disorder is the same for both sexes. Stigmas associated with certain disorders compound the problems of women, and the poverty and lack of control over other resources mean that ancillary services may be a prerequisite to treatment.

BARRIERS TO SERVICE

The lack of coordination and cooperation among health, mental health, and social service delivery systems create major barriers to women who need mental health care. Incorporating alternative services such as feminist counseling collectives, birthing centers, health clinics, rape crisis centers, and shelters for battered women in coordination efforts is essential.

A recent evaluation (Naierman, 1979) of health and human development programs points to several gaps between services needed and services offered in various types of delivery systems. For drug and alcohol projects, five basic services especially important for female substance abusers were identified: (1) treatment for prescription drug abuse; (2) counseling for incest victims; (3) counseling for battered women; (4) medical and nutritional care for pregnant women; and (5) women's support groups.

For mental health centers, services identified as particularly important for women include grief therapy, treatment for postpartum depression, sex-fair counseling with respect to changes in sex roles in the family and society, treatment for victims of spouse abuse, and comprehensive services for rape victims. The comprehensiveness of services to rape victims was considered essential, and included counseling of victims, training of emergency room personnel, and interfacing with the police and the court. Here inappropriateness of services also became an issue, and the need for special training for counselors of rape victims was noted.

Interconnection with nursing homes and protective living environments is crucial for chronically mentally ill women. The longer life span for women, combined with a disproportionate incidence of severe mental illness in later years, means that special consideration must be given to the needs of elderly women.

The hospital is the major focus of care for the elderly mentally ill. For that population, psychiatric hospitalization terminates in death almost as often as in discharge. When discharge does happen, it is most often to nursing homes (Minkoff, 1978).

APPROPRIATENESS OF SERVICES

One outcome of sex role stereotyping that cuts across the problems of women is overmedication. In 1974, 78 million new and refill prescriptions for Valium and Librium were written (Subpanel, 1978). Two-thirds went to females. Approximately 60 percent of these prescriptions were written by general practitioners or internists, not mental health specialists. Statistics on emergency room use and mortality rates related to these tranquilizers are disproportionately weighted toward women. One survey showed that for every 10,000 Valium prescriptions made to women, there were 30 emergency room episodes, while men maintained a rate of 21 episodes per 10,000 prescriptions (Naierman, 1979). Approximately 60 percent of drug-related visits to emergency rooms are by women, about two-thirds of whom have attempted suicide (Fidell, 1978).

Among the reasons offered to explain the relatively high incidence of psychotropic drug use among women is that "legal" drug use is more socially sanctioned and less deviant for women than alcohol abuse or drug addiction. Doctors may be subtly encouraged by drug companies to prescribe such drugs to their female patients. In addition, sex-role stereotypes may influence the physician's evaluation of patients and selection of treatment. In one study, 87 percent of male physicians judged daily use of Librium as legitimate for housewives, but only 50 percent approved such use of Librium for students (Linn, 1971).

We have seen how physicians may avoid confronting alcoholic women by offering them a prescription for tranquilizers (Sandmaier, 1980). Similarly, depressed menopausal women may receive hormonal therapy or psychotropic medication rather than counseling to deal with their role loss (Bart & Grossman, 1978). One study of women in prison reported that at least 50 percent of the inmates in jails for women in California were receiving tranquilizers (Sobel, 1980).

THE TRAINING OF MENTAL HEALTH SERVICE PROVIDERS

Sex bias has been part of the personal and professional socialization of mental health service providers. The processes are subtle, and many remain unaware of their role in the perpetuation of sex-role stereotyping as they train others, conduct research, influence mental health policies, and engage in clinical practice. We have seen how such biases can lead to the denial and neglect of women's needs and the tendency to respond inappropriately to women's problems with medication. Since biases stem from personal values and beliefs regarding the attributes and roles of women and men (Gilbert, 1979), training must be designed to deal with such values and beliefs (cf. Rawlings & Carter, 1977).

The need for staff education is partially due to the myths that they were taught in their early professional training (cf. Subpanel, 1978). For example, Marian Sandmaier (1980) has eloquently described the impact of two leading psychological theories on the cause of alcoholism that were based on early research that included only male subjects. One held that alcoholics drank to satisfy hidden dependency needs that they were forbidden to express in adult society. The other held that alcoholics who were unwilling or unable to dominate others turned to alcohol to quell the "unmanly feelings that they found unacceptable in themselves" (Sandmaier, 1980, pp. 86-87). The application of these results to women who exhibit dependent behavior as part of the female role and whose feminine identity does not depend on exercising power over others is spurious.

Clinical theories of personality have taught therapists that woman's innate nature is passive, dependent, masochistic, and childlike. All too often psychological treatment is focused on reducing complaints about the quality of life and promoting adjustments to a traditional sex role. Anger in women is viewed as a sign of pathology rather than as a consequence of the devaluation of status. The problem of sexual abuse of patients suggests that therapists also need to be educated about revisions in professional codes of ethics that now prohibit sexual contact between therapist and client (Subpanel, 1978).

These are but a few ways that sex biases in earlier research, theory, and professional training have contributed to sex bias in service delivery. They demonstrate the need to integrate the new information (Sherman & Denmark, 1978; Unger, 1979) on sex roles and the psychology of women throughout the training and education of mental health personnel. The use of nonsexist language can also serve as a consciousness-raising device, as well as a means to stimulate nonsexist thinking. Therapists have been found to be particularly uncomfortable in dealing with erotic attraction in therapy settings and female clients' unwillingness to fulfill the traditional role of mother (cf. Gilbert, 1979; Russo, 1979). Training experiences should include special attention to these two issues.

One model for introducing clinical personnel to sociocultural information and integrating it into supervision is presented by Baum and Felzer (1964). They held several brief in-service seminars on the life styles, needs, and expectations of lower-class patients and made sure that supervisors continued to discuss them in supervision of specific cases. With such a training program, they found lower-class patients remained longer and received better care. This model can obviously be used for any underserved population, such as women.

EVALUATION OF SERVICES TO WOMEN

If mental health services are to be responsive to women, data must first document their service needs. The Subpanel recommended that all programs be evaluated for (1) criteria for determining their target population; (2) the reality of the assumptions that are made about women's lives; (3) the degree to which program objectives are related to women's needs; and (4) the degree to which the special needs of women are met in the delivery of the services (Subpanel, 1978).

Program evaluation must be considered in the context of the values and goals of the evaluators. At each stage of data gathering, storage, and retrieval, the values and biases of the evaluators affect what is or is not considered relevant. An evaluation of a facility's services to women requires a commitment to identifying women's needs and an understanding of how sex bias and sex role stereotyping can subtly pervade every step of evaluation.

A major problem has been the omission of questions relating to women. Simple comparisons between the sexes in terms of utilization rates have been lacking. Access to services can be assessed by determining the type and quantity of services available for women, and the number of types of visits by sex. Specifying kinds of services offered exclusively to one sex is a relatively straightforward question that, unfortunately, still must be asked. Sex differences in types of services (outpatient and inpatient), modes of service (individual, group, or other therapy), and the nature of indirect and support services (outreach, child care, transportation) will suggest possible barriers to accessibility.

Structural barriers to access can be indirect (no public transportation, no child care services, limited hours of available services) or direct (no program in existence, inappropriate admission criteria, long waiting time before first appointment). The practice of giving preference to males in the scheduling of evening appointments is just one example of how sex-biased assumptions about work roles can create barriers to intervention. Admission procedures are also affected by sex bias. The role of insurance coverage should be examined, since men often have more comprehensive coverage than women. As a result, admission criteria tied to insurance coverage can have a differential impact on accessibility. Facilities that set fees on a sliding scale often use sex-biased criteria. A man might be allowed to deduct child support payments from income before his fee is set, but a divorced working woman with children may not be allowed to deduct child care fees. Woman may be more uninformed than men about their rights with regard to insurance coverage: for example, a woman may not realize that the insurance policy issued in her husband's name may not require his signature on the payment forms.

An important aspect of services utilization is client flow, that is, the analysis of client movement through the service system. The ability to distinguish between new and repeat visits is particularly important since there are sex differences in rates and duration for many disorders. Such an analysis may also serve to insure that sex-role stereotyping does not prolong the dependency of women clients on therapy and medication.

Often such data are coded and stored in a way that makes them useless for secondary analyses related to women's issues. Broad categories are often broken down by sex but not by subcategories such as by marital status or income level. We know that rates of mental disorder vary by race and sex. Disorders with the highest incidence for white women are not the same as those disorders with the highest incidence for black women, and the same holds for men. For example, black females tend to be diagnosed as schizophrenic more frequently than any other race/sex category. Data must be collected and stored so that they can be analyzed at the same time by sex and race in terms of length of treatment, mode of treatment, inpatient versus outpatient status, marital status, work status, medication, and duration of treatment. All of these variables have been demonstrated to vary with both sex and race (Subpanel, 1978).

STATUS AND FUNCTION OF WOMEN IN THE MENTAL HEALTH SYSTEM: WOMEN AS PROVIDERS

Women are well represented in the mental health delivery system. Based on a sample of 321 federally funded community mental health centers (CMHCs) in 1976, women represented 82.7 percent of the clerical and maintenance staff, 61.6 percent of the paraprofessional staff, and 53.2 percent of the professional staff (Bass, 1978). The percentages of women increase as the broad category of occupations decrease in training, prestige, and income. The same trend is evident when the specific professions within the "professional staff" category are examined. Women represented 11.9 percent of the psychiatrists, 17.3 percent of the nonpsychiatric physicians, 28.3 percent of the psychologists, 56.2 percent of the social workers, and 94.1 percent of the nurses (Bass, 1978). In one study of federally funded projects comprised of alcohol projects, drug projects, CMHCs, comprehensive health centers, family planning clinics, and vocational rehabilitation, 80 percent of the projects were directed by men (Naierman, 1979).

Whenever one perspective dominates a system, its operation will tend to be biased irrespective of the good intentions of its members (Kiesler, Cummings, & VandenBos, 1979). Many of the assumptions that pervade our mental health system have reflected the natural tendency of the white male physician to make judgments about the lives of others based on his own life experiences. All levels of a delivery system should be represented by varying perspectives and life experiences. Thus, there should be individuals with different professional degrees, a balance of males and females, and representation of varying cultural perspectives.

WOMEN AS ADVISORY/GOVERNING BOARD MEMBERS

Women providers and consumers are underrepresented on the advisory and governing boards of mental health agencies, even in those cases where there is a legislative mandate to ameliorate the underrepresentation. In a state-wide sample of mental health governing boards, Silverman (1979) found that 70 percent of board presidents were male. The overrepresentation of males may also reflect a bias toward male dominated occupations: 55 percent held executive or managerial positions.

Hausner (1979) reports that women as consumers are underrepresented on Health Systems Agency (HSA) Boards, comprising only 33.1 percent of the members and 28.7 percent of those on executive committees. Among provider board members, women on the average constitute 18 percent of the membership of both HSA Boards and executive committees. Thus, the percentages for provider members are even lower than those reported for consumer members. For the entire governing board, which is composed of both providers and consumers, women constitute 26 percent, reflecting a nationwide problem with regard to the representation of women at the policy level.

Similarly, in the study of federally funded projects previously cited, 90 percent of the boards of directors had more male than female members, at an average ratio of 5 to 2. Three of the boards were totally male and 90 percent of the boards were chaired by males (Naierman, 1979).

Increasing women's access to the informal network of communication among professional men is one step toward a solution to the problem of underrepresentation of women on advisory and governing boards. The Committees on Women of the professional associations and the coalitions of professional women's groups, such as the Federation of Organizations for Professional Women, play an important role in identifying and training women in strategies needed to enter male networks. The increasing political participation of women in society at large may also facilitate such representation. However, the status of women in the mental health delivery system is tied to the status of women in the larger society. Efforts to pass the Equal Rights Amendment and eliminate sex bias in employment, education, and the media may hold the key to the solution of the problem (Hilberman & Russo, 1973).

CONCLUSION

In summary, sex bias and sex-role stereotyping continue to detract from the quality of mental health services to both sexes, but particularly to women because of their disadvantaged status. Understanding how such processes can at the same time create barriers to service access and facilitate inappropriate service delivery is essential to insuring quality mental health services to all clients. If the design and utilization of mental health services are to be comprehensive and truly responsive to community needs, evaluation efforts must consider the extent to which the needs of women are met. Ameliorating the problems of women as providers and consumers in the mental health delivery system will require a sophisticated understanding of the nature of those problems and a firm commitment to seek creative solutions to them.

The elimination of sex bias and sex-role stereotyping can be seen as a crucial preventative strategy for the mental health problems of women. One must recognize the ethical obligation to go further, however. Prevention also means attention to societal institutions and norms that reinforce the powerlessness and devaluation of women's roles and are so destructive to their mental health. Any strategy for promoting mental health and preventing mental illness must have as one of its basic goals eradication of sexism in the larger society. As a step toward this goal, the Subpanel on the Mental Health of Women endorsed the National Plan of Action developed at the Houston Women's Conference (Subpanel, 1978). Two of the recommendations of that conference—passage of the Equal Rights Amendment and establishment of programs to insure reproductive freedom—were identified as priorities for prevention efforts. The ethical mandate to address sexism in the larger society extends to all persons who play decision-making roles in the mental health delivery system.

REFERENCES

Bart, P., & Grossman, M. Menopause. In M. T. Notman & C. C. Nadelson (Eds.), The woman patient: Sexual and reproductive aspects of women's health care. Vol. 1. New York: Plenum Press, 1978.

Bass, R. D. CMHC staffing: Who minds the store? National Institute of Mental Health, Series B, No. 16. DHEW Publication No. (ADM) 78-686, Washington, D. C.: Superintendent of Documents, U.S. Government Printing Office, 1978.

Baum, O. E., & Felzer, S. B. Activity in initial interviews with lower class patients. Archives of General Psychiatry, 1964, 10, 345-353

Cheadle, A. J., Freeman, H. L., & Korer, J. Chronic schizophrenic patients in the community. British Journal of Psychiatry, 1978, 132, 221-227.

Ericksen, J. A. An analysis of the journey to work for women. Social Problems, 1977, 24 (4), 428-435.

Etaugh, C. Effect of maternal employment on children: A review of recent research. Merrill-Palmer Quarterly, 1974, 20, 71-98.

Farran, D. C., & Ramey, C. T. Infant day care and attachment behaviors toward mothers and teachers. Child Development, 1977, 48, 1112-1116.

Fidell, L. S. Sex differences in psychotropic drug use. Working paper prepared for the Subpanel on the Mental Health of Women of the President's Commission on Mental Health, April, 1978.

Gilbert, L. A. An approach to training sex-fair mental health workers. Professional Psychology, June 1979, 10, 365-372.

Gordon, N. M. Institutional responses: The federal income tax system. In R. E. Smith (Ed.), The subtle revolution: Women at work. Washington, D. C.: The Urban Institute, 1979.

Gordon, S. Y. Occupational hazards include sexual harassment. Jobs Watch, 1980, 1(2), 12-13.

Hausner, A. Minorities and women on boards of health agencies. In Alvarez, R., Lutterman, K. G., and Associates (Eds.), Discrimination in organizations. San Francisco: Jossey-Bass Publishers, 1979.

Hilberman, E. The rape victim. Washington, D. C.: American Psychiatric Association, 1976.

Hilberman, E., & Russo, N. F. Mental health and equal rights: The ethical challenge for psychiatry. Psychiatric Opinion, August 1973, 15(8), 11-19.

Hofferth, S. L., & Moore, K. A. Women's employment and marriage. In R. E. Smith (Ed.), The subtle revolution: Women at work. Washington, D. C.: The Urban Institute, 1979.

Hoffman, L. W. Effects of maternal employment on the child: A review of the research. Developmental Psychology, 1974, 10, 204-208.

Homiller, J. D. Women and alcohol: A guide for state and local decision-makers. Washington, D. C.: Alcohol and Drug Problems Association of North America, 1977.

Kiesler, C. A., Cummings, N. A., & VandenBos, G. R. Psychology and national health insurance. Washington, D. C.: American Psychological Association, 1979.

Linn, L. Physician characteristics and attitudes toward legitimate use of psychotherapeutic drugs. Journal of Health and Social Behavior, 1971, 12, 132-140.

Minkoff, K. A map of chronic mental patients. In J. A. Talbott (Ed.), The chronic mental patient. Washington, D. C.: American Psychiatric Association, 1978.

Moore, K. A., & Hofferth, S. L. Women and their children. In R. E. Smith (Ed.), The subtle revolution: Women at work. Washington, D. C.: The Urban Institute, 1979.

Naierman, N. Sex discrimination in health and human development services (A final report to the Office of Civil Rights, Division of Planning, Budget and Research). Cambridge, Mass.: ABT Associates, Inc., Contract no. HEW-100-78-0137, 1979.

Portnoy, F. C., & Simmons, C. H. Day care and attachment. Child Development, 1978, 49, 239-242.

President's Commission on Mental Health. Report to the President: Volume I. Washington, D.C.: U.S. Government Printing Office, 1978.

Rawlings, E. E., & Carter, D. K. (Eds.). Psychotherapy for women: Treatment toward equality. Springfield, Ill.: Charles C. Thomas, 1977.

Russo, N. F. The motherhood mandate. Psychology of Women Quarterly (Special issue), Fall 1979.

Sandmaier, M. The invisible alcoholics: Women in alcoholic abuse in America. New York: McGraw-Hill Book Company, 1980.

Segal, S. P., & Aviram, U. The mentally ill in community-based sheltered care. New York: John Wiley, 1978.

Sherman, J. A., & Denmark, F. L. (Eds.). The psychology of women: Future directions in research. New York: Psychological Dimensions, Inc., 1978.

Silverman, W. H. A statewide assessment of mental health governing board training needs. Paper presented at the Rocky Mountain Psychological Association Meeting, Las Vegas, April, 1979.

Smith, R. E. The movement of women into the labor force. In R. E. Smith (Ed.), The subtle revolution: Women at work. Washington, D.C.: The Urban Institute, 1979.

Sobel, S. B. Women in prison: Sexism behind bars. Professional Psychology, 1980, 11(2), 331-338.

Subpanel on the Mental Health of Women. Report to the President, President's Commission on Mental Health: Volume III. Washington, D.C.: U.S. Government Printing Office, 1978, 1022-1116.

Test, M. A., & Berlin, S. B. Issues of special concern to chronically mentally ill women. Professional Psychology, in press.

Unger, R. K. Female and male: Psychological perspectives. New York: Harper and Row, 1979.

V

PLANNING
AND
ACCOUNTABILITY

Systematic planning and accountability are relatively new responsibilities in the field of mental health. Before the advent of the community mental health model, private practitioners and clinics simply chose clients on a first-come first-served basis. When the caseload was filled (according to professional judgment), waiting lists were drawn up. Other than professional pride, incentives to perform duties more effectively or efficiently were rarely in place.

Prior to the 1960s, financial resources earmarked for mental health were relatively limited and fixed in the public sector. Clients and third-party payers seldom, if ever, questioned the quality of services delivered or how funds were spent. Thus, there was no need to plan activities, only to schedule them. When more dollars entered the health and mental health fields through such government programs as Medicaid, Medicare, and Community Mental Health Centers, politicians began to pressure for accountability. At first, professional groups lobbied to keep these activities at a minimum. However, as government expenditures increased dramatically during the 1970s, accrediting and regulating bodies began to carry out their functions seriously.

Currently, many of us criticize regulatory agencies because they complicate our efforts at documentation. Notwithstanding the validity of these claims, systematic planning and accountability have been a boon to taxpayers and recipients. Cost-effective mental health care is both a right and a responsibility.

In my chapter, I emphasize that accountability can only be achieved by acting as knowledgeable agents of mental health boards in the community. Accountability entails two separate functions, representation and monitoring. Recruitment is the first step in valid representation. The board must then continually engage all segments of the community in as many settings as possible. Monitoring means assuring quality and cost-effective distribution of resources. To accomplish these goals, boards must develop a basic philosophy, acquire the power and willingness to impose sanctions, and commit themselves to learning new skills. Crucial resources for achieving accountability are appropriate staff, information on service area populations, their utilization rates and service outcomes, and a model for decision making.

Levy offers some basic principles to follow for planning. Most people in need of mental health care require brief intensive contact. Few need hospitalization. Those using 24-hour residential care should be treated on a voluntary basis for as short a duration as is feasible. CMHCs should cultivate community support systems and closely monitor and carefully evaluate their activities; they can offer a broad array of services structured into a consortium. Promotion of mental health and prevention of mental disorders are as important responsibilities of CMHCs as are treatment and rehabilitation. Levy outlines a system of comprehensive services so that the reader can grasp the elements that should be recognized during planning.

Surely the highly technical and complex skills associated with program evaluation are the most difficult to understand for professionals and boards. Krause explains that evaluation performs four basic functions: (1) it helps to avoid destructive crises of service; (2) it provides the facts for resource allocation; (3) it fosters cost-effectiveness; and (4) it provides information for public relations purposes. Evaluation systems can be set up to detect problems, compare programs, generate cost-effectiveness trends over time, and respond to accrediting and funding bodies. Evaluation systems compile data from many sources: service statistics, management reviews, and follow-up samples. Krause warns that the basis for selecting models and procedures for evaluation is dependent upon subjective rather than empirical judgment. What sort of questions need to be answered? How much staff time and money is the board willing to allocate? What are the particular concerns of the agency at a given time? Because organizations and communities are in constant flux, an evaluation system may be redesigned at a future date.

As governmental and accrediting bodies demand greater fiscal and program accountability, we must never neglect our basic responsibility to respect the rights and integrity of the individual. Soskin delves into the basic issues concerning the legal rights of clients and cites landmark cases. Citizens have won the right to treatment in the least restrictive setting, the right to refuse treatment and to choose alternatives (such as, drugs or psychotherapy), and the right to privacy and confidentiality. Nondiscrimination on account of socioeconomic background and type or degree of disability are issues currently being raised at both federal and state levels. Soskin concludes that an awareness of clients' legal rights by board and staff can augment available services, make them more accessible, and reduce stigmatization and abuse of clients.

While the concept of accountability is almost uniformly accepted, most boards and staff are frustrated at the varied and occasionally conflicting requirements placed upon them. Cagle reminds us that centers may have as many as 20 external organizations to which they are responsible. Since most of the larger external organizations augment agency reports with an on-site visit, it is vital that centers are thoroughly familiar with the on-site process and are adequately prepared for it. The center should understand the regulations and procedures of the organization conducting the visit and have available for inspection documents that will be requested during the survey. Cagle lists several of the most commonly used documents. He recommends that key staff and board members be on call to offer information and accompany the survey team.

27

ACCOUNTABILITY
Wade H. Silverman

A myriad of rules and regulations—public and professional, local, state, and federal—are designed to control the functioning of community mental health centers (CMHCs). They are continually amended and reintroduced. Most are unknown to the service recipients. While many safeguards have been instituted with the best of intentions, few are enforced with the same degree of care and concern with which they were created. For it is not the designers, funders, or service deliverers, but the recipients, who are most affected by the types and quality of available mental health services.

Accountability must ultimately emanate from a knowledgeable and active citizenry: mental health center boards and clients. This chapter is an attempt to provide a framework within which advisory/governing boards can perform activities that will realize accountability. It focuses on board roles and responsibilities in representing the community and in monitoring agency performance. The basic resources and information that boards must possess in order to make careful, intelligent judgments are described. The last section discusses a rational process for decision making in which board members construct an ideal model for their agency, factor in realistic constraints, and then judge the effectiveness of the service delivery system. Resource allocation emerges from the results of monitoring.

RESPONSIBILITIES OF BOARDS TO COMMUNITIES: ACCOUNTABILITY BEGINS AT HOME

During the turbulent 1960s and into the early 1970s, it was common to see community people and center staff confront each other over center control. Many directors lost their positions, and a large number of staff retreated to private practice offices and halls of ivy. The most strident community residents accused professionals of mental health colonialism, and the most reactionary professionals accused these public voices of paranoia and power grabbing. As we enter the 1980s, the period of confrontation has ended and both groups now realize that each is essential to the success of the community mental health movement. Citizens are vital as advocates for CMHCs; public service, in turn, deserves the best available professional expertise.

It is the community and not the professionals, however, that must assume responsibility for overseeing its public institutions. For expertise can be expressed in many forms, some of which are irrelevant or inconsequential to the majority of residents. Other types of services may be too expensive or too experimental. Who makes these judgments and on what basis? In community mental health it must be the advisory/governing board that acts as the agent of the community. No external official or institution can ever speak for or protect the welfare of a given community as well as can its own residents. Because of this, a board must be first and foremost accountable to itself. As community agent, the board possesses two basic responsibilities: community representation and agency monitoring.

REPRESENTATION

The board is the representative of the community in establishing program priorities. As such, it is essential that the board's demographic characteristics mirror those of the catchment area. Unfortunately, mental health boards have not been inclined to recruit members on this basis, raising valid arguments about the legitimacy of their status (Silverman, 1979). Too often the case has been that boards represent the interests of the executive director, staff, or local influentials rather than those of the catchment area. There is the mistaken notion that a board is supposed to function as an auxiliary to the center through volunteer and fund raising activities. These tasks are valuable but not germane to the responsibility of community representation. It is also important that the interests of minorities (defined as those populations with smaller frequencies residing in the catchment area) are also represented. Indeed, this classification of being different from one's neighbors in and of itself defines an at-risk group (Wechsler & Pugh, 1967).

Recruitment is but the first step in establishing valid representation. The board must then ensure that its ear is continually turned toward the voices of community need. How is this achieved? First, the membership identifies all the key institutions and grass-roots groups in its catchment area. The groups are invited to meetings to share information and resources and, in turn, board representatives visit them. Second, public meetings are arranged, information programs with question-and-answer formats are held, and entertainment programs such as fairs and art shows are offered. These events place residents in contact with board members, not only to sound out the community but also to make residents aware of available services and to recruit membership. Third, membership procedures must be designed to bring in as many residents as possible on the board. Terms of both officers and the general membership should be limited, and active recruitment should be the cornerstone of board activity.

MONITORING

The monitoring process involves two separate issues: quality assurance and selection of program priorities. Quality assurance can be accomplished with evaluation techniques and can generally be applied across centers. These will be addressed in greater detail later in this chapter and in the chapter on evaluation.

Program prioritization is a much more individualized and complicated process. Not only must it take into account program costs relative to benefits (a technology only recently introduced to CMHCs), but the process also involves value judgments about the relative needs of community residents. Questions such as "whom do we serve first?" and "on whom should we spend the most money?" will be answered differently by each community. No external guidelines for this process exist because vital interests differ dramatically as a function of demographic characteristics, economics, politics, and even geography. A sparsely populated but large catchment area in Montana has vastly different needs than a densely populated, multiethnic neighborhood in an urban setting like Chicago.

Community Development versus Direct Services

Although there are no guidelines for establishing priorities, it is possible to identify two ideologies, community development versus direct services, to which a board may adhere in making its decisions. Though the terms are arbitrary, they do identify two different approaches to serving the community. The direct service ideology assumes that the purpose of a CMHC is to offer the same sort of services in kind and quality available to the private sector. Direct service providers are sensitive to the criticism that CMHCs are guilty of giving second-class service, particularly to the poor. Consequently, their basic goals are the availability and accessibility of quality care. In comparison, the community development ideology emphasizes prevention and quality of life issues. Community developers assume that, at best, traditional forms of service delivery do not address or ameliorate causative factors, and, at worst, are irrelevant to the concerns of the vast majority of recipients. They address recipients as visitors and clients rather than as patients, and view their symptoms as natural reactions to iatrogenic environments rather than as mental disorders. Their basic goal is to improve the quality of life of all residents by altering institutions that affect them and increasing available choices.

Using Sanctions

Effective monitoring requires the capacity and willingness to impose sanctions. But what right does the board have to act? In the case of governing boards, this power is formal. The fact that advisory boards often use their informal status as an explanation for inaction is inexcusable. Since it is the prime responsibility of the citizen representative to protect the rights of all residents, an advisory board can and should be as effective as a governing board. There is no difference between an advisory board that does not seize the power to ensure accountability and a governing board that does not exercise its formal power to do so.

Whom does the board hold accountable for center operations? The executive director is responsible for program implementation; the ultimate sanction is the power to hire and fire. While the board must be willing to use this authority for it to be taken seriously, it is an action of last resort.

All too frequently, boards invade the domain of the executive director, rendering him or her impotent. For example, boards tend to involve themselves in personnel management. If the executive director cannot replace the staff, then the directorship becomes a sinecure. Boards too often are caught in the middle of a fight between two departments or a director and a staff member. The board responds to complaints rather than referring them to the director. If the director is accountable for program implementation, then he or she must have the latitude to perform as an administrator with full control over allotted resources. While directors at times tend to blame wayward staff or inadequate resources for their own failures, these reasons are just excuses for improper management.

Acquiring New Skills

A final and essential aspect of monitoring is the acquisition of knowledge and skills. Board members must participate in training experiences to be effective. All boards need orientation programs for new members and continuing education experiences for veterans to keep current with the latest knowledge in the field (Silverman & Mossman, 1978; Silverman, in press). The membership committee might also consider recruiting residents with particular skills such as accounting or law to aid the board in the monitoring process.

RESOURCES FOR EFFECTING ACCOUNTABILITY

If the setting of priorities is to be based on rational decision making rather than on fads, prejudice, or selfish motivation, then the board needs factual information. A system for collecting this information must be devised before it can be used by the board. At some CMHCs, sophisticated computer programs called Management Information Systems are employed (see Elpers & Chapman, 1977). For other CMHCs, data must be collated arduously by hand. Regardless of the collection method, three different structures are needed for proper implementation: a bookkeeping team, a research and evaluation (R & E) team, and a liaison person linking center and board.

The Bookkeeping Team

State and federal regulations, accrediting bodies, and third-party payers require that records be kept of the center's fiscal and operational activities. This necessitates the employment of a book-keeping team to log the daily activities of the center. This team usually assembles the raw data necessary for the R & E team to conduct their activities. The number of employees required depends on the number of staff hours it takes to provide systematic auditing of the CMHCs activities. More help is needed if the following questions are answered negatively: Do all accrediting boards and governmental agencies receive the information they require on time; does the board receive regular and complete information on CMHC functioning; and, are specific answers given to specific questions, such as how much did the outpatient department spend on overhead costs last quarter? Effective monitoring demands a wide variety of information. (Three basic types of information critical to a board's functioning will be discussed in detail in a later section.)

The Research and Evaluation Team

Until recently, not much emphasis had been placed by NIMH or by CMHCs in general on research and evaluation. With the imposition of "two percent money" for R & E by the 1975 amendments, the importance of this activity has finally been officially recognized. It is impossible to find and rectify deficiencies in the service delivery system without R & E and, needless to say, all CMHCs have deficiencies. A CMHC may experience a high dropout rate, or a particular intervention program may be unsuccessful. A vulnerable population may be underserved, or the inpatient service used too much. Given such problems, an R & E team not only points out mistakes but tests potential solutions. The team also acquires and disseminates new knowledge. New interventions can be tested for their potential benefits, and various relationships between types of problems and their causes can be examined.

The R & E department requires a professional who has expertise in research design and the ability to communicate effectively to colleagues and laypersons. Not only must the R & E head devote full time to R & E, have access to a computer, and employ support staff to collect the required data, but he or she must be able to communicate vital information to the executive director without going through channels. The R & E head must also be responsible solely to the executive director to avoid the potential interference of program directors who may be threatened by negative feedback.

The Liaison Person

While the R & E head is the primary information source for the executive director, a liaison person is needed to perform the same function for the board. How this liaison works is dependent upon the board's preference. At most centers, the executive director is the liaison. However, there are two fundamental drawbacks to this arrangement. The director is probably too busy with administrative duties to honor the varied and numerous requests made by the board to be adequately informed. It is also difficult for any administrator to be objective about his or her programs to a monitoring body.

Another common liaison relationship involves program chiefs reporting to the board. Unfortunately, this method is subject to the same problems as those of the first arrangement. It also sets the stage for competition for board attention, often degenerating into "dog and pony shows." Each of the program chiefs would be hard-pressed to develop a systems perspective based upon a balanced view of his or her own programs in relation to others.

The most workable liaison relationship is to assign a staff member to this responsibility in order to avoid a potential conflict of interest. A specially designated liaison person would have no administrative duties at the center. His or her primary function would be to serve the board as an information provider—to be in contact with all programs and obtain the necessary information. The liaison person could be a therapist in the outpatient department or a specialist in consultation and education who works an allotted amount of time per week for the board.

INFORMATION A BOARD REQUIRES TO EFFECT ACCOUNTABILITY

In this section, we will consider the information a board requires to make rational decisions about program priorities and judgments about service quality and productivity. It cannot be emphasized enough that this information is the bare minimum. Without these data, staff cannot determine the types of problems in their community or the effectiveness with which they solve them. Without such data, the board will be unable to lend any validity to its ranking of priorities.

Demographic Data

The first set of required information, demographic data on the catchment area, answers the question "who lives in the community?" These data describe socioeconomic status, age, and sex of residents. Not only can demographic data be used to indicate potential for mental health problems (Redick & Goldsmith, 1971), but they can also be employed in setting program priorities (Beech, Fiester, & Silverman, 1976).

Since demographic statistics are usually obtained from the census taken once every ten years, it is necessary to update them, particularly for rapidly changing communities or in years beyond the midpoint of the ten-year cycle. Updating is accomplished with field data in which direct observations of the community and its institutions are made. For instance, visits to schools provide an excellent estimate of the latest populations to move into the service area. A perusal of the major shopping thoroughfare will determine to whom the stores are advertising and gearing their merchandise. Since movement into an area begins along the geographic borders, observation of perimeter streets help to determine the rapidity of population change.

Utilization Data

While demographic data offer an unbiased estimate of the
population we expect to come to the center, we need to know who is
actually showing up at the door. Information about actual recipients
is called service utilization data. These data answer the following
questions: what are the demographic characteristics of those who
come to the center? when do they come? for what reasons do they
seek assistance? where are they placed in the service-delivery
system? how long do they stay? and to whom are they referred?
Too often, the types of problems encountered are fit into available
treatment procedures, rather than vice versa. This utilization can
be remedied by employing data to decide what, when, and where
services are to be offered. In an ideal world with an infinite supply of money and staff, we would tailor interventions to individuals;
but in the real world of limited resources, we must decide on
strategic placement of intervention programs to maximize successful outcome in the most cost-efficient manner.

Since utilization data are typically unavailable to boards, let
us review some specific examples of how they can assist board
decision making. A classic case showing the benefits of answering
"who is coming?" was done by Hollingshead and Redlich (1958),
who found that service systems were biased against lower socioeconomic clients. In general, answering the "who is coming" question informs us about the availability and accessibility of services
to subpopulations, such as minorities, the elderly, or the poor.
This is because the demographic characteristics of the service area
residents should be essentially the same as those of the client population, except for the overrepresentation of vulnerable groups.
Discrepancies between expected and actual use should be carefully
studied to insure that there are no barriers such as prejudice toward
a particular group. Traditionally, minorities, the elderly, children,
and the chronically mentally disabled have been victims of bias.

Program hours also have a direct bearing upon deployment of
staff. Outpatient departments have often been accused of a "9 to 5"
mentality. Although program hours are frequently established at
the convenience of the staff, few professionals support this kind of
functioning. On the other hand, it is unreasonable and economically
impossible to expect "Las Vegas" coverage. Evening and weekend
work is more costly, particularly in unsafe areas requiring protection. Utilization data can indicate when clients and referral agents
are taking unfair advantage of CMHC resources. In one study,
Fiester, Silverman, and Beech (1975) report a dramatically increasing use of off-hour CMHC services over a two-and-a-half year
period because the host hospitals increasingly called upon CMHC

staff for hospital crisis cases. As a result, utilization rates at the CMHC were actually higher for nonresidents than for residents! Mendell and Rapport (1969) note that clients enter service systems at off-hours because of fewer barriers for acceptance at these times. CMHC programs should not be required to see all clients any time they want to be seen; a compromise can be struck between available resources and realistic client needs.

Another reason for having utilization data handy is to determine whether a client's program is being addressed by the center. In theory, the reason for which the client seeks service determines whether intervention is appropriate and what type is needed. Specifically, a direct relationship has been found between clients' presenting problems and CMHC response on four variables: mode of intervention, total number of contacts, disposition of cases, and institution to which referred (Silverman & Beech, 1980). At many centers, service gaps exist. There may be plentiful substance abuse complaints with no service program; persons with psychotic symptomatology may be turned away at the door; and particular modes of intervention, such as group therapy, may be underutilized.

Where clients are placed in the service delivery system is often a function of economic or political issues rather than the welfare of the client. The most frequent improper placement is inpatient referral. Hospital bed usage is big business. In our upside-down world of health economics, reimbursements are greater and easier to obtain for hospital than for ambulatory care. There is a great temptation, therefore, to keep as many beds filled as possible, even if it requires an inappropriate admission. Another common cause of inappropriate placement is a program's refusal to admit clients because its criteria are too specialized or it feels overworked: clients are then "dumped" somewhere else. Silverman and Val (1975) describe this problem vis-à-vis day hospital use. Also closely identified with the issue of inappropriate placement is the concept of continuity of care, defined as the relatedness between past and present care in conformity with client need. A continuity of care index has been developed that takes into account length of involvement and movement in the system (Bass & Windle, 1972).

Length of stay continues to be a highly controversial issue in community mental health. If the client is kept in the system for too great a time, dependency is fostered and valuable manpower resources are wasted. This usually occurs with inpatient or day care services. If the client terminates prematurely (unilaterally), it is often assumed that intervention is a failure; thus the dropout rate continues to be an embarrassing statistic at many CMHCs. In a study of 20 CMHCs involving over 13,000 clients, Sue, McKinney, and Allen (1976) determined that 40 percent of the clients terminated after only one session. However, Silverman and Beech (1979) later found that unilateral termination is not necessarily an indication of poor intervention. Of the clients interviewed who dropped out after one session, 70 percent expressed satisfaction with the service they received and 79 percent reported that the problem for which they came to the mental health center had been solved. Despite these findings, inordinately high dropout rates, particularly in specific intervention modalities such as group and family therapy, are indicative of either inappropriate placement, inadequate therapeutic skills, or therapist and programmatic bias.

Still another benefit of utilization data is illumination of referral patterns. Where clients go in conjunction with or upon termination of CMHC participation indicates the comprehensiveness of the service delivery system in meeting clients' needs. Community mental health has been frequently criticized for overstepping its bounds by working on social problems (see Serban, 1977). Critics maintain that mental health professionals do not have the right or the expertise to be involved in changing society. While it is true that a CMHC cannot be "all things to all people," it is unrealistic to assume that mental health service can exist independently of the cooperation and assistance of other human service agencies. As pointed out by the Joint Commission on Accreditation of Hospitals (1979a):

> The mission of a mental health system is also influenced by differing interests and criteria of other sectors of the human service system and by varying expectations of the system's three constituent groups: patients/clients, providers, and social institutions. [p.5]

The realities of intervention, particularly in poor or minority neighborhoods, dictate bringing together many resources for multiproblem clients. The richness of the referral network can be inferred by the data on the types of agencies in the network and the extent to which they are used.

Outcome Data

Many readers who have patiently read the chapter up to this point are beginning to wonder if the author will ever get to the question, "How do we know if we are meeting the needs of our clients?" The bottom line in service delivery is not availability, accessibility, or even cost—it is outcome. How do you find out if clients have benefited from your services? The first method is to ask them!

This logical step is infrequently taken and often criticized. One board member told me that you cannot ask clients because they are crazy. While there may be some truth to criticisms of reliability and validity, consumer satisfaction measures are vital to the implementation of successful intervention.

Irrespective of the expertise of the staff and the amount and variety of available resources, if clients do not like the center they will not come and they will tell their friends and neighbors to avoid it too. Dissatisfaction is as dependent upon local values and preferences as on professional expertise. To illustrate, a CMHC outpost located in a poverty area in Chicago could not attract clients. In order to feel that they were part of the community, the staff furnished their offices in "early slum." Residents reacted by avoiding an agency with no class. When new office furniture was installed, business picked up dramatically. There are many different client satisfaction questionnaires available. McPhee, Zusman, and Joss (1975) provide an overview of their use.

Ways of measuring outcome include personality assessment scales, adjustment scales, goal attainment scales, symptom checklists, and systematic follow-up interviews. Resource Materials for Community Mental Health Program Evaluation (Hargreaves, McIntyre, Attkisson, & Siegel, 1977) not only discusses all of these measures, but also contains an appendix on particular inventories. Fiester and Fort (1978) present a case study of the implementation of the goal attainment scale at a CMHC, a technique for rating the effectiveness of specifically designated outcomes.

BOARD DECISION MAKING

To be entrusted with the power to choose what is best for a given community in terms of mental health service is not an easy burden to carry. Board members must be familiar with community residents, center functioning, and administrative staff. The first step in decision making is for the board to define a raison d'etre, the purpose of the CMHC.

Agreeing on an Ideal Agency toward Which
the Board Can Work

Each CMHC must develop its own philosophy of purpose. Such a philosophy will involve the basic tenets of the community mental health movement filtered through the value and belief systems of local residents. What are the basic tenets of the movement? Bloom

(1973) has listed nine characteristics, which I shall paraphrase:
(1) work in the community rather than in institutional settings; (2) work with the total community (catchment area) rather than on individual clients; (3) emphasize prevention and early intervention; (4) emphasize indirect rather than direct services; (5) use innovative intervention strategies to serve the largest number of people in the shortest possible time; (6) use rational planning based upon objective evidence; (7) make innovative use of manpower; (8) encourage community control, and (9) place emphasis upon stress producers rather than psychopathology. At some centers, the philosophy will be more in line with a community development approach, while in others it will be oriented toward direct service. Regardless of its emphasis, the philosophy should be written so that it can serve as the basis for operating principles—for example, (1) all clients will be served regardless of financial circumstances, (2) services will be accessible to all residents in the community, and (3) we are particularly committed to services for the elderly.

Operating principles are used to design an ideal CMHC model, one that will best serve residents. The model produces goals that the staff attempts to accomplish. Goals are concrete statements that can be measured: We will serve X number of clients in our outpatient department; we will contact X percent of schools in our catchment area this year; or, we will spend X dollars for each direct service hour. One certainly does not expect to accomplish all the goals generated from an ideal model. However, the extent to which they are achieved is the basis on which decisions about priorities and resources are made.

The Problem of Constraints

Before making judgments about a CMHC's actual functioning compared to its ideal model, one must weigh realistic constraints under which the CMHC must operate. Agranoff (1975) refers to constraints as "the other face of opportunities." He lists numerous sources of constraints, including federal, state, regional, and local government and organizational idiosyncrasies. We are probably most familiar with the federal Community Mental Health Centers Amendments of 1975, which list 12 services each center should furnish. Other federal requirements derive from Medicare and Vocational Rehabilitation, which identify certain populations and services for federal reimbursement. National accreditation and certification bodies set high standards of performance necessitating much time and cost to attain, and they can even demand alterations in delivered services. For instance, the survey instrument of the

Joint Commission on Accreditation of Hospitals (1979b) used to ac-
credit community mental health service programs contains standards
that cut across direct services, support functions, and facilities.

State constraints include regulations defined in mental health
codes and licensure agencies, and requirements for matching money.
Regional constraints are primarily concerned with joint planning and
implementation. (Agranoff and Mahler, in Chapter 19, describe
these thoroughly.) Finally, there are local constraints. The nature
of the problems indigenous to a particular catchment area will determine how flexible a center can be in its operations. A poverty
area will probably require more direct services and linkages with
social agencies than a more economically affluent area. In particular, prevention programs will be much more difficult to initiate and
maintain in a poverty area.

In a sense, constraints are our "excuses" for not functioning
as our ideal CMHC model. We now must examine our information
data to ascertain whether constraints are sufficient explanations for
our failures. We can expect to find, of course, that constraints
cannot justify all of our failures. In those cases where they are
valid explanations, our ideal model will then be modified to conform
with reality.

Prioritizing Programs and Allocating Resources

Our ideal CMHC model defines our ultimate objectives, but the
data obtained from our bookkeeping and R & E teams describe our
current effort. Discrepancies between ultimate goals and current
outputs determine our priorities. First to be examined are issues
of availability, accessibility, and appropriateness. They should be
solved before quality of care issues. If the most sophisticated intervention is given at an inopportune time or to inappropriate targets,
the intervention serves no purpose. "Whom shall we serve?" is the
highest priority question, followed by "how shall we serve them?"
and "when shall we serve them?"

A preeminent concern in light of the present fiscal environment
is "how much shall we spend?" Since Rydman discusses this in
Chapter 11 (above), we need not discuss it here. However, I do want
to emphasize that economic considerations should be entertained
only after first considering who shall be served. To do otherwise
is to violate our own principles and the basic tenets of community
mental health. Also we should never put the center's need for dollars
ahead of the residents' need for services. There are circumstances
under which it is best not to accept grants and matching funds. (Both
Elpers and Levin address this point. See Chapters 8 and 16, above.)

Setting program priorities has usually been a joint function of granting institutions and agency administrators. If public mental health is to suceeed, this task must be taken over by those who are to be served. Governmental waste and bureaucratic insensitivity are the products of an uninterested and uninformed public. Grass-roots participation in those decisions affecting the allocation of public resources is the only mechanism for solving these problems.

SUMMARY AND CONCLUSIONS

Citizen participation is the cornerstone of community mental health. It requires an active and representative citizenry in advocacy, planning, and public education. However, it is at the local level that participation has the greatest effect upon community mental health service delivery. CMHC advisory/governing boards have the ultimate responsibility and authority to affect types and quality of available public mental health services.

As agents of the mental health needs of their residents and protectors of the resources of the community, boards must perform two main functions. First, members must represent the needs of their community by soliciting information from all its segments and recruiting membership to reflect demographic characteristics. The second main function is to monitor the functioning of the center to establish program priorities and to assess quality of service delivery. The executive director is held responsible for center operations and must be given the freedom to execute his or her administrative functions. In turn, board members need orientation programs for new members and continuing education for veterans in order to perform their monitoring duties.

There are at least three separate administrative structures involved in assembling information to effect accountability. A bookkeeping team collects the information, a research and evaluation team analyzes and disseminates it to the executive director and appropriate staff, and a liaison person retrieves it for board use.

The basic information a board requires to make rational decisions about program priorities and judgments about service quality and productivity includes demographic data, utilization data, and outcome data. Demographic data inform us about who resides in the catchment area, thereby giving us an estimate of the types of problems with which we might expect to work. Utilization data indicate who is actually being served at the center. These data aid us in a variety of ways. They point out biases in serving subpopulations, suggest strategies for deployment of staff, indicate appropriateness of offered services, and measure continuity of care and

richness of the referral network. Outcome data are used to determine if clients have benefited from center interventions. There
are many different measures of outcome including satisfaction ratings, adjustment scales, personality assessment scales, goal
attainment scales, symptom checklists, and follow-up interviews.

The decision-making process for quality control and program
prioritization begins with a basic statement of the purpose of the
CMHC. It is based upon the values and belief systems of the local
residents and the values of the community mental health movement
as applied to the mental health needs of the catchment area. The
statement of purpose can then be translated into a set of operating
principles, which are used to design an ideal CMHC model. This
model generates goals that can be measured. Discrepancies between ultimate goals and current outputs determine our program
priorities and quality control objectives. Realistic constraints,
such as economic and political considerations, may cause us to
amend our model. It may be tempting to alter a basic operating
principle of a CMHC, particularly under economic pressure. However, grass-roots representation is useful only to the extent that it
serves the needs of the public and not the center or its board.

REFERENCES

Agranoff, R. Political constraints on the mental health budgetary
process. Journal of Mental Health Administration, 1975, 4(7),
38-57.

Bass, R. D., & Windle, C. Continuity of care: An approach to
measurement. American Journal of Psychiatry, 1972, 129,
196-201.

Beech, R. P., Fiester, A. R., & Silverman, W. H. The utilization
of demographic data for mental health planning. Administration
in Mental Health, 1976, 3, 166-173.

Bloom, B. L. Community mental health: A historical and critical
analysis. Morristown, N.J.: General Learning Press, 1973.

Elpers, J. R., & Chapman, R. L. Statistical subsystems I: Man-
agement information for mental health services. In W. A.
Hargreaves and C. C. Attkisson (Eds.), Resource Materials for
Community Mental Health Program Evaluation. Department of
Health, Education and Welfare Publication # (ADM) 77-328.
Washington, D.C.: U.S. Government Printing Office, 1977,
112-122.

Fiester, A. R., & Fort, D. J. A method of evaluating the impact of services at a comprehensive community mental health center. American Journal of Community Psychology, 1978, 6, 291-302.

Fiester, A. R., Silverman, W. H., & Beech, R. P. Problems involved in delivering emergency services in a hospital-based community mental health center. Journal of Community Psychology, 1975, 3, 188-192.

Hargreaves, W. A., McIntyre, M. H., Attkisson, C. C., & Siegel, L. M. Outcome measurement instruments for use in community mental health program evaluation. In W. A. Hargreaves & C. C. Attkisson (Eds.), Resource Materials for Community Mental Health Program Evaluation. Department of Health, Education and Welfare Publication # (ADM) 77-328. Washington, D.C.: U.S. Government Printing Office, 1977, 243-250.

Hollingshead, A. B., & Redlich, F. C. Social class and mental illness. New York: Wiley, 1958.

Joint Commission on Accreditation of Hospitals. Principles for accreditation of community mental health service programs. Chicago, Ill.: Joint Commission on Accreditation of Hospitals, 1979(a).

Joint Commission on Accreditation of Hospitals. Program review document: Community mental health service programs. Chicago, Ill.: Joint Commission on Accreditation of Hospitals, 1979(b).

Mendell, W. M., & Rapport, S. Determinants of the decision for psychiatric hospitalization. Archives of General Psychiatry, 1969, 20, 321-328.

McPhee, C.B., Zusman, J., & Joss, R. H. Measurement of patient satisfaction: A survey of practices in community mental health centers. Comprehensive Psychiatry, 1975, 16(4), 399-404.

Redick, R. W., & Goldsmith, H. F. 1970 census data used to indicate areas with different potentials for mental health and related problems. Chevy Chase, Md.: NIMH Report, PHS #2171, 1971.

Serban, George (Ed.). New trends of psychiatry in the community. Cambridge, Mass.: Ballinger, 1977.

Silverman, W. H. Some aspects of advisory board functioning in a large urban area. Journal of Social Service Research, 1979, 2, 323-334.

Silverman, W. H. Self-designed training for mental health advisory/ governing boards. American Journal of Community Psychology, in press.

Silverman, W. H., & Beech, R. P. Are drop-outs, drop-outs? Journal of Community Psychology, 1979, 7, 236-242.

Silverman, W. H., & Beech, R. P. Primary presenting problem and mental health service delivery. Journal of Community Psychology, 1980, 8, 125-131.

Silverman, W. H., & Mossman, B. Knowledge assessment of mental health advisory boards. American Journal of Community Psychology, 1978, 6, 91-96.

Silverman, W. H., & Val, E. Day hospital in the context of a community mental health program. Community Mental Health Journal, 1975, 11, 82-90.

Sue, S., McKinney, H., & Allen, D. B. Predictors of the duration of therapy for clients in the community mental health center system. Community Mental Health Journal, 1976, 12, 365-375.

Wechsler, H., & Pugh, T. F. Fit of individual and community characteristics and rates of psychiatric hospitalization. American Journal of Sociology, 1967, 73, 331-338.

28

SOME BASIC PRINCIPLES IN PLANNING
FOR SERVICE DELIVERY
Leo Levy

INTRODUCTION

As the reader will immediately understand from the title of
this essay, the scope of the subject is more fit for a book-length
manuscript than for the few pages allotted here. Thus I would like
at the outset to explain that what follows is a highly abbreviated exposition of a few theoretical principles that I believe should guide
the mental health planner setting out at this time to develop a set of
comprehensive mental health services. I will not venture beyond
what is currently accepted as falling within the boundaries of mental health services, though the reader should certainly be aware that
I am describing a portion of a spectrum of necessary human services
that extends to education, vocational, health, legal, welfare, and
family services with which mental health services necessarily interact and interconnect.

I should point out as well that while the attempt here is to be
systematic and comprehensive, there is no attempt to be encyclo-
pedic, nor is this a methodological treatise. Often a consensus of
opinion is referred to without the documentation, referencing, and
bibliographic citation that a more scientific paper would offer.
While this is a deficit from a scientific point of view, it makes for
a more readable document for a general audience.

PLANNING FOR SERVICE DELIVERY—PRINCIPLES

1. <u>Twenty-four-hour residential care is unnecessary and undesirable
   for the great bulk of persons experiencing a mental disorder.
   Hospital beds should be allocated sparingly.</u>

A large, venerable, formidable, and conclusive literature indicates that hospital treatment of the mentally disordered person carries with it considerable dangers for the client. Basically, the argument boils down to the recognition that severing the client's ties with the community, pronouncing him sick and disabled, and depriving him of his personal liberty (often against his will) are overwhelming liabilities associated with 24-hour residential care. Beyond this there is good evidence that care of emotionally disordered clients is in most instances better accomplished without the coercion and confinement implicit in hospital care. Emotionally disordered persons are, after all, for the most part not physically ill or totally incompetent to care for themselves, and the placement of such individuals in a bed in a hospital becomes a highly questionable practice. True, there exist a small number of persons whose symptoms are so severe and grotesque that protection of themselves or the community in which they reside becomes an issue of some relevance. In these cases, brief hospitalization may be a useful phase of the treatment process. One should note, however, that even in these cases, chemotherapy has advanced to a sufficient degree that, although in no sense "cured," the mentally disordered person may still, with the aid of psychoactive drugs, avoid the onerous and potentially stigmatizing experience of being placed in a hospital.

2. Where 24-hour residential care is indicated, it should be voluntary and of brief duration. Custodial care is no longer a valid mental health enterprise.

Civil commitment is a procedure to be avoided, and truly voluntary consent should be obtained when hospitalization appears unavoidable. Such hospitalization should be accomplished in a local community hospital rather than a distant, massive state mental hospital. Duration of hospitalization should be measured in days and weeks rather than months and years. Severely and permanently disabled persons may ultimately (all else failing) be cared for in a nursing facility, but mental hospitals should be regarded and consciously utilized as brief, intensive treatment facilities and in the end the concept of the lunatic asylum (state mental hospital) should be stricken from our professional response repertoire, along with civil commitment and forced involuntary administration of treatment.

3. Treatment in the mental health arena should be conceived of flexibly, ranging from brief outpatient contact through extended outpatient contact, partial hospitalization (day and night treatment centers) and, finally, inpatient care.

Options for treatment of emotionally disordered clients should be many and broadly conceptualized. Flexible and eclectic modes

of treatment are to be preferred. The primary tools of treatment
are group and individual psychotherapy, psychopharmacology, and
rehabilitative techniques such as milieu therapy, occupational therapy, and industrial therapy (sheltered workshop). These treatments
are accomplished in a variety of settings, ranging from simple offices and meeting rooms to highly equipped workshop settings, mental
hospitals, and residential hotels. In planning a comprehensive set
of mental health services, one should make provision for accommo-
dating persons ranging in severity of problems and intensity of intervention from the person seen for a few times in an office to persons who will be active in various sectors of the program continuously for many years. A consortium approach to mental health services
is here being advocated, where the various elements may disperse
throughout a considerable geographic area. This dispersion is tol-
erable, provided two conditions are met. The first is that all elements are in good communication with each other, will freely exchange information, and will share responsibility for intervention
with clients. This linkage insures that mental health services are
physically and psychologically accessible, and it conveys to clients
the (correct) impression that the services comprise—conceptually,
if not legally—a system of care, any element of which is open to
them. Finally, this consortium of mental health services should
interface with a broad system of human services not traditionally
identified as falling under the rubric of mental health, for example,
health, educational, vocational, and welfare services.

4. Mental health services should be conceptualized as going considerably beyond formal treatment for those officially classified as
   mentally ill. The promotion of mental health and prevention of
   mental disorders are legitimate and important concerns of any
   mental health enterprise.
   The network of mental health activities should encompass indirect services to the client population (community), such as consultation, mental health education, community organization, and genetic
counseling. Mental health professionals should be available to consult with a variety of community institutions, such as schools, police,
courts, family service agencies, welfare departments, departments
of public health, clergy, departments of housing and urban affairs,
and so on. This consultation should be conceived of as introducing
mental health expertise into the working of these organizations to
enable them to function better in their traditionally defined roles,
and possibly also to expand their range of functions to include certain kinds of service to emotionally disordered persons. Mental
health education should range from activities of a general educational
nature (for example, presentations on mental health topics to groups
such as PTAs) to highly focused programs of anticipatory guidance

for groups at high risk of mental disorders (for example, adolescent "rap" sessions on topics of strong concern, such as appropriate sexual behavior). Classes for parents of young children focusing on child development and educational programs on alcohol and drug abuse would fall in this category. Concern with the structure and functioning of the community should be expressed by the support of community organizations, self-help groups, and the active solicitation of advice concerning direction of mental health activities through the formation of a citizen mental health advisory board. With the accumulation of knowledge concerning the genetic components of various forms of mental disorder and mental retardation, genetic counseling services should begin to play an increasingly prominent role in the mental health system.

5. The vast bulk of people in need of services are those undergoing periods of severe stress (crises). They require brief intensive contact with a mental health worker and possible involvement with self-help groups.

By far the most common type of appeal for relief from emotional distress issues from persons undergoing a period of acute stress resulting from some immediately identifiable crisis in the person's life. Intake and reception services should be so constructed that such persons have immediate and ready access to the mental health system. They frequently profit from contact with one or another predicament-oriented self-help group in the community (for example, Widow-to-Widow program, or Parents-without-Partners). These self-help groups should be well known to mental health professionals and generously used by persons facing various life crises. From the mental health worker's point of view, intervention with such clients will appear much like brief intensive psychotherapy. Intervention should be intensive, highly supportive, and sharply goal-focused. Such intervention will seldom run beyond two months but may require many visits, involvement of significant others in the client's life, and flexibility on the part of the worker, who may be accessed at odd times for sessions of varying length in person and by telephone. These clients should not be regarded as "mentally ill" but rather as normal persons facing difficult circumstances, and the crisis should be viewed as an opportunity for personal growth and enhancement of mental health.

6. The second largest group of persons in need of services comprises those with continuing adjustment problems, most of whom can be helped by long-term (though not intensive) outpatient care.

There is a large number of persons with chronic problems, who require mental health services over substantial periods of time. These are frequently ex-mental hospital patients who carry the diagnosis of chronic schizophrenia, though other types of persons also fall in this group. Many of these persons need continuing medication that must be constantly monitored for effectiveness and adverse side effects. Frequently, this group will be quite passive with regard to treatment, and the stance of the mental health worker must become correspondingly active. These persons simply cannot be closed out as unmotivated and forgotten. Outreach programs, home visitation, and linkage with various support systems in the community are important aspects of successful intervention programs with such persons. Where medication is being used, at least monthly visits should be planned to renew the prescription, check for effectiveness and undesirable side effects of the medication, and to counsel the client regarding his day-to-day problems in living. Frequently, home visits by public health nurses are very helpful to the chronic schizophrenic client. Other categories of persons who may be helped by this long-term nonintensive approach are certain kinds of depressed persons and those with so-called character problems.

7. Many persons with mental health problems profit little from professional psychiatric care and need instead the development of community support systems to keep them functional.

   Mental health professionals have frequently overvalued and oversold their services. Most people with adjustment problems do not consult a mental health professional. They frequently take their problem to friends, their clergyman, or family doctor. In addition, over the past two decades, there has been a truly phenomenal growth of self-help groups, which are becoming an increasingly important resource for persons with adjustment problems of many varieties. The common problems of dislocation and isolation are quite readily addressed by these groups, which offer emotional support, good role models, and social learning experiences—functions that simply cannot be matched by traditional mental health services. From the mental health worker's point of view, these groups are to be encouraged to develop and grow. Liberal use of these programs should be made by clients who may or may not be using professional mental health services concurrently. One should not overlook, in this connection, the centrality of certain basic human needs such as work, membership in a familial (or surrogate) group, adequate housing, and stable income, all of which must be concerns (however indirect) of the mental health service consortium. It becomes rather academic to talk of mental health when these basic needs are unmet.

8. The mental health service system should be conceived of in an aggregative, confederative sense. The consortium approach to provision of services should be considered the ideal.

It should be clear that the mental health service delivery system must extend over many different types of programs to fit the needs of a vastly heterogeneous group of clients. All of the required services need not be offered by a single organization, but integration of effort must be accomplished. Contractual arrangements among the various organizations that contribute programs of service to the consortium are desirable. The accompanying diagram lays out an illustrative consortium using the public health concepts of primary, secondary, and tertiary prevention. (Primary prevention refers to the effort to decrease the rate of new cases in the community or, alternatively, to promote positive mental health. Secondary prevention refers to the effort to decrease the rate of existing cases in the community. Tertiary prevention refers to the effort to minimize disability in chronic mental disorder.) The consortium of services should be comprehensive, interconnected, and highly accessible through a 24-hour a day, 7-day a week Intake and Reception Service. Treatment decisions should be made flexibly, and multiprogram use should be made possible by the presence of the large number of modalities of service represented.

9. Mental health personnel are many and varied. Arbitrary divisions along professional and paraprofessional lines should be avoided.

It follows from the above that many and varied personnel are required to mount such a program of services. They range from "street-wise" community residents with little formal mental health training to extensively schooled professionals such as psychiatrists, psychologists, social workers, and psychiatric nurses. It appears clear that titles and certificates do not infallibly determine functions in the system. Psychiatrists obviously will be making the medication and other organic treatment decisions. Aside from this function, however, the boundaries among the various professional and paraprofessional groups represented are not clear and are not determined by title. As in any organization, people should do what they like to do and what they do well. Defined leadership and structural hierarchical relationships are necessary, but not a caste system based on title or kind of previous training or university degree possessed. Often, decisions about contacts with clients will be determined by extra-professional considerations such as language and ethnicity and, sometimes, sex and social class. Mental health workers need to feel comfortable with their clients and their clients must feel comfortable with them in order for effective intervention to take place. From the point of view of hiring and retaining personnel, one must attend to salary and career development potential. Realistically, one must recognize that large salary differentials will obtain among various categories of personnel (often performing similar

FIGURE 28.1

A System of Comprehensive Community-Based Mental Health Services
Delineating Programs of Primary, Secondary, and Tertiary Prevention

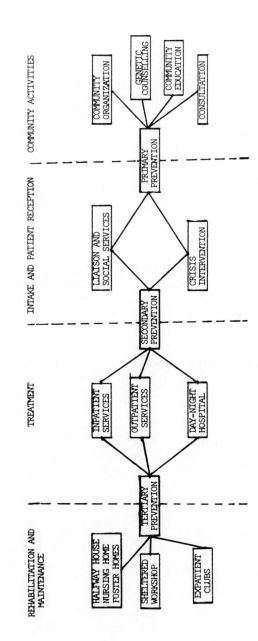

functions); still, one should at least be attentive to the status problems of the lower-paid personnel and see to it that salary floors are high enough to make the job attractive and that advancement upward in the organization is possible for all personnel.

10. <u>Continuous monitoring and evaluation of activities is essential to this enterprise. All programs and services should be considered experimental and potentially dispensible or improvable.</u>

All programs of service in the mental health arena are to one degree or another unvalidated and thus experimental. This permits, indeed demands, a highly flexible innovative stance with regard to provision of services. Programs that have promise and that threaten no damaging consequences or risk to clients should be instituted on a time-limited, experimental basis. But with this opportunity to try out new approaches comes the forthright obligation critically to evaluate service modalities, and an institutionalized decision process must be continuously in effect either to drop, modify, or continue programs. Nothing in this area is to be held as self-evident; all programs must be continuously examined. This process is aided by provision in the budget for research personnel who are free of client treatment responsibilities and thus charged with this task as their sole function. Continuous monitoring of programs of service entails a detailed system of record keeping, monitoring of both service and community demographic data, and specific research studies of selected programs that may entail considerably more and different types of data.

It is fitting to close on this cautionary note. The field of mental health practice has undergone revolutionary changes in the past 25 years. We have seen the emptying of the state mental hospitals, the emergence of effective chemotherapy for psychosis, the emergence of comprehensive community mental health centers, a monumental increase in sensitivity to the civil rights of severely emotionally disturbed persons, the proliferation of a variety of community-based human services for persons with mental disability, and the generally emerging concern with social and environmental determinants of emotional disorder. The entire field is in a state of growth, and new knowledge is accumulating at a rapid rate. This places a heavy responsibility on the purveyors of service in the mental health area who must critically absorb and judiciously apply this new knowledge while at the same time adding to it through rigorous examination of the outcomes of all offered services.

SUGGESTED READINGS

Bloom, B. L. Community mental health: A general introduction. Monterey, Cal.: Brooks/Cole, 1977.

Caplan, G. Principles of preventive psychiatry. New York: Basic Books, 1964.

Dannenmaier, W. D. Mental health: An overview. Chicago: Nelson-Hall, 1978.

Denner, B., & Price, R. H. (Eds.). Community mental health. Social action and reaction. New York: Holt, Rinehart and Winston, 1973.

Goffman, E. Asylums. Garden City, N.Y.: Anchor Books, 1961.

Mechanic, D. Mental health and social policy. Englewood Cliffs, N.J.: Prentice-Hall, 1969.

29

FUNCTIONS, MODELS, AND ORGANIZATIONAL DESIGNS OF EVALUATION: AN INTRODUCTION TO PROGRAM EVALUATION FOR CMHC BOARD MEMBERS
Merton S. Krause

In order for a group of people who are not regularly involved in the daily operations of a mental health center sensibly to assume responsibilities for the center, they must have some means of objectively appraising how the center is operating. This is so whether they are responsible for overseeing, advising, or financially supporting the center, and in each case the center's management can be seen as exercising the day-to-day authority for carrying out these very responsibilities. Evaluative data systems and special evaluation projects are an important means of making such an appraisal. The terms in which this appraisal should be done are the same terms as would be appropriate for managing the center, because inasmuch as management receives its authority by delegation from its board, both board and management properly share the same values and point of view on the center's operations. Where they do not share these, it is desirable to work out or at least be aware of the differences before undertaking evaluations. Thus, I will address myself to the functions, models, and organizational design of evaluation relevant to the exercise of management and so also board responsibilities.

FUNCTIONS OF EVALUATION

The fundamental consideration in constructing management-oriented evaluation systems is to determine for what sorts of decisions or functions they are to be relevant. The role of management in mental health service organizations involves at least four functions that depend on service evaluative data. These are (a) the

450

avoidance of destructive crises of service, (b) the allocation of resources to organizational functions, (c) the evolution of more cost-
effective service to meet competition, regulatory standards, or service goals, and (d) the favorable presentation of the organization to
sponsors, clients, and staff (cf. Attkisson et al., 1974). I should
like to clarify and illustrate these four management functions. The
illustrations might be greatly varied, but I will limit them to just
three aspects of organizational work for our illustrations: (1) intake
demand and the selection of clients from these requests, (2) those
aspects of service directed toward resettling disturbed patient-client
systems (families, networks) in the community, and (3) the subsequent services needed or obtained by the organization's closed cases.
As our focuses of interest, we can use these to contrast the four
management functions.

(a) The Avoidance of Destructive Crises of Service. Looking
for organizational problems that may affect service, so that management can intervene to avoid or reduce the trouble, was the first management function. What this involves depends upon what specific
area of organizational work we are considering.

1. A downward trend of intakes could imply an insufficient
caseload in the future. A burst of referral or linkage problems
with a particular state facility could lead to pressure from a state
administrator to absorb more "inappropriate" cases. A wave of
deflections of request to serve delinquent juveniles can create
serious community resentment.

2. An increasing rate of patient extrusions from the community can indicate a staff weakness or a shifting toward a more
difficult kind of case.

3. An increasing recidivism rate can call for some internal
changes at intake or in programming, or for a review of back-up
institutions before things deteriorate too far.

(b) The Allocation of Resources to Organizational Functions.
Each organizational service function contributes something to survival and success, and some allocation patterns of resources to those
functions may be better than others. For example, shifting some
staff from extended outpatient services to an intake crisis-interven-
tion team may increase the annual case count, the percent of those
discharged from mental hospitals who are given follow-up services,
or even the percent of planned closings. Or a couple more staff on
inpatient liaison and after-care may improve cost-effectiveness
markedly in terms of subsequent hospitalization.

1. An intake overload and a great number of extended-service
missed appointments or slack times at intake, such as early

mornings, and lots of reopening cases trying to bypass the in-take staff suggest, respectively, reallocations of staff time to intake coverage and consultation on intake issues with extended-service staff.

2. One geographical area team may have a better cost-effec-tiveness or longer waiting list than another and so might better have some of the other's staff reallocated to it.

3. The low staffing of a follow-up unit for closed cases may be allowing a much higher recidivism rate than would more sus-taining relationship and crisis intervention work with these clients, perhaps suggesting a reallocation from regular treatment units and intake.

(c) The Evolution of More Cost-Effective Service. Sometimes the solutions to organizational problems are not presently available and no reallocation among current services appears very promising, but the organization could certainly afford to be more cost-effective and so new services need to be evolved. Perhaps staff is experi-encing failure, other agencies and groups are agitating about under-served clients, or there are doubts about management's serious com-mitment to providing comprehensive service to its catchment area.

1. How much good could better screening do for us and what could we try? Would a team to specialize on those discharged from mental hospitals increase the number of these cases in the caseload and thus please certain funding sources?

2. Is work on getting patients settled in residences and roles in the community really consistent with seeing them only in the therapist's office and with concentration on only the family-identi-fied client? Would home-visiting family-treatment teams be better?

3. How might we maintain some minimal contact with ex-clients and learn how to improve our programming from our clients' subsequent careers? Would a follow-up team be worth trying?

(d) The Favorable Presentation of the Organization. Regard-less of all the preceding, a service organization must also be able to present itself as having been cost-effective enough in the terms convincing to its various important constituencies: number and pro-portion of the State Mental Health Department's and NIMH's high priority cases served, professional standards of work with patients or clients, the cases disturbing to important members of the com-munity settled expeditiously, and so forth.

1. The proportion of intake accepted or deflected by satisfactory rules, its volume, and some documented quality controls on it may do for intake accountability.

2. The follow-up data on completed cases can speak to questions of the efficacy of resettlement efforts.

3. Clients' service history since first admission/opening over an extended period, such as five to ten years, is clearly relevant data on recidivism.

The needs for information to carry out and to evaluate management functions, such as service crisis avoidance, resource allocation, program evolution, and presentation of the organization to its constituencies, are also the logical bases for models of evaluation. Each model applies to a particular management function.

MODELS OF EVALUATION

The models of functionally specialized evaluation are those of problem detection, program comparison, outcome extrapolation, and organizational accountability. They may use information of overlapping sorts, but they use it differently to answer different sorts of questions or, in the case of accountability, to address different audiences.

(a) Problem Detection. To monitor the critical processes of organizational functioning so as to detect limit-exceeding incidents or trends that might endanger the agency's funding or morale (as might staff improprieties or falling caseload or number of service hours per staff member), an evaluation system ought ideally to be connected continuously to all these processes and reliably transmit information about all problems that are real and serious. A lot of this sort of information—for example, the possibility that a staff member is coming in drunk, a contract with another agency is not being honored, or a client suicide could have been averted—is transmitted verbally, informally, much like gossip, and is responded to without being recorded, so its formal, process-evaluative properties may go unmarked. But trends requiring the aggregation of data and the self-conscious formulation of "safety limits" for them cannot be managed so informally: "Is our demand rising and being translated into inappropriate deflections?" "Is the Westside office hospitalizing proportionally more of its case openings every month?" "Why are so many fewer acting-out adolescent cases reopening this year?"

(b) Program Comparison. To compare the several service programs and units in an organization, so as to be able to decide on somewhat objective grounds on the allocation of resources among them (resources in the form of position and hour assignments, pay raises, transportation and recording equipment, supervisory time, and so on) an evaluation system must produce periodic outcome evaluation data summarizing the cost-effectiveness of each program or unit in fairly comparable terms. The object is to optimize the total organization's cost-effectiveness, usually by shifting available resources among current programs, but also by adding or substituting programs that have been developed elsewhere and have already been evaluated for cost-effectiveness, or by changing the organization's size and resource total to a more cost-effective level (for example, see Karon & VandenBos, 1976; Scharfstein, Taube, & Goldberg, 1977). The emphasis here is on comparisons instead of safety limits.

(c) Outcome Extrapolation. To trace and promote the cost-effectiveness evolution of a service program or unit by documenting its developmental history and its concurrent trend of cost-effectiveness performance, an evaluation system (or formative evaluation) must maintain the historical continuity of these data, of development costs (and its process-benefits, like staff morale, R & D income, reputation, and so on), and make extrapolations of the gains plausible for the various directions of feasible future development (such as staff training or additions, more reliable medication administration, family training in crisis management, and so on).

Such research and development efforts should themselves be allocated to programs and patient populations of the greatest probable total cost-effectiveness improvement for the organizations: to programs for the most frequent type of case (for example, family crisis with chronically high levels of strain, alcohol problems, children's behavior problems, old peoples' social survival), and for the most costly type of case (for example, protracted addiction, socially unconnected patients—such as chronic schizophrenics—who do not take adequate care of themselves, and the moderately or severely retarded), and/or for cases that are the most amenable to available or adaptable service technology such as pharmacotherapies or behavior modification (for example, the anxious, the phobic).

(d) Organizational Accountability. To present its record to its important constituencies in order to increase or maintain their support, an organization must be clear about whom it must be accountable to and just what service processes or outcomes each of these constituencies values. The evaluation system required will be some combination of those depicted in the preceding three models. So, for example, accrediting bodies may demand monitoring of the agency's standards of practice in its provision of services, funding sources may also want outcome effectiveness data to use in making their allocations, and some client, professional, or community groups may be impressed by evidence of certain program improvements.

ORGANIZATIONAL DESIGNS FOR EVALUATION

Specific evaluation or evaluation system research designs must translate these models into concrete operations for producing, transmitting, coding, analyzing, reporting, and using data to serve each model's management function. These designs must also assure that the data are valid for the interpretations that are wanted of them, so that what we see are really indications of service problems, not normal seasonal variations in demand; of differences in service unit efficacy, not the units' intake differences; of program evolution, not better adjunctive services by other agencies. (See Cook & Campbell, 1975, for the logic of how this can be done.)

I shall limit myself here to three omnifunctional or broad-spectrum organizational arrangements for routine evaluation-research that differ in their means of data production and transmission. These are (1) staff produced service statistics, (2) periodic process and outcome reviews by management, and (3) a continuing follow-up team taking a random sample of cases from each service program and unit.

(a) Service Statistics. If staff understands the statistics and is sympathetic with their use, and they are all obviously used, then the critical trends, cost-effectiveness levels, and program development indicators can be routinely estimated from collations of service statistics. For example, these statistics might derive from (1) pre-coded intake records indicating the nature of each request for service (but tell nothing about the service itself): demographics, diagnostics, intake processes, dates, effort in hours, costs, disposition of case, follow-up; (2) pre-coded extended-service records, focused on the resettlement of the client's life in the community, which do describe the service provided (but tell little about its long-term effectiveness): living circumstances, problems, resettlement processes, dates, effort, costs, disposition or closing status, follow-up; (3) pre-coded reopenings records for intake, for extended-service units, and for the interagency records clerk (scanning State Mental Health Department data and certain key referral partners' openings), which do indicate something about long-term effectiveness and use portions of (1) and (2) above, as relevant.

Without computerization of these data, however, they will be of little practical use (because hand calculations are expensive), and so a person comfortable with numerical data analysis (accounting

and statistics), computers, and familiar with management use of
the data as well as with its production by service staff is also needed.
The interpretation of the data calls for additional knowledge, essentially of the "interrupted time-series" "quasi-experimental design"
(see Cook & Campbell, 1975), especially to be sensitive to what
other events than program developments might be affecting organizational costs or results (for the evolution-extrapolation model) and
how staff is reacting to or biasing the statistics they produce. This
may require someone with the necessary research training. (See,
for example, Breedlove & Krause, 1966, and Krause & Howard,
1976, for an idea of the sorts of topics that should be covered.)

(b) Management Reviews. By selecting a random sample of
all requests for service over the past three years, say, and reviewing their service records, getting staff reports on the cases, and
searching out the present status of some (a random subsample),
some rough trends, comparisons, and extrapolations can be made
(though with considerable management and staff effort and distress),
especially by comparing the results of a series of such reviews over
several years. Investigations by new management teams or supervisors, by accrediting bodies, and for annual reports often approxi-
mate this design.

(c) Follow-Up Samples. A regular follow-up operation on case
applications, openings, and closings may be more costly and, at
least initially, as distressing as management reviews. Also, because of the necessity for resorting to very small samples of cases,
it may yield only rough estimates of trends, comparisons, and extrapolations. But the data need not have the biases of service statistics, can be of very high quality and reliability, and can provide information on clients' lives, especially after case closing, which the
other designs cannot. Recontacting every twentieth or fiftieth application, opening, or closing three months after that point in the case
for a half-hour interview about what has happened since then and
how things are now is the sort of thing that is involved here. It permits the discovery of service problems experienced by clients, more
valid comparisons and extrapolations, and more extended efficacy of
service estimates.

I suggest that service statistics, management review of service, and a small follow-up team together constitute an optimal practical design. (See Binner, 1973, on this issue also.)

REDESIGNING EVALUATION

It is not likely that an organizational design for evaluation-
research can be settled once and for all. An organization's evalua-

tion resources (including its tolerance for evaluation research) are not a constant. Budget, staff time and skills and sympathy, management interest and vulnerability and capabilities, constituency pressures, client acceptance and capacity all vary. The importance of the four management functions to which evaluation research is relevant (avoiding crises, allocations, evolution, and presentation) also vary. Various components of the organization may react against the evaluation arrangements from time to time because, for example, management is swamped with data, there have been foul-ups in data production or analysis, an evaluation coordinator has alienated people, some strong staff factions have been offended or unconvinced by certain unfavorable comparisons or extrapolations, there are new management personnel unsympathetic to the current design, and so forth.

Therefore one must decide just what is worth evaluation (see Zusman & Bissonette, 1973), and one must expect to redesign an organization's evaluation system every so often, though, hopefully, without too much loss of continuity for rational program evaluation. (If more technical knowledge would be of use, Ozarin, 1977, provides a review of the relevant evaluation research and several books concern how it is done, for example, Attkisson et al., 1978; Coursey, 1977; Schulberg et al., 1969.)

SUMMARY

There are at least four functions the evaluation projects and systems can serve for community mental health center boards and management, and for each function there is a particular model of evaluation that is most appropriate. A problem detection model can help to avoid destructive crises in the provision of service. A program comparison model can be useful in deciding on the allocation of resources to programs. An outcome extrapolation model can aid in the evolution of more cost-effective services. And an organizational accountability model can assist in making favorable representations of the agency's work. These models can be embodied in various organizational designs, including those of routine service statistics, management reviews, and follow-up teams.

REFERENCES

Attkisson, C. C., McIntyre, M. H., Hargreaves, W. A., Harris, M. R., & Ochberg, F. M. A working model for mental health program evaluation. American Journal of Orthopsychiatry, 1974, 44, 741-753.

Attkisson, C. C., Hargreaves, W. A., Horowitz, M. J., & Sorensen, J. E. Evaluation of human service programs. New York: Academic Press, 1978.

Binner, P. Program evaluation. In S. Feldman (Ed.), The Administration of Mental Health Services. Springfield, Ill.: Thomas, 1973, 342-383.

Breedlove, J. L., & Krause, M. S. Evaluative research design. In L. G. Gottschalk & A. H. Auerbach (Eds.), Methods of Research in Psychotherapy. New York: Appleton-Century-Crofts, 1966, 456-477.

Cook, T. D., & Campbell, D. T. The design and conduct of quasi-experiments and true experiments in field settings. In M. D. Dunnette (Ed.), Handbook of Industrial and Organizational Research. New York: Rand McNally, 1975, 223-326.

Coursey, R. D. (Ed.). Program evaluation for mental health. New York: Grune & Stratton, 1977.

Karon, B. P., & VandenBos, G. R. Cost/benefit analysis: Psychologists versus psychiatrists for schizophrenics. Professional Psychology, 1976, 7(1), 107-111.

Krause, M. S., & Howard, K. I. Program evaluation in the public interest. Community Mental Health Journal, 1976, 5, 291-300.

Ozarin, L. Community mental health: Does it work? Review of the evaluation literature. In W. E. Barton & C. J. Sanborn (Eds.), An Assessment of the Community Mental Health Movement. Lexington, Mass.: Heath, 1977.

Scharfstein, S. S., Taube, C. A., & Goldberg, I. D. Problems in analyzing the comparative costs of private versus public psychiatric care. American Journal of Psychiatry, 1977, 134, 29-32.

Schulberg, H. C., Sheldon, A., & Baker, F. Program evaluation in the health fields. New York: Behavioral Publications, 1969.

Zusman, J., & Bissonette, R. The case against evaluation (with some suggestions for improvement). International Journal of Mental Health, 1973, 2, 111-125.

30

THE RIGHTS OF CLIENTS IN COMMUNITY MENTAL HEALTH CENTERS
Ronald M. Soskin

The past decade has witnessed a radical change in perception
of the legal rights of persons seeking mental health treatment.[1]
The seemingly unending growth of large, isolated mental institutions
was halted, and the focus of attention shifted initially to conditions
of confinement. More significantly, increased emphasis has been
placed upon locus of treatment. Through litigation, legislation, and
growing public awareness, a dedication to providing mental health
treatment in community-based facilities has emerged.

Any discussion of clients' rights in community mental health
centers must center about this major change in philosophy from custodial care in long-term, large institutional settings to treatment in
short-term, community-based facilities. As an essential perspective to the understanding of clients' rights, this chapter will first
review the development of two principles: right to treatment and
least restrictive alternative. Later sections will discuss the right
to refuse treatment, rights of adolescents, privacy and confidentiality, and nondiscrimination.

It is not sufficient for the boards running community mental
health centers or for the professionals working within the centers
to see their roles merely as service providers for the community.
The provision of services, especially in an area as complex and potentially stigmatizing as mental health services, places an obligation
upon boards and professionals to the best of their abilities to ensure
that the rights of clients are protected and that the abusive aspects
of the impersonal system are minimized.

RIGHT TO TREATMENT

Right to treatment develops from two sources, constitutional doctrine and legislative authority. The doctrine emerged constitutionally against the background of an awakening to the vast abuses occurring in mental hospitals. To a large extent, persons were being warehoused, receiving custodial care with little pretense of active treatment designed to return the individual to the community. Not only did they fail to receive needed treatment: they were locked away against their wills and routinely deprived of all basic rights. What then was the purpose or rationale for hospitalization?

The courts have asked this very question. They conclude that the primary rationale for removing an individual from his community and locking him away in an institutional setting is to provide treatment designed to alleviate the disability and return the individual to an acceptable community functioning level. The state's power lay in either parens patriae, acting in the best interest of an individual who as a result of his mental illness is unable to so act, or its police power, intervening in a person's life to alleviate the mental illness that represents a danger to the community. However, as the Supreme Court has stated: "at the least, due process requires that the nature and duration of commitment bear some reasonable relation to the purpose for which the individual is committed."[2] Since commitment entails "a massive curtailment of liberty,"[3] the only justification for a state's intervening in a person's life via commitment is to provide needed treatment. In the absence of treatment, "the hospital is transformed into a penitentiary where one could be held indefinitely for no convicted offense."[4]

The importance of establishing a right to treatment under the United States Constitution must be underscored. While federal and state statutes may provide for a right to treatment, the constitutional right has a special significance. First, the United States Constitution is the "last line of defense" for individual rights, and the existence of a constitutional right to treatment means that this right can be enforced independently of any statutory right that may or may not exist. Secondly, the existence of a constitutional right to treatment means that statutes that might not otherwise explicitly provide a right to treatment will be interpreted to provide such a right in order to avoid constitutional challenge.[5]

The landmark right to treatment decision is Wyatt v. Stickney.[6] Confronted with the abysmal conditions at Bryce State Hospital and Partlow State School in Alabama, Judge Frank Johnson issued a clear judgment:

> The purpose of involuntary hospitalization for treat-
> ment purposes is <u>treatment</u> and not mere custodial
> care or punishment. This is the only justification
> from a constitutional standpoint, that allows civil
> commitments to mental institutions. [7]

The decision in this case outlined the minimum constitutional standards for adequate treatment of the mentally ill. The three basic
components of these standards are a humane psychological and physical environment, qualified staff in numbers sufficient to administer adequate treatment, and individualized treatment plans.

Since the <u>Wyatt</u> decision, there have been numerous lower
court decisions upholding a right to treatment (habilitation) for mentally ill (mentally retarded) persons not only upon the due process
rationale utilized in <u>Wyatt</u> but also upon the constitutional rights to
equal protection under the laws and to freedom from the imposition
of cruel and unusual punishment. [8] The United States Supreme Court,
however, has not yet ruled upon this issue: while scores of state
courts, federal district and federal appellate courts have found such
a right, the Court avoided the issue when squarely confronted with
it in <u>O'Connor v. Donaldson</u>. [9] Instead, the Court chose to issue a
narrow ruling (with other implications to be discussed <u>infra</u>), limited to the facts of the case: "A State cannot constitutionally confine, without more, a nondangerous individual who is capable of surviving safely in freedom by himself or with the help of willing and
responsible family members or friends."[10] Given the overwhelming case law existing on right to treatment, this right must be recognized until and unless the Supreme Court expressly rules otherwise.

Many of the cases discuss a right to treatment in terms of involuntarily committed individuals. Does this preclude the implementation of the right for voluntary patients? Several courts, in considering the voluntary/involuntary distinction, have ruled that the
label applied is not a basis upon which to withhold a right to treatment.[11]

First, there would be no rational basis on equal protection
grounds to have a facility in which some individuals received treatment (those involuntarily committed) while others were denied treatment and were merely provided custodial care (those labeled voluntary patients).[12] Second, many admissions labeled "voluntary" are
in no real sense voluntary on the part of the person admitted to the
facility. Studies have shown a marked lack of understanding on the
part of a large majority of "voluntary" patients as to their status or
rights.[13] Thus, courts have established specific procedures to protect the rights of voluntary patients[14] and have placed a heavy burden
on the state to show actual voluntariness.[15] Finally, the concept of

voluntariness may be meaningless given the circumstances of commitment. An individual may enter a facility under extreme pressure or coercion, or due to the absence of any state-created alternatives, or based upon the substituted voluntary consent of a parent
or guardian.[16] Given the closed nature and physical confinement of
the facility, the lack of informed voluntary consent, the nature of
substituted consent, and the total lack of community services as a
meaningful alternative, most courts have simply found that no real
distinction for treatment purposes exists between those labeled voluntary or involuntary.[17]

Other chapters in this book discuss legislation in detail, but
some statutes should be mentioned here. Various statutes such as
the Community Mental Health Centers Construction Act of 1963 and
Amendments of 1975,[18] Titles XIX[19] and XX[20] of the Social Security
Act, the Developmentally Disabled Assistance and Bill of Rights
Act,[21] and the Special Health Revenue Sharing Act of 1975[22] provide
for basic treatment rights. Section 504 of the Rehabilitation Act of
1973[23] is especially promising legislation to guarantee individuals
basic rights by prohibiting discrimination against handicapped persons, including the mentally disabled. Section 504 states: "No
otherwise qualified handicapped individual . . . shall, solely by
reason of his handicap, be excluded from the participation in, be
denied the benefits of, or be subjected to discrimination under any
program or activity receiving Federal financial assistance."

Section 504 has been viewed as a codification of the constitutional right to equal protection.[24] The regulations provide that, to
be equal, services "must afford handicapped persons equal opportunity to obtain the same result, to gain the same benefit, or to
reach the same level of achievement, in the most integrated setting
appropriate to the person's needs."[25] In applying Section 504,
courts have emphasized the prohibition on unnecessarily separate
services and the duty to integrate the handicapped into the community by providing services. In Halderman v. Pennhurst State School
and Hospital, the court held that Section 504 gave a "federal statutory right to habilitation in a non-discriminatory manner."[26] Thus,
once basic services are being provided, either to nonhandicapped
persons or to other handicapped persons, these services cannot be
denied to a class of handicapped persons due to their handicapping
condition.

The significance of all this to community mental health centers
is clear. The obligation of the centers, whether functioning with inpatients or outpatients, is to provide treatment. If the center has inpatients, then the constitutional and statutory rights to treatment
bind the center in its operations. Similarly, if treating outpatients,
the center is statutorily required to provide treatment and constitu-

tionally is tied to a mandate of treatment under the least restrictive alternative principle.

LEAST RESTRICTIVE ALTERNATIVE

The cases discussed previously do not stop with the finding of a right to treatment in an institutional setting. Rather, the courts have applied a principle, first enunciated by the Supreme Court in Shelton v. Tucker: "even though the governmental purpose be legitimate and substantial, that purpose cannot be pursued by means that broadly stifle fundamental personal liberties when the end can be more narrowly achieved."[27] As an adjunct to right to treatment, the application of this least restrictive alternative principle has radically altered the service system. No longer can restrictive institutions be the only basis for treating the mentally handicapped; rather, on an individual basis, less restrictive community services must be utilized.

The results have been staggering. The court in Dixon v. Weinberger[28] ordered the District of Columbia to plan for, fund, and create sufficient alternative community placements for at least 43 percent of the patients at St. Elizabeth's Hospital, patients whom the staff of the hospital had identified as unnecessarily hospitalized. Other courts have ordered the virtual closing of institutions and the movement of all (or almost all) patients or residents into community service systems.[29] Courts hearing petitions for civil commitment have required a full exploration of all existing, less restrictive community alternatives prior to authorizing commitment,[30] and some courts have gone beyond existing services and have ordered the creation of less restrictive community alternatives which, though possible treatment settings from the individual's perspective, did not as yet exist.[31] Even the Supreme Court in O'Connor v. Donaldson, supra, cited Shelton v. Tucker favorably in relation to its least restrictive alternative language.[32] Mental health centers, along with other community residences and services, obviously have become a key element of this deinstitutionalization process.

Are community mental health centers, in fact, living up to this obligation and providing individuals with a right to treatment in the least restrictive alternative? In his report to the Congress,[33] the Comptroller General of the United States found that community mental health centers have had a positive but limited impact on the prevention of unnecessary admissions to public mental hospitals or in providing aftercare or follow-up treatment to released patients. The report concludes that one factor contributing to a high readmission rate is the lack of appropriate facilities and services in the community, a fault that can be placed directly on the community mental health centers.

Much more directly critical of the centers is the book by Ralph Nader's Study Group. [34] The report raises questions concerning the shipping of patients from the centers to state hospitals, the relationships between mental health centers and state hospitals, and the utilization of ability to pay as a basis for lack of care in community centers. The authors find that, due to financial considerations, many centers rely upon private paying clients. The result is often to exclude poor and ethnic minorities from receiving treatment and to operate as an inpatient facility for patients of private psychiatrists. Instead of becoming an integral and progressive component of the deinstitutionalization process and providing access to meaningful treatment in the least restrictive alternative, the centers tend to function as traditional psychiatric hospitals and "tend to involve only a renaming of conventional psychiatry." The centers utilize traditional methods of care which, if not effective, preclude any further attempts at treatment. Such findings, if valid, illustrate that community mental health centers are, when viewed in an overall context, violating the right to treatment in the least restrictive setting as envisioned by numerous courts in their interpretations of the constitutional and statutory authorities.

RIGHT TO REFUSE TREATMENT

The right to treatment does not mean that treatment can be provided solely upon the discretion of the professionals within a center. The positive right to treatment is a right of access to treatment; the individual still retains the right to be consulted on alternative treatments and the power to reject or refuse certain treatments. As with any other patient receiving treatment, the consent of the client is of paramount concern. Treatment without consent or over the individual's objections can constitute an illegal battery upon the person, invading his bodily integrity.

Traditionally, it was believed that once an individual entered a community mental health center or another facility, he surrendered all decision-making rights. If at the center voluntarily, he was considered to have contracted away his choices as to treatment. If at a center involuntarily, he was considered to be incompetent to decide upon treatment. Courts have recently rejected this reasoning in no uncertain terms, [35] as illustrated by the following cases.

In Rogers v. Okin, [36] the court enjoined the use of medication or seclusion without the patient's consent or the consent of his guardian, except in emergency situations. The court first recognizes that treatment may be forcibly administered when failure to do so results in a substantial likelihood of physical harm to that patient, other patients, or to staff members of the facility. However, in all other nonemergency situations, informed consent must be obtained. The court rejects the notion that involuntary patients are legally incompetent to decide, and bases their right to refuse treatment upon the right to privacy and upon the First Amendment right to prevent interference with mind and thought processes. The court rejects the notion that voluntary patients waive their right to refuse treatment once they agree to treatment; rather, the court views this treatment agreement to permit patients the right to play an integral role in exploring alternate treatments and in deciding upon the desired treatment(s) and refusing other treatment(s). Of course, if an individual is incompetent, the court recognizes the power of a legal guardian in most instances to consent to or refuse treatment upon the patient's behalf.

Another court has similarly confronted this issue but has varied somewhat its practical approach.[37] The court recognizes in nonemergency situations the absolute constitutional and state statutory right of voluntary patients to refuse medication and the qualified right of involuntary patients to do so. However, instead of relying upon guardianships in order to pursue treatment for nonconsenting and incompetent involuntary patients, the court establishes due process procedures to be followed. In nonemergency situations, an involuntary patient cannot be given psychotropic medication unless a consent form has been signed and he or she makes no oral objection. However, if the individual is legally incompetent, then the consent of a guardian is sufficient; if he or she is functionally incompetent, medical certification will suffice. Both instances are subject to review by an independent patient advocate with the power to request a due process hearing review through an independent psychiatrist established for that specific review purpose. Decision to medicate would turn upon the patient's physical threat to other patients and to staff, the patient's capacity to make a decision, the existence of less restrictive treatments, and the risk of permanent side effects.

While the growth of effective community mental health center treatment as opposed to institutional care has been spurred by the discovery and use of psychotropic medications, the development of a legal right to refuse such treatment has resulted from the recognition of individual rights and by the dangers inherent in the use of those medications. The courts deciding these issues have focused upon the growing research data evidencing the adverse side effects that can develop.[38] Among the most undesirable results are tardive dyskinesia, a neurological side effect involving involuntary motor

movements, particularly of the face, lips, and tongue, and extra-
pyramidal effects, consisting of akathesia (motor restlessness),
akanesia (physical immobility), dystonia (spasmodic muscle reaction),
and pseudo-parkinsonian syndrome (mask-like face, rigidity of the
hand).[39] While some of these reactions are reversible, the danger
of irreversibility of others, as well as the discomfort and stigmatization that occur, form a sound foundation for many individuals to
refuse these medications.

While the prime focus here is upon medications, the right to
refuse treatment extends to various other treatment forms, such as
seclusion, restraints, behavior therapy, electroconvulsive therapy,
and psychosurgery. Informed consent remains the key to any of
these processes. In many instances, as the "treatment" becomes
more radical, substituted consent will not be accepted, and even
the individual's own consent will be deemed insufficient.[40]

Similar rights of consent and refusal are involved in the area
of research and experimentation. One of the major hazards of being
identified as an individual who is seeking treatment or is mentally
ill is the easy availability for researchers. Fortunately, the federal
government has become increasingly involved to prevent abuses, and
much of this area is now governed by federal regulations.[41]

ADOLESCENTS

When the patient is an adolescent, even more difficulties arise.
While the Supreme Court has recently approved the initiation of institutional mental treatment for minors based upon parental consent,[42] a frequent occurrence in a community mental health center
may be an adolescent's request for treatment without a parent's consent or knowledge. The traditional need for parental consent for
medical treatment and the inability of minors to enter a binding contractual relationship constitute impediments to the adolescent's access to treatment.[43] In the mental health context, short of the drastic situation in which the parent believes institutionalization is required, the parent may be unwilling to utilize community center
treatment due to fears of societal stigma, admission of failure in
accepting responsibility for a child's problems, sense of guilt, or
reluctance to have family secrets revealed during treatment.[44] On
the other hand, the child may not wish to have parents know of his
or her problems.

In many instances treatment can be provided in the absence of
parental consent. This can occur in emergency situations, when
minors are emancipated statutorily, under a judicially created mature minor rule, under a specific state mental health statute, or in

special situations in which society encourages adolescents to seek care (for example, with birth control, abortion, pregnancy-related problems, venereal disease, and drug addiction).[45] Potential problems of financial payments for services and liability for treatment, however, still operate as deterrents to needed treatment services for these adolescents. State legislation will in most instances be the key in resolving the right of adolescents to obtain treatment in community mental health centers voluntarily.

PRIVACY AND CONFIDENTIALITY

The process of treatment in a community mental health system involves an individual's revelations of intimate personal information. This information is received and digested by a therapist, entered into records, disseminated to other treatment personnel, including professional and nonprofessional staff, made accessible to outside treatment and other relevant agencies, and ultimately given to and stored by government authorities in complex, computerized data retrieval systems. What rights of privacy and confidentiality can an individual expect to possess in these circumstances?

Privacy refers to the right of a person to keep information about himself/herself out of the hands of other persons, including government and agency sources. This information includes identifying characteristics of the individual, disabilities or handicaps, measurements on test scores, financial transactions, medical treatment or services, and contacts with agencies or groups. Confidentiality, on the other hand, deals with information once it is gathered and a commitment to withhold from unauthorized users information obtained from or about an individual.[46]

Privacy has become a major concern due to several developments within the past century. These include the increased interdependence and interaction of individuals, development of complex communications technology, growth of large, unresponsive institutions, and the contemporary revolution in computer technology.[47] For individuals seeking treatment at community mental health centers, these concerns are intensified. Traditionally, the rights of privacy and confidentiality of this class of persons have been routinely ignored, while services have steadily increased. The result has been a rapidly growing and uncontrolled service system. Control over information and potential users has been under assault and significantly weakened. Potential dangers include the misuse of information disclosed to service providers through inappropriate means, the ill effects of being labeled, which has resulted in massive discrimination especially in employment and the criminal justice system, and an identification of the individual as a fit subject for research.

The right to privacy has been recognized in two legal concepts. The first is a general constitutional right to privacy, developed through case law. The second is a right established and defined through legislation.

The Supreme Court has carved from the Constitution a zone of privacy that encompasses "personal rights that can be deemed 'fundamental' or 'implicit in the concept of ordered liberty.'"[48] This privacy right has been utilized to uphold individual rights in varied personal matters, including use of contraceptives,[49] private possession of obscene matter,[50] abortion,[51] and marriage and family life.[52] Within this zone of privacy, the government lacks any justification to interfere.

The statutory privacy right includes the concept of privilege as well as the rights afforded in statutes such as the Privacy Act,[53] the Education for All Handicapped Children Act,[54] the Developmentally Disabled Assistance and Bill of Rights Act,[55] and various state statutes governing mental health treatment and medical records. The concept of privilege is a key safeguard in the transmittal of information in community mental health centers.

To be effective, treatment must be based upon the development of a relationship of trust between patient and therapist. The prime source of information relevant to treatment lies with the patient: he or she controls what is or is not conveyed. Yet in the absence of trust or if filled with doubts about the usage of the information, an individual will be extremely hesitant to convey significant data.

The physician-patient privilege has "emerged because society has a significantly greater interest in encouraging those who need medical care for either physical or mental conditions freely to obtain it than in soliciting information which may be important for the resolution of a civil or criminal action."[56] Thus, relevant information conveyed to a physician in the process of treatment is privileged, that is, the physician cannot convey that information without the patient's consent. Most states apply this privilege to psychiatrists as physicians. However, a real concern within a community mental health center is the needed application of this resultant confidentiality to other therapists and treating personnel.[57]

Only some states extend the privilege to psychologists, nonmedical therapists, and social workers. Courts, for example, upon the reasoning that an individual will reveal his most intimate thoughts to a psychiatrist or licensed psychologist but not to a social worker or counselor, have excluded the latter categories from the operation of the privilege.[58] The patient, therefore, if he is concerned about

protecting his privacy, must be extremely careful to whom he talks
and what he says.

Once information is conveyed to a medical person in a center,
what are the individual's legitimate expectations ? In obtaining consent for treatment from the individual, all uses of the information
must be explained. This includes the discussion of the patient's
case with other professionals at the center, the access of nonprofessionals to the information, and the potential access of third parties to the records that are maintained. Unfortunately, all of this
is often not explained to the patient, and thus true, informed consent
is not obtained. The intake process is especially troublesome since
the individual often feels helpless, not knowing what is to happen or
what to expect at this interview. [59]

In an interesting study at the Georgia Community Mental Health
Center in Athens, in response to a state reporting requirement to
transmit social security number, personal background data, primary
disability, diagnosis, and previous mental health services into a
computerized information system, it was found that the type and
form of the medical information release played an important part in
obtaining the client's consent. [60] When clients were given a release
form, all signed. When clients were given a release form that
stated they could sign if they wished, again all signed. However,
when a clerk read them an option providing that if the release form
were not signed then the information would be kept locally and not
sent to the state and would not affect their services, only 41 percent
signed. Finally, when this option was read by a clinician (with assumed authority), only 20 percent signed. Many spontaneously re-
marked of their concerns over the effect this information could have
on their current jobs and future employment opportunities, the future
custody of their children, or the denial at a later time of various
services, benefits, or opportunities. The author of the study concluded that a significant number of individuals would withhold consent for the dissemination of their personal information to the
state if they were aware of their right to do so and felt that it would
not jeopardize mental health services. [61] Affirming a client's right
to this decision would strengthen the treatment and make the client
more willing to cooperate and trust the professional staff at the
center.

If the state requires the collection of such information and its
maintenance in a central computerized system, the individual's
rights are less clear. Though the dangers become greater as information gets into the hands of more and more agencies and into more
and more data storage sources, such as computers, the individual
may have less and less control and no rights to contain this flow of
information. In Whalen v. Roe, [62] the Supreme Court ruled that an

individual has no constitutional protection of privacy interests in his own medical records. Thus, a New York law requiring copies of prescriptions of certain dangerous drugs to be sent to a centralized state source was upheld. In Gotkin v. Miller,[63] the court found no constitutionally protected property right in direct and unrestricted access to one's own medical records. However, several lower courts have enjoined the collection of records of sensitive and probing information that invaded individuals' privacy.[64]

Mental health center clients must be aware of a major exception to the accepted right of privilege. In Tarasoff v. Regents of the University of California,[65] the court held that a psychotherapist who knows or should know that a patient poses a "serious danger of violence" to a third party must exercise "reasonable care to protect the intended victim against such danger," including warning the victim. Privilege in most instances provides more safeguards to the individual than confidentiality statutes since, while the statute is subject to numerous exceptions including court ordered disclosure, privilege overcomes even a court order.[66] However, the Tarasoff ruling may undermine the client's trust in the therapist/patient relationship as well as adversely affect the functioning of the therapist.[67]

NONDISCRIMINATION

Society is moving away from the notion that an individual who seeks or obtains treatment is incompetent or must have numerous rights curtailed. The process for guardianship and especially limited guardianship has developed recently with substantive and procedural safeguards.[68] Access to treatment is now recognized as being unrelated to competency. Only a judicial proceeding based upon strict standards and with full procedural protections can result in an individual's being held incompetent and limited as to certain rights.

Similarly, federal legislation now supports many state statutes that attempt to eliminate widespread discrimination occurring as the result of treatment and consequent labeling. Section 504 of the Rehabilitation Act of 1973[69] prohibits discrimination by all federal recipients against qualified handicapped persons, while Section 503 of the Rehabilitation Act[70] prohibits discrimination and requires affirmative action in employment by all employers with federal contracts in excess of $2,500. Thus, while the fears of discrimination are still real and justified, legal tools exist to battle this disrimination and to have individuals judged equally based upon their abilities and not their disabilities.

CONCLUSION

Community mental health centers play an integral role in the radical changes that have occurred in the provision of mental health services to the population. With this integral role comes a distinct responsibility to recognize and to respect the integrity of the individual. Community mental health centers must not only fulfill their legislative purpose and help guarantee the constitutional right to treatment in the least restrictive setting but also ensure that individual rights and individual consent are not sacrificed in this process. By maintaining an awareness of the legal rights of their clients, the boards and staff of community mental health centers can maximize their role in providing a service readily accessible to the community, and without the dangers of stigmatization and abuse of their clients.

NOTES

1. The issues discussed in this chapter pertain to all mental handicaps, including mental illness and mental retardation. While these conditions are distinct and not to be confused, many of the legal principles apply equally to all individuals with mental handicaps. In addition, terms such as client and patient are used interchangeably.

2. Jackson v. Indiana, 406 U.S. 715, 738 (1972).

3. Humphrey v. Cady, 405 U.S. 504, 509 (1972).

4. Wyatt v. Stickney, 325 F. Supp. 781, 784 (M.D. Ala. 1971), aff'd sub. nom., Wyatt v. Aderholt, 503 F.2d 1305 (5th Cir. 1974).

5. Judge Bazelon's dicta in Rouse v. Cameron, 373 F.2d 451, 453 (D.C. Cir. 1966).

6. Wyatt v. Stickney, 325 F. Supp. 781 (M.D. Ala. 1971), 344 F. Supp. 373, 344 F. Supp. 387 (M.D. Ala. 1972), aff'd sub. nom., Wyatt v. Aderholt, 503 F.2d 1305 (5th Cir. 1974).

7. Wyatt v. Stickney, 325 F. Supp. at 784.

8. See Johnson v. Solomon, Civ. No. 76-1903 (D. Md. Aug. 17, 1979); Michigan Association for Retarded Citizens v. Smith, 475 F. Supp. 991 (E.D. Mich. 1979); Wuori v. Zitnay, Civ. No. 75-80-SD (D. Me. July 14, 1978); Evans v. Washington, 459 F. Supp. 483 (D.D.C. 1978); Halderman v. Pennhurst State School and Hospital, 446 F. Supp. 1295 (E.D. Pa. 1977), aff'd in part, remanded in part, Nos. 78-1490, 78-1564 and 78-1602 (3rd Cir. Dec. 13, 1979); Gary W. v. Louisiana, 437 F. Supp. 1209 (E.D. La. 1976); Woe v. Mathews, 408 F. Supp. 419 (E.D.N.Y. 1976), remanded in part,

dismissed in part sub nom., Woe v. Weinberger, 556 F.2d 563
(2nd Cir. 1977); Saville v. Treadway, 404 F. Supp. 430 (M.D.
Tenn. 1974); Davis v. Watkins, 384 F. Supp. 1196 (N.D. Ohio 1974);
Welsch v. Likins, 373 F. Supp. 487 (D. Minn. 1974), aff'd in part,
remanded in part, 550 F.2d 1122 (8th Cir. 1977); Horacek v. Exon,
357 F. Supp. 71 (D. Neb. 1973) and No. 72-6-299 (D. Neb. 1975);
Rouse v. Cameron, 373 F.2d 451 (D.C. Cir. 1966); Kesselbrenner
v. Anonymous, 33 N.Y.2d 161, 305 N.E.2d 903 (N.Y. 1973); Nason
v. Superintendent, Bridgewater State Hospital, 233 N.E.2d 908
(Mass. 1968). In New York State Association for Retarded Children
v. Rockefeller (Carey), 357 F. Supp. 752 (E.D.N.Y. 1973) and 393
F. Supp. 715 (E.D.N.Y. 1975), the court utilized an Eighth Amendment right to protection from harm basis to reach similar results
as the right to treatment cases.

    9. O'Connor v. Donaldson, 422 U.S. 563 (1975).

    10. Ib. at 576.

    11. See Halderman v. Pennhurst State School and Hospital,
supra note 8, at 1131; Wyatt v. Stickney, supra note 6, at 390 n.5;
New York State Association for Retarded Children v. Rockefeller,
357 F. Supp. at 764-65; Griswold v. Riley, Civ. No. 77-144 (D.
Ariz. July 15, 1977).

    12. See Mason, B. and Menolascino, F., The right to treat-
ment for mentally retarded citizens: An evolving legal and scientific interface, Creighton Law Review, 10, 124, 1976, p. 148, n. 74.

    13. See Gilboy, J. A. & Schmidt, J. R., Voluntary hospitali-
zation of the mentally ill, Northwestern Law Review, 66, 429, 1971;
Olin, G. B. & Olin, H. S., Informed consent in voluntary mental
hospital admissions, American Journal of Psychiatry, 132, 938,
1975; Palmer, A. B. & Wohl, J., Voluntary admission forms:
Does the patient know what he's signing?, Hospital & Community
Psychiatry, 23, 250, 1972.

    14. In re Buttonow, 244 N.E.2d 677 (N.Y. Ct. App. 1968).

    15. Wyatt v. Stickney, 344 F. Supp. at 390 n.5.

    16. While the Supreme Court has recently upheld the concept
of substituted consent for the commitment of children by parents or
guardians, Parham v. J.R., 99 S.Ct. 2493 (1979) and Secretary of
Public Welfare v. Institutionalized Juveniles, 99 S. Ct. 2523 (1979),
this in no way alters the analysis for right to treatment purposes.

    17. See for example, Halderman v. Pennhurst State School
and Hospital, supra note 8, at 1311:

> Thus, the notion of voluntariness in connection with ad-
> mission as well as in connection with the right to leave
> Pennhurst is an illusory concept. Few if any residents
> now have, nor did they have at the time of their admission,

any adequate alternative to their institutionalization.
As a practical matter, Pennhurst was and is their
only alternative.

18. 42 U.S.C. §2689.
19. 42 U.S.C. §1396 et seq.
20. 42 U.S.C. §1397 et seq.
21. 42 U.S.C. §6001 et seq. (1975). The Third Circuit Court
of Appeals in Halderman v. Pennhurst State School and Hospital,
supra note 8, has just relied heavily upon the D.D. Act to find a
right to treatment for institutionalized mentally retarded persons.
The Court is the first to place real teeth in the Act which, it is generally expected, will be followed by other courts.
22. 42 U.S.C. §246.
23. 29 U.S.C. §794.
24. Halderman v. Pennhurst State School and Hospital, supra
note 8.
25. 45 C.F.R. 84.4(b)(2).
26. 446 F. Supp. at 1323.
27. Shelton v. Tucker, 364 U.S. 479, 488 (1960).
28. Dixon v. Weinberger, 405 F. Supp. 974 (D.D.C. 1975).
29. See Michigan A.R.C. v. Smith, supra note 8; Evans v.
Washington, supra note 8; Halderman v. Pennhurst State School and
Hospital, supra note 8; Brewster v. Dukakis, C.A. No. 76-4423-F
(D. Mass. December 7, 1978).
30. See Eubanks v. Clarke, 434 F. Supp. 1022 (E.D. Pa.
1977); Stamus v. Leonhardt, 414 F. Supp. 439 (S.D. Ia. 1976);
Suzuki v. Quisenberry, 411 F. Supp. 1113 (D. Haw. 1976); Lynch v.
Baxley, 386 F. Supp. 378 (M.D. Ala. 1974); Davis v. Watkins,
supra note 8; Welsch v. Likins, supra note 8; Lessard v. Schmidt,
349 F. Supp. 1078 (E.D. Wis. 1972), remanded, 414 U.S. 473 (1974),
reinstated, 379 F. Supp. 1376 (E.D. Wis. 1974), remanded, 421
U.S. 957 (1975), reinstated, 413 F. Supp. 1318 (E.D. Wis. 1976);
Dixon v. Attorney General of the Commonwealth of Pennsylvania,
325 F. Supp. 966 (M.D. Pa. 1971).
31. See Morales v. Turman, 383 F. Supp. 53 (E.D. Tex.
1974), vacated and remanded on procedural grounds, 535 F.2d 864
(5th Cir. 1976), rev'd and remanded, 430 U.S. 322 (1977); New York
State Association for Retarded Children v. Carey, No. 72-C-356,
Memorandum and Order (E.D.N.Y. March 10, 1976); Michigan Asso-
ciation for Retarded Citizens v. Smith, supra note 8; In re Joyce Z.,
No. 2035-69 (C.C.P. Allegheny County, Pa. 1975); In the Interest
of Stephanie L., No. J-184924 (C.C.P. Phila. County, Pa. 1977);
In the Matter of Deborah Philbeck, No. 76-2650 (C.C.P. Probate
Div., Pickaway County, Ohio 1977).

32. O'Connor v. Donaldson, supra note 9, at 575.

33. Comptroller General of the United States, Returning the Mentally Disabled to the Community: Government Needs to Do More (Washington, D.C.: U.S. Government Printing Office, 1977).

34. Chu, F. D. & Trotter, S., The Madness Establishment (New York: Grossman Publications, 1974).

35. For a general discussion of the right to refuse treatment, see Plotkin, Limiting the therapeutic orgy: Mental patients' right to refuse treatment, Northwestern Law Review, 72, 461, 1977.

36. Rogers v. Okin, C.A. #75-1610-T (D. Mass. Oct. 29, 1979).

37. Rennie v. Klein, 462 F. Supp. 1131 (D.N.J. 1978) and 476 F. Supp. 1294 (D.N.J. 1979).

38. See Sovner, R., DiMascio, A., Berkowitz, D., and Randolph, P., Tardive dyskinesia and informed consent, Psychosomatics, 19, 172, 1978; Crane, G. and Cole, J., Two decades of psychopharmacology and community mental health: Old and new problems of the schizophrenic patient, Transactions of the New York Academy of Sciences, 36, 488, 1974; Gardos, G. and Cole, J. O., Maintenance antipsychotic therapy: Is the cure worse than the disease?, American Journal of Psychiatry, 133, 32, 1976.

39. Rogers v. Okin, supra note 36, slip opinion at 37-39.

40. See Kaimowitz v. Michigan Department of Mental Health, No. 73-19434-AW (Cir. Ct. Wayne County, Mich. July 10, 1973), holding that a mental patient could not give informed consent to psychosurgery.

41. See Federal Register, 43, 53950, Nov. 17, 1978 (Proposed Regulations on Research Involving Those Institutionalized as Mentally Disabled); Federal Register, 43, 31786, July 21, 1978 (Proposed Regulations on Research Involving Children); final rules to be issued in early 1980 (C.F.R., 45, Part 46). Controversy does exist as to the degree of protection provided by these regulations. See Bersoff, D., Handicapped persons as research subjects, Amicus, 4, 133, May/June 1979.

42. Parham v. J.R. and Secretary of Public Welfare v. Institutionalized Juveniles, supra note 16.

43. Wilson, J. P., The Rights of Adolescents in the Mental Health System (Lexington, Mass.: Lexington Books, 1978), p. 123.

44. Ib. at 124.

45. Ib. at 125-26.

46. See generally, Pfau, M., Engstrom, K., and McDonough, P., Privacy and the Law: An Overview (Belmont, Mass.: Contract Research Corporation, 1978).

47. Ib. at 1-2.

48. Roe v. Wade, 410 U.S. 113, 152 (1973).

49. Carey v. Population Services, Inc., 431 U.S. 678 (1977); Eisenstadt v. Baird, 405 U.S. 438 (1972); Griswold v. Connecticut, 381 U.S. 479 (1965).

50. Stanley v. Georgia, 394 U.A. 557 (1967)

51. Roe v. Wade, supra note 48.

52. Moore v. City of East Cleveland, Ohio, 431 U.S. 494 (1977).

53. 5 U.S.C. 552 a (1974).

54. P.L. 94-142, 20 U.S.C. 1401 et seq.

55. P.L. 94-103, 42 U.S.C. §6001 et seq.

56. Tancredi, L. R., Lieb, J., & Slaby, A. E., Legal Issues in Psychiatric Care (Hagerstown, Md.: Harper & Row, 1975), p. 52.

57. See generally, Laves, M., Confidentiality in the community mental health center, in Shore, M. F., and Mannino, F. V. (Eds.), Mental Health and Social Change: Fifty Years of Orthopsychiatry (New York: AMS Press, 1975), pp. 199-202.

58. See Allred v. State, 554 P.2d 411 (Alaska 1976). See also Belmont v. California State Personnel Board, 111 Cal. Rptr. 607 (Ct. App. 1974).

59. See Laves, supra note 57, at 203.

60. Rosen, C. E., Signing away medical privacy, Civil Liberties Review, 3, 54, October/November 1976.

61. Ib. at 58.

62. Whalen v. Roe, 429 U.S. 589 (1977).

63. Gotkin v. Miller, 514 F.2d 125 (2nd Cir. 1975).

64. See Phoenix Place v. Michigan Department of Mental Health, No. 77-737-260 CZ (Cir. Ct. Wayne County, Mich. June 20, 1978); Merriken v. Cressman, 364 F. Supp. 913 (E.D. Pa. 1973).

65. Tarasoff v. Regents of the University of California, 551 P.2d 334 (Cal. Supr. Ct. 1976).

66. See Ennis, B., and Emery, R., The Rights of Mental Patients: An American Civil Liberties Union Handbook (New York: Avon Books, 1978), p. 176.

67. See Wise, T. P., Where the public peril begins: A survey of psychotherapists to determine the effects of Tarasoff, Stanford Law Review, 31, 165, 1978.

68. See American Bar Association Commission on the Mentally Disabled, Guardianship and Conservatorship (Washington, D.C.: Developmental Disabilities State Legislative Project, 1979).

69. 29 U.S.C. §794. Section 504 has been amended by the Rehabilitation, Comprehensive Services, and Developmental Disabilities Amendments of 1978 to include executive agencies and the United States Postal Service.

70. 29 U.S.C. §793.

31

THE ON-SITE VISIT PROCESS
A. Brooks Cagle

In the course of conducting their daily operations, community mental health center staff and governing boards face numerous and complex accountability requirements. It is not unusual to find centers giving accountability reports to 20 or more external organizations. These organizations consist of such groups as licensing bodies, funding agencies, accrediting programs, governmental organizations at local, state, and federal levels, and community fund raising groups. No doubt the number of external accountability organizations will increase because centers are continually searching for funding sources in order to maintain or expand services.

Many of these organizations require on-site visits by evaluators and surveyors as well as written materials and data. The on-site visit is most frequently found as part of the accountability requirements of larger funding agencies, including the National Institute of Mental Health (NIMH), the Health Care Financing Administration, state mental health authorities, accrediting organizations such as the Joint Commission on Accreditation of Hospitals (JCAH), The Council for the Accreditation of Rehabilitation Facilities, and the recently formed Accreditation Council of Mental Retardation and Developmental Disabilities Programs. Licensure agencies rely heavily on site-visit findings to render their decisions, which ultimately have far-reaching impact for center functioning and fee collection.

Site visits are often perceived as time-consuming since many hours of preparation and documentation are required. On occasion, both the center staff and the site-visit team place themselves in unnecessary defensive postures. And, too frequently, benefits that flow from the experience are lost. In this chapter, I will explore

the purpose of site visits, review techniques and procedures followed
by site visitors, comment on the kind of preparation to be accomplished by center staff, and suggest ways of utilizing the expertise
of the site visitors.

WHY ARE SITE VISITS CONDUCTED?

The primary reasons for site visits are quality assurance
monitoring and the determination of compliance with regulatory and
funding requirements. Schulz and Johnson (1976) point out that external accountability agencies are an integral part of the quality assurance and compliance effort. The health care industry, of which
community mental health is a part, is too large and costly to be completely unregulated.

Efforts to assure quality must be given priority for the sake
of the consumer. Consumers are generally uninformed, and may
not be able to judge the type of service they need. They are sometimes even unable to evaluate the quality of the service they receive
(Schulz & Johnson, 1976).

Funding agencies are concerned about utilization of their contribution. The free enterprise system does not work well in the
health care industry because service providers rather than consumers control demand. In this climate, considerable opportunity exists for inappropriate utilization of resources. For this reason,
caution must be exercised within community mental health to guarantee that those consumers requiring services do, indeed, receive
them, that those no longer in need are not unnecessarily served, and
that all services provided are selected on the basis of identified need.
External monitoring then determines the appropriateness of the utilization of resources within the program.

Certain external accountability agencies such as NIMH provide
monies to develop specific programs and services. NIMH expects a
center receiving an operations grant to offer within 90 days inpatient,
emergency, outpatient, screening, follow-up, and consultation and
education services. These centers must also have a timetable for
phasing in, within three years of receipt of the initial grant, partial
hospitalization, specialized services for children and the elderly, and
transitional halfway house services (unless determined to be unnecessary). To determine compliance with these requirements, NIMH relies almost exclusively on site visits conducted by its regional offices.

WHAT DO SITE VISITORS DO?

Most site visitors and surveyors are not professionally trained
program evaluators. Instead, they are usually clinicians or admin-

istrators who have been chosen to perform survey functions because of their past performance in their fields. In order to prepare the surveyors for the work to be performed, voluntary agencies such as JCAH and government agencies such as the Health Care Financing Administration provide intensive training.

Surveyors are particularly alert to the confidential aspects of their work. While they must have access to data on the facility, personnel, consumers, and agency operations, they are cautioned in their training to recognize their critical responsibility in protecting the confidential nature of the information and documentation they see. It is clearly recognized that assurance of confidentiality is a matter of professional conduct and is supported by state and federal laws. An agency being surveyed should recognize that an external accountability agency will protect confidential information and, consequently, it should cooperate by providing such information when requested. However, special concerns should be discussed with the survey organization prior to the site visit.

Techniques and methods of data collection are also taught in the orientation of surveyors. While in most instances the final assessment of the center's performance is subjective, surveyors are introduced to methods and techniques that help them arrive at a justifiable decision based on their observations. For instance, in the Health Facility Surveyor Training Orientation Program utilized by the Health Care Financing Administration, surveyors are taught to review the provider's policy and procedure manuals, and then to check whether procedures are being carried out by staff. JCAH surveyors are also instructed in methods of evaluating existing policies and their congruence in practice.

Surveyors are capable of consulting with the staff and board on procedures to follow in complying with standards. The training and orientation given to JCAH surveyors highlight this aspect of their work. Similar expectations can be placed on surveyors from other organizations. In using such consultation, center staff and board members should be alert to the possibility that surveyor bias will be presented; in some instances, a surveyor's personal preferences may not be relevant to the standards of the external accountability agency. Under these circumstances, they should ask the surveyor to give specific references to the applicable standards or procedures.

PREPARING FOR THE SITE VISIT

A local agency should not enter into an on-site visit without adequate preparation, including an understanding of the regulations and procedures of the organization conducting the visit. One should know how many surveyors will be involved in the visit, how the division of labor will occur, and which sites will be visited. If this information is not provided well in advance, the local agency should request it.

Site visits depend on the availability of source documents, which give the surveyors data upon which to base their findings. Each external accountability body defines the source documents in different ways; nevertheless, certain ones are generally found to be necessary for all surveys. The remainder of this section describes particular source documentation found in JCAH training materials for community mental health surveyors.

Governing Board and Advisory Council Records

Items in this source documentation consist of the bylaws, resumes of members of boards and councils, and minutes of all full board and committee meetings. In the actual on-site survey process, the records of the governing board and advisory councils will be reviewed to determine the frequency and regularity of meetings, the level of activity of the board and councils, the degree of representativeness of the membership when compared to the community served, and the relationship of the chief executive officer to the governing board. A number of documents are collected in order to provide the necessary data. In addition, management staff and governing board members, preferably the chairperson, should be available to discuss the operations of these boards and councils with the surveyors.

Budget

JCAH survey procedures expect a detailed presentation of budget information since its approach gathers data on all resources (land, labor, and capital) by service activity. The other external accountability agencies are not this detailed in their budget reviews. However, they do expect data regarding the availability of resources.

The budget should be perceived as a part of the current short-range plan of the program. During the actual survey, persons familiar with the budget should be available in order to explain how and why resources are allocated and to answer questions about budget procedures.

Policy Manual

A policy and procedure manual should be written that addresses such functional areas as service delivery, administration, citizen participation, staff development, and research and evaluation. All policies should be approved by the governing board of the program and reviewed and updated annually.

Not only should wide distribution of the manual be evident within the center, but procedures must exist that insure that staff know about policies relevant to their work performance. Site visitors and surveyors will be looking for consistency of application.

Personnel Records

Complete personnel records should be kept for all staff. These records contain evidence of licensure for those staff who are licensed to perform their duties, evidence of staff training and development for each employee, and all necessary processing materials such as withholding statements.

In reviewing personnel records, surveyors will usually ask staff to provide a sampling. Personnel records are reviewed to determine the adequacy of their content; most survey procedures require specific records to be reviewed in addition to the sample. For example, the record of the chief executive officer is examined to check compliance with minimum qualifications, persons in food handling positions for compliance with local, state, and federal food handling and health clearance requirements, and licensed personnel for the presence of licensure.

Planning Documents

An agency should have a current comprehensive plan of its specific service area. Such a plan should identify other agencies in the area with similar services, their hours of operation and relationships, and the number of individuals at risk in the various age and disability groups. An organizational plan is separate from the comprehensive plan, and it describes the internal operation of the program. Other planning documents show procedures followed by the organization in developing plans, time frames, and specification of what planning activity will occur at the various organizational levels.

Planning documents take a considerable amount of time and effort to complete. As with other aspects of the site visit, the surveyors attempt to ascertain the extent of congruence between plans and current operation. Survey experience has shown that planning and design is an area in which many agencies perform poorly, probably because most senior staff are clinicians by training and not well prepared for planning.

Minutes of Staff Meetings

Records in the form of minutes of all executive, middle management, and program staff meetings should be kept. These minutes should be shared so that all levels within the organization are aware of important events as they occur. A good set of minutes will contain the date, time, and place of the meeting, names of members present and absent, an account of all items discussed, and the signature of the individual responsible for the meeting.

Many community mental health agencies fail to keep adequate records. As a result, the management effort tends to be fragmented and information documenting performance is lost. Agencies should have a policy stating that minutes of the meetings of all staff groups be kept, outlining the minimum format and content of all such minutes, and describing how the minutes will be exchanged.

Service Records

The service record or client record should contain all assessment data regarding the consumer being served, a fully developed service plan, activity notes, progress summaries, medication records, and other data. For the purpose of site visits, the service record is the major source document for reviewing service delivery. Local agencies should develop mechanisms for continuous monitoring of the quality of the service record so that last minute review and updating of service records can be avoided.

Preparing Records

Every site visit will require that time and effort be given to preparation. In order to accomplish this task effectively, responsibility for coordinating the work should be vested in a single staff member. The designated person should be familiar with all aspects of the local center's programs and should be aware of procedures generally followed in a survey. The organization conducting the site visit will, in most instances, provide a listing and description of the needed source documents. However, when such listings are unavailable, a review of the on-site procedures used by the surveying agency will allow staff to identify these documents.

In order to assist the individual assigned responsibility for preparation, a task force can be organized and assigned responsibility for coordination. For example, one task force member may be assigned responsibility for ensuring that all agency policies are current, another for life safety and therapeutic environment, and a third for clinical services. Each reports back to the coordinator chairing the task force.

It is a mistake to schedule every minute of the survey team's time. Overscheduling tends to produce the appearance of a "show and tell" situation in which inadequate and inaccurate data are collected. This often works toward the detriment of the agency being surveyed.

WHAT HAPPENS DURING THE SURVEY?

Prior to the beginning of the actual survey, the surveyors convene to organize their work. During this meeting, they review the pre-survey materials supplied to the external accountability agency. These materials include such items as the application, description of the program and service area, and other materials. From these data, unique features are identified and assignments are made to survey team members.

Once the survey team arrives at the site, a short meeting with executive staff will probably take place. During this meeting, the team leader describes how the survey will be conducted and explains the work of each team member. At this time, it is important to set the times for key events during the visit. For example, a clinical records workshop is conducted during a JCAH survey. By specifying the hour and place for this workshop at the beginning of the survey, participating staff are informed well in advance and the necessary space for the workshop is reserved. In addition, executive staff and the surveyors should agree on a time and location for the exit interview since it too requires ample time for notification of all interested persons.

It is recommended that key staff be available to survey team members during the entire survey process. The chief administrator can be assigned to accompany the survey team member reviewing administration and management, while a senior clinician can work with the surveyor on clinical services. The staff member responsible for building upkeep can be available when a surveyor visits facilities and checks compliance with safety requirements.

As the survey progresses, program staff can keep notes of surveyor comments and observations. Not only will notes be of value when making changes to enhance compliance, but they can be useful if a dispute over survey outcome develops.

During the entire survey, the presence and involvement of board members should be encouraged. Their active participation tends to impress surveyors since it demonstrates community investment in the center's programs. When board members are introduced to survey procedures and source documents are reviewed with them, they are able to respond to questions in a knowledgeable manner.

The on-site survey concludes with the exit conference, during which the survey team presents its findings and recommendations. Since content of the exit conference is important in any appeal of adverse findings, staff should not hesitate to ask questions and point out areas where potential disagreement might exist. A complete record of the summation should be made with a tape recorder to ensure that nothing is missed.

It is suggested that agencies not invite news media to report on the findings presented at the exit conference. Such conferences tend to focus on deficiencies and the press may unnecessarily highlight them. Press releases prepared by the agency immediately following the completion of the survey are more suitable.

REFERENCES

Affeldt, J. E. Accreditation problems: Confidentiality of survey report. Hospitals, 1979, 53(6), 44.

Cagle, A. B. CMHC monitoring package and AP/PF requirements for community mental health programs. Washington, D.C.: National Council of Community Mental Health Centers, 1976.

Gaver, K. D., & Franklin, J. L. A review of the recent literature: Accountability in public mental health organizations. Community Mental Health Review, January-February 1978, pp. 3-11.

McCleary, D. How to prepare for a JCAH evaluation. Hospitals, September 1979, 53(18), pp. 189-190, 192, 194.

O'Malley, N. When hospitals and JCAH surveyors disagree. Hospital Peer Review, February 1978, 32(2), p. 22.

Program review document: Community mental health service programs, PF-337. Chicago: Joint Commission on Accreditation of Hospitals, 1979.

Schultz, R., and Alton, C. J. Management of hospitals. New York: McGraw Hill, 1976.

U.S. Department of Health, Education and Welfare. Health Care Financing Administration. Health facility surveyor training orientation program. Washington, D.C., January 1980.

INDEX

acceptability of services: board/ director role in, 70, 150; measures of, 150

accessibility of services, 6, 26, 149, 344-48, 411, 423, 427; board role in, 293

accountability, 1, 11, 421-22, 424-38; board's role in, 15, 22, 30, 31, 35, 424-53; community representation, 425-26; cost of, 437; governing board's role, 31; history in mental health, 421; monitoring, 426-28; politics of, 421; and program evaluation, 454; reports, 476; required information for, 430-34; required resources, 428-30; using sanctions, 427

accrediting bodies, 421, 435, 476 (see also Joint Commission on Accreditation of Hospitals)

acculturation, 364, 365-66

administration (see management of mental health organizations)

adolescents' legal rights, 466

adult service delivery, 231-46; anxiety disorders, 237; diagnostic evaluation, 236; drug treatment, 237-40; electroshock, 237; hospitalization, 244-45; mood disorders, 239-40; partial hospitalization, 244; psychotherapy, 241-43; psychotic disorders, 238-39

advisory board (community): accountability, 424-38; and allocating resources, 436-37;

authority of, 29-30, 45, 48-49, 67-68; characteristics of, 20, 45, 47, 67-68, 122; Chicago All-City Board, 46-59; and the community, 45-47, 55-56, 58; compared to governing boards, 12, 30, 32, 47, 67-68; conflict with agency, 47-49, 55-57; and constraints, 435-37; in consultation and education, 188-89; coordination responsibilities, 292-95, 306-07; decision making, 434-37; and evaluation of programs, 450-57; and the federal government, 48-49, 53, 58; in financial management, 148-49, 162-64; in funding, 122-23, 139-47; history, 46; independence from agency, 49-50; as lobbyists, 140; and mental health services for the mentally retarded, 391, 396; monitoring, 426-28; need for alliances, 46-47; and the on-site visit, 479, 482; and partial hospitalization, 291; and planning, 444; politics of, 48, 50-55, 58; and prioritizing programs, 436-37; and professionals, 51-54; and public administrators, 51-52, 56-57; and public education, 288; recruitment, 426; and representation, 425-26; required information, 430-34; and the research and evaluation team, 429; and services for the chronically mentally ill, 360;

484

ABOUT THE EDITOR

WADE H. SILVERMAN is Associate Professor at the University of Illinois School of Public Health and Executive Director of Continuing Education in Mental Health.

Dr. Silverman has published widely in the area of community psychology and community mental health. His articles and reviews have appeared in the <u>American Journal of Community Psychology</u>, <u>Journal of Community Psychology</u>, and <u>Professional Psychology</u>.

Dr. Silverman holds a B.S. from the University of Pittsburgh, and an M.S. and Ph.D. from Kent State University, Kent, Ohio.